REHABILITATIVE AUDIOLOGY FOR CHILDREN AND ADULTS

COMMUNICATION DISORDERS

REHABILITATIVE AUDIOLOGY FOR CHILDREN AND ADULTS

Julia M. Davis
University of Iowa

Edward J. Hardick
Ohio State University

with a chapter by
Dianne J. Van Tasell
University of Minnesota

JOHN WILEY & SONS
New York • Chichester • Brisbane • Toronto

Library of Congress Cataloging in Publication Data:

Davis, Julia M., 1930–
Rehabilitative audiology for children and adults.

(Wiley series on communication disorders, ISSN 0271-6240)
Bibliography: p.
Includes index.
1. Deaf—Rehabilitation. 2. Audiology.
I. Hardick, Edward J., 1930– . II. Van Tasell, Dianne J. III. Title. IV. Series: Wiley series on communication disorders.
RF297.D38 362.4′283 81-7427
ISBN 0-471-03560-2 AACR2

Printed in the United States of America

10 9 8 7 6 5 4 3 2 1

FOREWORD

Those who read this book expecting another run-of-the-mill text on "aural rehabilitation" will be disappointed. *Rehabilitative Audiology for Children and Adults* does not focus on the "the ear" as books of the aural rehabilitation type have done in the past, but devotes its attention to the consequences of hearing impairment on people, the evaluation of problems faced by persons who are hearing impaired, and the management of problems of the hearing-impaired person as they are manifested in their educational, social, psychological, and communication milieu. Davis and Hardick have brought clearly into focus the special knowledge and skill of the audiologist in the management of the person with hearing impairment. Both within and between the lines of their contribution are found implications for redefining the future directions in which audiologists will have to consider moving if they are to be devoted to the whole of the person with a hearing impairment. *Rehabilitative Audiology for Children and Adults* is a skillfully woven fabric whose fibers are research data, clinical experience, and insightful consideration of special needs when established evaluation and management methods are applied to persons with hearing impairment. Those who have come to realize the importance of contemporary studies of language development to the understanding of the problems of hearing-impaired children will find in this book one of the most thorough and sophisticated discussions of this important factor assembled anywhere under one cover. One comes away from this book with a distinct impression that much of the two-way street between basic science and clinical application has been traveled by Davis and Hardick. The reader will find the work an enlightening, scientifically based journey through an important clinical topic.

THOMAS J. HIXON
ADVISORY EDITOR IN COMMUNICATION DISORDERS

PREFACE

This book is intended as a text for an introductory course in the rehabilitation of hearing-impaired people. Our experience indicates that such courses are usually taken by undergraduate seniors or first-year graduate students of speech-language pathology or audiology and, to a lesser extent, by students in education of the deaf. Because courses in aural rehabilitation occur as part of a sequence of professional courses, students have usually had previous coursework that provides the necessary background for the understanding of communication problems and the principles underlying treatment programs assigned to overcome them. For example, coursework in anatomy and physiology of the speech and hearing mechanisms usually precedes the study of specific disorders and their effects on the functioning of these mechanisms.

In the case of hearing impairment, the areas of prerequisite knowledge are so varied and numerous that it simply is not possible to review each of them in a text such as this. Therefore, the authors assume that readers have previously acquired information in the following areas: anatomy and physiology of the speech and hearing mechanisms, an introduction to normal language development, audiometric testing (terminology and procedures), and basic speech and hearing sciences regarding the speech signal and how it is processed.

The purpose of this text is to familiarize students with the issues involved in the rehabilitation of hearing-impaired children and adults. The effects of hearing impairment on communication, linguistic, educational, and social behavior are described and guidelines for their assessment and remediation are provided. To help accomplish these goals, a large body of related literature is reviewed. We have two reasons for including a rather extensive literature review: (1) to provide a resource for students that can be used as an overview of the topics under discussion and (2) to provide a basis for the procedures recommended. There exist serious disagreements among professionals who serve hearing-impaired clients as to the remedial procedures to be employed, the settings in which treatment should occur, and the identity of the professionals who should provide the disputed services. It is important for students to be aware of these disagreements and their sources, and a review of pertinent literature may help in this.

The topics in this book have been influenced by our teaching and clinical experiences and by the existing curriculums of our academic institutions. The topics represent what we consider to be minimal information required by anyone who engages in the remediation of hearing-impaired children and adults through speech and language therapy, hearing aid orientation, auditory training, speechreading, and counseling. Like almost everyone else involved in these activities, we have biases and preferred procedures that will become clear to the reader. For example, we strongly support the audiologist's role as a dispenser of hearing aids; we do not advocate an extended period of treatment for adults; we have serious doubts about the teaching of lipreading per se; we take a linguistic approach to the habilitation of children; and we favor an eclectic approach toward the treatment of hearing-impaired children, including the use of manual communication when it appears warranted.

Certain activities involved in the management of the hearing impaired will not be discussed in depth in this book. An example is hearing aid selection, an important aspect of rehabilitation, but one that requires special training and knowledge beyond that necessary for assisting people in learning to use a hearing aid. Because of space limitations we have not included a detailed discussion of programs for deaf adults or multiply handicapped individuals. The omission of these topics does not imply that they are not important, only that they pose difficult questions that deserve a more complete coverage than is possible here.

Because of their usefulness in remediation, the Northampton Chart symbols have been used throughout the book when orthographic representation of phonemes is necessary. Readers who are unfamiliar with that symbol system are referred to Figures 8.3 and 8.4 of Chapter 8. We have also included materials in appendixes that are not easily available to clinicians, including copies of several hearing handicap scales and lists of materials for parents.

We are indebted to a number of people who have contributed to the development of this book in various ways. Our thanks go to Tom Hixon, Advisory Editor in Communication Disorders, for his advice and encouragement as we struggled with the writing; to Carol Luitjens, editor, for restoring our faith in editors just in time; and to Margaret Seemuth, Varena Wade, Pam Mueller, Margie Watkinson, and Joanne Littell for their tireless typing and organizing.

We are most deeply grateful to Dianne Van Tasell for sharing her considerable knowledge of speech perception and hearing impairment in Chapter 2.

Finally, we want to thank our students for their interest in hearing impairment. Without that, this book would never have been conceived.

JULIA M. DAVIS
EDWARD J. HARDICK

TABLE OF CONTENTS

PART One

COMMUNICATION AND HEARING IMPAIRMENT

CHAPTER 1

Introduction

I. Development of Rehabilitative Audiology
II. Characteristics of Hearing-Impaired Listeners

The rehabilitation[1] of hearing-impaired individuals has been attempted by various types of professionals for several hundred years. The activities involved have depended on the characteristics of the persons being served and the professional identification of those providing the services. Educators have focused on the teaching of academic subjects, speech-language pathologists have emphasized the development of oral communication skills, and audiologists have stressed the use of amplification. Before the development of modern hearing aids, lipreading schools were common and popular, especially among hearing-impaired adults in urban communities. Until relatively recently, however, the relationships among the hearing, language, educational, and social problems experienced by hearing-impaired children and adults were not well understood. At least they were not used commonly

[1]The term *rehabilitation* is used here in its generic sense to refer to programs for both children and adults. The term *habilitation* will also be used to refer to programs for children when they represent initial attempts to overcome the effects of hearing impairment.

as the basis for a multifaceted treatment program designed to address the variety of needs experienced by hearing-impaired individuals.

DEVELOPMENT OF REHABILITATIVE AUDIOLOGY

Several factors have contributed to the remedial philosophies presently in use. The development of the profession of audiology, rapidly expanding knowledge about the nature of language and its acquisition by children, the recent emphasis on the psychological impact of physical impairments on individuals and families, and technological advances in hearing aid design have all contributed to changes in the procedures employed.

Prior to World War II, the habilitation of children consisted of educational programs located primarily in residential schools for the deaf. Few children wore hearing aids, making the use of residual hearing rare. Consequently, remedial procedures stressed the use of vision to receive messages. Preschool programs were rare. Children often reached school age without learning language beyond a few simple words. Instruction in language structure and vocabulary preceded the teaching of academic material, which often proceeded at a very slow pace. All aspects of management of children with any significant degree of hearing loss were the responsibility of teachers of the deaf whose training had prepared them to teach primarily through the visual sense. Lipreading[2] instruction was the cornerstone of the educational process in most schools; manual communication was used in others but was usually not introduced in the classroom until the child had been in school for several years.

During the same period, adult rehabilitation was limited to lipreading instruction. Between 1875 and 1930 several "methods" of lipreading were developed. Lipreading schools flourished, specializing in teaching visual skills to adults who were losing their hearing. Most of the developers of the methods were young professionals whose own hearing had been lost recently. Although little is published about the socialization aspects of these schools, they often resulted in the establishment of hearing societies and newsletters for hearing-impaired adults. At least one of the founders of a method, Edward Nitchie, recognized the psychological impact of hearing impairment and the need for adults to share their experiences and frustrations.

Following World War II two events occurred that caused profound changes in the kinds of rehabilitative procedures recommended for hearing-impaired adults. First, programs were developed in Veterans Administration hospitals for persons who had suffered hearing loss during military service. These programs were called *aural rehabilitation,* and consisted of a triad of services: auditory training, lipread-

[2]The terms *lipreading* and *speechreading* are used interchangeably to refer to the use of the visual information available in speech as an aid in speech perception.

ing, and speech conservation. Attempts to devise better ways of testing hearing and remediating the effects of hearing loss were made by speech-language pathologists and psychologists. As knowledge grew and personnel specialized in the problems caused by hearing impairment, the profession of audiology emerged, resulting in a sharp increase in the time and effort expended in the study of hearing impairment and its effects on communication.

About the same time, the electronics industry experienced enormous growth in knowledge and technology. Wearable hearing aids were developed and their fidelity and convenience steadily improved. The use of residual hearing could now be enhanced by amplification, and the use of vision, although still important to the reception of speech, was no longer the primary means through which speech could be processed by hearing impaired people.

The habilitation of hearing-impaired children was also affected by the growth of the profession of audiology and improvements in wearable amplification, but a third development also influenced it appreciably. Research into the nature of language and its acquisition by young children has contributed to a large body of knowledge about normal language development and the effects that various disorders may have on it. Because language is learned primarily through audition, hearing impairment affects its development directly. These effects can and have been quantified and analyzed, resulting in knowledge that can be used in planning programs for hearing-impaired children.

As a result of these developments, programs for children and adults have undergone many changes during the last three decades. The procedures employed, the location of services, and the identity of those providing them are different in many respects from those that existed previously. These differences are reflected in the procedures recommended in the following chapters. Emphasis is on the linguistic and communicative deficits imposed by hearing impairment and the effects of the linguistic deficit on other aspects of development, including educational achievement and social interaction. The contribution of audition to communication and the use of vision as an adjunct to it will be stressed. The role of various professionals will be discussed, but the audiologist is described as the primary provider of rehabilitative services to hearing-impaired persons, from the selection and dispensing of hearing aids to the coordination of remedial and educational services.

The management process begins as soon as hearing loss is confirmed. The adult or the child's parents should be informed of the characteristics of the hearing loss and the rehabilitative options available. For some adults, a discussion of the ways in which communication can be enhanced is sufficient treatment of the loss, particularly if the adult is a hearing aid user. For others, extensive remedial procedures are necessary to enhance communication skills. It is the responsibility of the audiologist to determine (1) whether remediation is needed and (2) what the components of an appropriate program should be for a given individual. Some of the recommended procedures (such as academic tutoring, speech remediation and language therapy), may be provided by other professionals, but they should be conducted only by persons who have special knowledge and training in hearing impairment.

CHARACTERISTICS OF HEARING-IMPAIRED LISTENERS

All hearing-impaired listeners have at least one characteristic in common: they do not hear normally. Beyond that basic fact, however, hearing-impaired people represent a heterogeneous population, varying on a large number of parameters. Degree of hearing loss, age of onset, use of amplification, exposure to remedial procedures, family support and/or resources, age of identification, and presence of a variety of other handicapping conditions may combine in numerous ways to determine the effects of a given loss on an individual. Common sense suggests that the more severe the hearing loss, the greater the handicap and the earlier in life the hearing loss occurs, the worse its effects will be, but even these logical assumptions are not always true. One of the authors evaluated two women during the same week who illustrated the difficulties involved in estimating the handicapping effects of a given loss. The first was a vigorous 78-year-old woman, active in social affairs and a leader in a small southern community. Her recently acquired hearing loss was mild; the pure tone average (PTA) in the poorer ear was 28 dB HL and her discrimination score for monosyllables was 92 percent in quiet. She complained of being unable to hear well enough to pursue her usual activities and elected to use a hearing aid. The second was a 40-year-old mother of five children whose PTA was 52 dB HL bilaterally and whose speech discrimination score was 72 percent. She elected not to use a hearing aid, stating that she heard "everything I need to hear. If someone wants me, they can always tap me on the shoulder!"

These cases illustrate the necessity of distinguishing between hearing *impairment* and hearing *handicap*. Impairment refers to the physical deficit associated with a loss of hearing. It can be expressed precisely in terms of decibels, speech discrimination scores, speech reception thresholds, frequency difference limen, or pressure in the middle ear. Stating that an individual has an average hearing loss of 50 dB is a description of the degree of impairment of the detection of pure tone signals. It says nothing about the degree to which the loss of hearing affects the individual's ability to communicate or to function socially, academically, or vocationally. When hearing loss interferes with these or other aspects of life, the result is *handicap*. Handicap is rarely describable in objective terms. Degree of handicap depends on many factors, most of which must be described subjectively. For example, when discrimination of speech is reduced, yielding a score of 70 percent, the person may be said to have "moderately poor" speech discrimination skills. The degree to which these skills actually interfere with daily life will depend on a number of factors not easily described. A pharmacist with such a problem is sure to be more affected by it daily than a farmer who lives alone. The degree of *handicap* would be quite different for these two people, and quantification of the difference can never be precise.

All people with hearing loss exhibit impairment; many exhibit handicaps. One of the first tasks of the audiologist is to determine if the loss is handicapping and, if so, under what circumstances. Treatment procedures can then be designed that will address directly the specific needs of the individual involved. For some, the selection of a hearing aid and/or counseling about how to manipulate environmental factors, such as light and noise sources or distance from the speaker, is sufficient to alleviate the handicapping effects of the hearing loss. For others, an intensive program of training may be required before the individual can communicate effectively. Therefore, rehabilitative plans and techniques must be based on a thorough knowledge of the individual to be served.

Factors Affecting Degree of Handicap

There are dozens of factors that may influence how handicapping a given hearing loss will be to the person who has it. These include personality factors, vocational choice, and the particular communicative tasks that make up the person's daily activities, to name only a few. It would be impossible to identify every conceivable factor, but there are several that are of primary importance and that can be easily described.

Age of Onset. Hearing loss can occur at any age. From a developmental point of view, the effects of a sensory deficit will depend on the stage of development that exists at the time the deficit occurs. Hearing is one of two distance senses that allow the reception and decoding of a vast amount of input beginning at birth. It is on the basis of sensory stimulation that cognitive development proceeds. Although they are functional at birth, sensory systems such as vision and audition undergo refinements over time; sensitivity and acuity develop rapidly, then combine with increased cognitive skills to allow more and more sophisticated discriminations to be made. As knowledge increases, the need for redundancy of input information is reduced. Observers are able to make discriminative or evaluative judgments using less information than was necessary at an earlier developmental stage. Consequently, the specific effects of hearing impairment, for example, will be influenced by the stage of development (sensory, linguistic, social and so on) that exists at the time of onset of the impairment.

Studies of the effects of sensory deprivation in young animals indicate that changes occur in the central nervous system fibers when sensory stimulation is withheld by blocking the visual or auditory receptors early in life. Studies have shown that animals never achieve complete development of sensory function after early deprivation (Bruner, 1961; Webster and Webster, 1977), even though the deprivation was temporary and mechanical and could be completely reversed later by removing the barriers to reception. These studies support the theory of critical periods of development, during which organisms are thought to be programmed to respond to certain types of stimuli and to incorporate them into development of the organism as a whole. If a given type of stimulation does not occur during its critical period, it may not be possible to process such stimuli efficiently when they are available at later stages of development. This issue is an important one in management of the hearing impaired. It indicates the importance of early identification of hearing loss and the necessity of providing as much early auditory stimulation as possible in order to foster the maximum possible development of auditory processing.

Effective use of the redundancy of the acoustic cues of speech probably depends on early exposure to these auditory events as a natural adjunct to experience with other stimuli. Once they become the basis of auditory processing and differentiation, their later absence affects speech perception. People who hear normally while language is being learned and then suffer hearing loss probably face an auditory task that is quite different from that encountered by people whose hearing losses are congenital. In the first case, auditory processing involves using the acoustic cues that remain available to make decisions about the ones that are now absent. This process is known as *auditory closure*. Visual cues may substitute for auditory ones because of associations between visual and auditory information that have developed over time. By contrast, people whose hearing losses occur before such associations are firmly established must learn to use fewer acoustic cues for speech recognition, many of which are not audible without the use of amplification. Intensive exposure within meaningful contexts is necessary before auditory and visual cues can be used as a *gestalt* and before the relationship among acoustic cues can be used as the basis of speech discrimination. Although the hearing losses for pure tones may be identical in both cases, the usefulness of the auditory information available and the perceptual basis on which it is processed may be quite different.

In addition to speech perception, other aspects of development are also affected by early onset of hearing loss. Because reduced hearing limits the understanding of speech, it affects language development. Delayed language development in turn affects academic achievement, social interactions, and, often, vocational choice. It is easy to see, therefore, that the earlier the onset of hearing loss, the greater the impact on future life-style is likely to be.

Children who experience hearing loss in infancy may require special educational placement and procedures, a situation that is unlikely for children whose onset of hearing loss occurs in late adolescence. Older children and young adults who develop hearing impairments often have to make changes in previous plans for vocational choices and training. Adults who experience severe damage to their hearing may have to change vocations as a result of inability to perform tasks associated with their professions or jobs. Some older adults find it necessary to retire early if the hearing loss is severe. In some cases, a hearing loss that might have resulted in handicap had it occurred in childhood, becomes only a nuisance when it occurs in adulthood. Therefore, age of onset is a primary factor in determining the handicapping effects of a given hearing loss.

Severity. The degree of hearing loss is an important factor influencing the handicapping effects of hearing impairment. Stated simply, the greater the hearing loss, the greater the reduction in loudness for some (or all) of the component frequencies of speech. This results in a decrease in the number of acoustic cues that are available to the listener. Normally hearing individuals perceive speech optimally when it is 25 to 40 dB above threshold and obtain their maximum speech discrimination scores in this range of sensation levels (SL). The average intensity level of conversational speech is approximately 50 dB HL, and the average threshold for speech in normal listeners is 0 to 10 dB HL, allowing for an SL for speech of 40 to 50 dB under ordinary circumstances. Conversely, a person with a hearing loss for speech of 40 dB HL will hear conversational speech at a significantly reduced loudness level (about 10 dB SL), which sharply reduces speech discrimination. The relationship between hearing loss and the audibility of speech is discussed in detail in Chapter 2.

Although a hearing loss of 40 dB is considered to be relatively mild, the individual with this degree of hearing impairment may be able to understand speech only if it is clearly enunciated and occurs in an exceptionally quiet environment. Less favorable communication situations will result in failure to hear and understand. When speech is softer than average or the environment is noisy, communication by audition alone may be impossible, and speech must be amplified even to be heard. More severe hearing losses limit even further the use of auditory input as a way of communicating, even under favorable listening conditions.

At the risk of oversimplifying the factors determining the loudness of complex sounds, the following statements may be helpful in understanding the relationships between intensity and the loudness perceived by the listener. A reduction of 10 dB in sound pressure level (SPL) results approximately in a halving of the loudness sensation. Therefore, an individual with an average threshold of 20 dB HL perceives speech only one-half as loudly as a normally hearing listener whose threshold is 10 dB HL. With a 30 dB HL threshold, an individual perceives speech as being approximately one-fourth as loud as the normal listener whose threshold is 10 dB HL. Significant reductions in redundancy occur as a result of the reduced sensation level. As the number of acoustic cues that can be heard diminishes, the difficulties encountered in understanding speech increase. Communication deficits occur that interfere with other aspects of development or daily functioning. Thus, the severity of the hearing loss directly affects the degree of handicap associated with hearing loss.

Degree of hearing loss is usually expressed in terms of the pure tone average (PTA) or the speech reception threshold (SRT). *Severity* of hearing loss is expressed by descriptive terms, such as *mild* or *severe*. The relationship between the degree of a loss and its severity is not clear cut. As a result, authors employ different terminology to express this relationship, primarily because the terms used are so imprecise and difficult to quantify. For example, hearing losses are referred to as being mild, moderate, severe, and profound. There is no general concensus among audiologists as to the criteria appropriate to each term. Another common way of expressing differences in severity is by use of the terms "deaf" and "hard of hearing," with the former usually indicating a severe to profound hearing loss and the latter referring to hearing losses ranging from mild to severe. Unfortunately, these terms are never self-explanatory and must be defined by those who use them.

We will use the term "deaf" primarily when reporting the work of others who use that terminology. Otherwise, severity of hearing loss will be indicated by the terms *mild, moderate, severe,* and *profound*. Because the ability to process speech is more important than sensitivity for pure tones, we prefer not to establish pure tone criteria as cutoff points for these descriptors. Nevertheless, it is necessary to provide a framework for mutual understanding of the terms used. Therefore, with reluctance, the following *general* guidelines are suggested.

Thresholds for Pure Tones and/or Speech (Degree)	*Description of Hearing (Severity)*
0–15 dB HL	Normal
16–40 dB HL	Mild
41–55 dB HL	Moderate
56–70 dB HL	Moderate–severe
71–90 dB HL	Severe
91 and above	Profound

If the thresholds listed are accompanied by unusually severe problems with speech perception or additional handicapping conditions, the terms may not be appropriate descriptors of the handicapping effect of a particular hearing loss. It is important, therefore, that these terms be used as general estimates for purposes of easy communication and not as diagnostic designations. People who have hearing losses of 40 dB seldom consider them mild. They often refer to themselves as "deaf" and "unable to hear anything." If we consider the fact that they are experiencing approximately *one-eighth* of the loudness associated with normal hearing, the relativity of the term *mild* becomes obvious.

Site of Lesion. The location within the auditory system of the condition causing hearing loss is the third important factor influencing the degree of handicap. Generally, the more peripheral the impairment the greater the possibility for successful auditory perception. Conductive hearing losses, involving the outer and middle ears, result primarily in reduced sensitivity for sound. Increasing the SPL of auditory input will overcome the effects of conductive hearing loss making habilitation of the communication deficits associated with it a simple matter.

By contrast, sensorineural hearing loss, resulting from problems in the inner ear or the auditory nerve leading to the brainstem, and central hearing losses resulting from lesions in the auditory pathways in the brainstem and beyond, usually involve some degree of *dysacusis* in addition to a reduction in sensitivity. Dysacusis refers to "any impairment of hearing that is not primarily a loss of auditory sensitivity" (Davis and Silverman, 1978). Dysacusis includes the following conditions: discrimination loss for words, syllables, or phonemes; phonemic regression (difficulty understanding speech that is unusual for the degree of hearing loss); auditory agnosia or central auditory imperception; recruitment (an abnormal sensitivity to loud sounds); and diplacusis (faulty pitch perception). Some of these conditions are common effects of sensorineural hearing loss; others occur only in hearing losses of central origin, especially phonemic regression and auditory agnosia. Therefore, persons with conductive hearing loss have an excellent prognosis for overcoming their communication deficits. People with sensorineural hearing loss have good potential for use of amplification and other conventional management procedures, whereas individuals with central hearing losses are the least likely to benefit from hearing aids and traditional remedial measures.

It is possible for an individual to exhibit hearing loss arising from any combination of these sites of lesion. Mixed hearing loss (conductive and sensorineural) is quite common among children. Central auditory problems that produce specific learning disabilities may be present in children with normal hearing and conductive or sensorineural losses. Some of the major causes of prenatal and prelingual hearing impairments are also among the leading etiologies of brain damage that results in other disabilities. These include maternal rubella, meningitis, prematurity, and Rh incompatability, all of which have been shown to contribute to both peripheral and central auditory deficits. The presence of more than one site of lesion significantly increases the degree of handicap associated with the resulting impairment and complicates the rehabilitative process as well.

Family Support. Although much more difficult to quantify than the factors discussed above, family attitudes and actions are important determiners of how well the hearing-impaired member of the family communicates both in and out of the home. The style of communication among family members can enhance or undermine attempts to use amplification or participate in family discussions, for example. Loud and boisterous families, in which people compete for the floor, all talk at once, or call to each other from room to room provide a very different communicative environment from families whose members are quiet, restrained communicators. The former may result in a situation that is too noisy to allow use of a hearing aid or optimal perception of speech. The latter may result in speech patterns that are too quiet for a hearing-impaired listener to understand. However, with some guidance and effort either type of family could provide strong support to its hearing-impaired member. Therefore, the most important family characteristic is the willingness of its members to try to understand the communication problems caused by hearing loss and to expend effort in modifying communicative behavior to the benefit of the hearing-impaired member.

This is easier said than done. Communicative behavior is usually well-established before a member of the family becomes hearing impaired. Most families encounter the problem in one of two ways. Either an elderly relative loses hearing or comes to live with the family after hearing has diminished, or a child with hearing impairment is born into the family. The two situations present quite different family adjustment needs and require different types of information and action on the family's part.

It is difficult to assess the degree to which families are able to provide the necessary support and assistance. Sometimes family members express open resentment toward the hearing-impaired member; usually they do not. Many families express bewilderment about their roles in rehabilitative plans. Some families seem unaware that they *have* a role to play. It is the audiologist's responsibility to obtain information about the level of knowledge, attitudes, and abilities of families to provide an atmosphere that is conducive to good communication and the achievement of other rehabilitative goals appropriate to each hearing impaired individual. Treatment procedures should then include whatever activities are necessary to improve family participation in the remediation process. Discussion of some of these activities appears in succeeding chapters.

Other Factors. The factors discussed above are only a few of those that influence the degree to which a hearing impairment may result in a handicap. Other important factors include the presence or absence of other impairments (visual or mental, for example), the availability of and response to special educational or remedial procedures, and many others. The audiologist must investigate the factors involved in each individual case by use of interviews, case histories, assessments by other professionals, and close observation. Provision of adequate services depends on a thorough knowledge of the person to be served and the collection of descriptive information should always precede the planning and execution of rehabilitative procedures.

REFERENCES

Bruner, J., The cognitive consequences of early deprivation. In P. Solomon, P. Kubansky, P. Leiderman, J. Mendelson, R. Trumbull, and D. Wefler (Eds.), *Sensory Deprivation*. Cambridge: Harvard University Press, 1961.

Davis, H. and Silverman, S., *Hearing and Deafness*. New York: Holt, Rinehart and Winston, 1978.

Webster, D. and Webster, M., Neonatal sound deprivation affects brain stem auditory nuclei, *Arch. Otolaryngol.*, 103, 392–396, 1977.

CHAPTER 2

Auditory Perception of Speech

by Dianne J. Van Tasell

The effects of hearing loss on the perception of speech are central to the remediation of hearing-impaired people. For adults with acquired hearing loss, the gradual or sudden decrease in their ability to comprehend the speech of others constitutes the major handicap produced by the loss of hearing. Consequently, the main thrust of rehabilitation with adults is to provide them with amplification, the primary purpose of which is to restore the speech information that has been ''lost'' by virtue of their impaired hearing.

For children with hearing loss that exists prior to the acquisition of language, the issues are different in many ways. The auditory speech signal is the main vehicle by which information about language is conveyed to developing children. Hearing-impaired children will be unable to extract all the language information from the speech signal that is needed to infer and ultimately master the complex rules that govern language form, content, and use. Hearing loss may also make it difficult for children to develop intelligible speech, since this requires hearing the speech of others well enough to imitate it and hearing their own speech well enough to monitor its intelligibility. The communication handicap imposed by hearing loss in early childhood is much more devastating than that caused by hearing loss acquired in adulthood, because the speech perception problems experienced by hearing-impaired children result in delayed acquisition of speech and language. These, in turn, may lead to profound educational, vocational, emotional, and social consequences.

Although both conductive and sensorineural hearing loss can disrupt the speech perception process, the problems caused by conductive hearing loss can often be overcome by medical/surgical means, or through the use of amplification. It is sensorineural hearing loss, specifically that caused by cochlear damage or abnormality, that most frequently causes serious speech perception difficulties. This chapter focuses exclusively on perception of speech by children and adults with sensorineural hearing loss, primarily of cochlear origin.

EFFECTS OF HEARING LOSS ON SPEECH PERCEPTION

One function of the peripheral auditory system is to convert the auditory speech signal into a neural code for input to the central nervous system. When this function is disrupted by sensorineural hearing loss, some or all of the information in the speech signal may be coded inaccurately or not at all. The inability of the abnormal auditory system to preserve speech information constitutes the speech recognition *impairment* caused by hearing loss.

The communication *handicap* that results from impaired speech perception ability is more difficult to define and evaluate. Spoken language is rich in information about the message it conveys. Consider the sentence, "Mary went to the pet store and bought two kittens." A listener who was asked to identify the final word of that spoken sentence could do so based on a variety of information. First of all, there would be the acoustic structure of the word "kittens." Even if that structure were unclear, there would be other clues. Because of its location in the sentence, the word has to be a noun. It has to be a plural noun, since it is preceded by the word "two." It has to be something that can be bought in a pet store. And if the listener knows that Mary has discovered mice in her house, chances are that the identity of that final word will be easy to guess.

A hearing-impaired listener with a good knowledge of language and some life experience may be able to use these kinds of contextual clues to aid in understanding spoken language. A very young hearing-impaired child or a hearing-impaired adult who has language problems, however, may not find them so helpful. Thus, it is quite possible for two persons to experience the same speech perception impairment, but to be communicatively handicapped to very different degrees.

There are two major types of variables that affect speech perception, but the exact contribution of each of them is difficult to determine. Acoustic variables such as the length of the speech unit, its phonetic context, the intensity at which it is delivered, and whether or not it is degraded by noise or filtering affect a listener's ability to perceive a message. Linguistic variables such as the vocabulary from which stimuli are taken and the length and complexity of the utterances (words versus sentences, for example) also affect performance. It is the combination of the effects of these variables that make monosyllabic words more intelligible than nonsense syllables and spoken digits more intelligible than spondaic words. The number of possible items from which the stimulus is taken is smaller for the easier stimuli. If a word is presented in a sentence it will be recognized more easily than if it is in isolation because of the clues in the rest of the sentence that help to identify the word. The effect of sentence context on intelligibility of single words is roughly similar to the effect of increasing the SPL of the word in isolation by about 6 dB (Miller, Heise, and Lichten, 1957).

Because of the influence of acoustic, linguistic, and other variables, the conclusions we can come to about any person's ability to perceive speech will depend heavily on the materials used to assess it and the conditions under which the materials are presented. This fact makes it difficult to determine how much the performance of a hearing-impaired individual is affected by the hearing loss itself and how much is affected by other variables. For example, many hearing impaired people score 100 percent correct on a list of spondaic words, but perform at a much lower level on a list of monosyllabic words presented at the same intensity. Which score most accurately reflects the effects of that individual's hearing loss on speech perception?

To answer that question, it is first necessary to isolate the effects of hearing loss from those of all other variables that influence performance on speech perception tasks. A logical point at which to begin to separate and define the specific effects of hearing loss is at the acoustic level. It is reasonable to assume that hearing loss somehow interacts with the acoustic structure of speech, resulting in the alteration of the speech signal so that certain aspects of it are either inaudible to or otherwise unusable by the hearing-impaired listener. This altered speech signal functions as the input to the central nervous system of the hearing-impaired listener; from it must be extracted linguistic information.

In a sense, it is the interaction of the hearing loss with the acoustic parameters of speech that is the limiting factor in speech perception. Any further use that the hearing-impaired listener can make of the degraded speech input will depend almost entirely on linguistic sophistication.

To understand the ways in which hearing loss may interact with the acoustic structure of speech, the acoustic characteristics of the speech signal must be considered.

The Speech Signal

Long-Term Characteristics. The acoustic waveform of conversational speech is complex and constantly changing. It is possible to specify average characteristics of this waveform, although this obscures the short-term characteristics of smaller segments of the signal that may be perceptually more important.

The average level of speech measured 18 inches from the lips of a male talker is approximately 74 dB SPL (Benson and Hirsh, 1953). However, segments of the waveform corresponding to individual phonemes may differ from each other in relative power by as much as 30 dB (Fletcher, 1970). This would be the case in the word "thaw," in which the relative power of the consonant **th** would be about 30 dB below that of the vowel **aw.** If the average rate of speaking in American English is 440 syllables per minute (Gerber, 1974), and each syllable comprises, on the average, two phonemes, then this translates to 880 phonemes per minute, or 15 phonemes per second. Thus, the speech waveform may actually fluctuate in level as many as 15 times per second.

The long-term average spectrum of conversational speech depicted in Figure 2.1 is familiar to most students of speech science. It shows clearly that the greatest energy, on the average, is to be found in the 500-Hz region. The spectrum level decreases toward the higher frequencies at the rate of about 9 dB/octave (Dunn and White, 1940). This average description of speech does not provide much information about the spectral characteristics of shorter segments of the speech waveform.

While it is possible to break down the speech waveform into segments of many different lengths, the one that lends itself most readily to acoustic analysis is that corresponding to the phoneme. The concept of phoneme is really a linguistic one, since the phoneme is defined as the smallest unit of speech that can signal a change in linguistic meaning. The actual perceptual unit that a listener uses for extraction of information from the signal may or may not be one of phoneme length. Nevertheless, phonemes can be separated into classes that do have sets of acoustic characteristics in common. The most obvious distinction is that which separates phonemes into vowels and consonants.

Short-Term Characteristics (Vowels). The sound source for all vowels is the complex, quasi-periodic waveform that is generated at the level of the larynx. This waveform contains its greatest energy at the vocal fundamental frequency, with energy decreasing at about 10 to 12 dB/octave above the fundamental frequency (Flanagan, 1958).

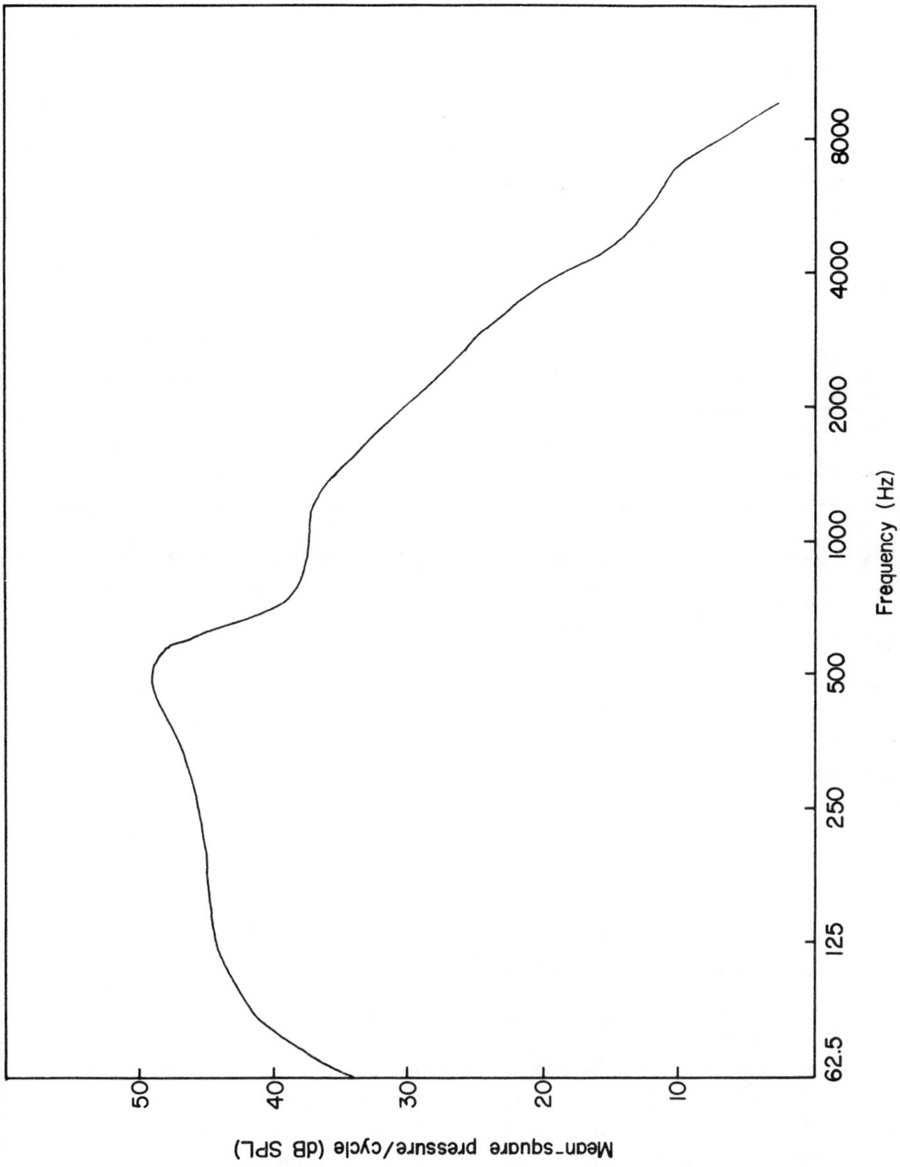

Figure 2.1. Long-term average power density spectrum of conversational speech measured 30 cm from the talkers' lips. (Adapted from H. K. Dunn and S. D. White, Statistical measurements on conversational speech, *J. Acoust. Soc. Am.*, 11, 1940, 278–288.)

The vocal tract acts as an acoustic resonator that modifies the spectrum of the laryngeal sound source. The frequencies, bandwidths, and amplitudes of the vocal tract resonances are directly dependent on the overall configuration of the tract, which can be changed via movements of various articulators such as the tongue, jaw, velum, and lips. For example, the spectrum of any vowel will contain energy at the fundamental frequency of the speaker's voice and its harmonics. Each vowel will be distinguished by certain peaks in the spectrum that result from the placement of the articulators and the size and shape of the vocal tract as it forms that particular vowel. These peaks of energy are called *formants*, and vowels can be defined in terms of the formant frequencies associated with them.

Although there may be as many as six or seven audible formants in a vowel, all vowels of English can be distinguished from each other on the basis of the lowest-frequency two or three. The lowest-frequency formant (F_1) corresponds roughly to the degree of tongue constriction employed during vowel production; those vowels that are produced with a relatively narrow constriction (high vowels) are characterized by relatively low-frequency F_1. Vowels produced with the tongue lower in the mouth have higher-frequency F_1.

The second formant (F_2) corresponds to the front-back place of major vocal tract constriction; the frequency of F_2 is high for front vowels, and decreases as the place of constriction moves to the back of the oral cavity. Of course, the frequencies of the vocal tract resonances are actually functions of the three-dimensional area of the entire tract; it is merely convenient to think of the lowest two formants as they relate to tongue height and place.

For male talkers, F_1 frequency ranges from roughly 270 to 730 Hz, the region in which most energy is concentrated in the long-term spectrum of speech (see Figure 2.1). F_2 frequencies range from 840 to 2290 Hz, and F_3 frequencies include 1690 to 3010 Hz (Peterson and Barney, 1952). As formant frequency increases, the amplitude of the formant peak in the vowel spectrum decreases by as much as 40 dB from F_1 to F_3 (for the vowel **oo**). This is largely a function of the decreased energy in the laryngeal waveform at high frequencies and is reflected in the high-frequency falloff seen in the long-term speech spectrum.

Short-Term Characteristics (Consonants). It is convenient to classify consonant phonemes according to their characteristic subphonemic features. Although many different and more elaborate sets of subphonemic features have been devised, it is possible to describe all consonants in terms of the three-feature set consisting of manner, voicing, and place. The manner feature describes the specific articulatory gesture used to produce the consonant. The voicing feature classifies consonants according to the presence or absence of the laryngeal tone as a sound source. The place feature relates to the point in the vocal tract at which the consonant is produced. Table 2.1 shows the classification of consonants according to this three-feature system. Note that semivowels and nasals are voiced consonants; the mem-

Table 2.1 Subphonemic Feature Classification of Consonants

	MANNER OF ARTICULATION					
			Stop		*Fricative*	
Place of Articulation	*Semivowel*	*Nasal*	*Voiced*	*Unvoiced*	*Voiced*	*Unvoiced*
Front						
Bilabial	w	m	b	p		
Labiodental					v	f
Middle						
Dental					$\overset{2}{\text{th}}$	$\overset{1}{\text{th}}$
Alveolar	j, l	n	d	t	z	s
Palatal	r				zh	sh
Back						
Velar		ng	g	k		
Pharyngeal						
Glottal						h

Adapted from J.M. Pickett, *The Sounds of Speech Communication*. Baltimore: University Park Press, 1980. Reprinted with permission.

bers of these two manner classes differ from each other only in terms of place of articulation. Stops and fricatives may be either voiced or unvoiced, and may differ in place of articulation.

Semivowels. Like vowels, the semivowels **r, l, w, and y** are the result of the modification of the laryngeal waveform by the vocal tract. They differ from vowels in that they are shorter in duration and are produced with a greater degree of vocal tract constriction. Vocal tract resonant frequencies vary in much the same way as they do for vowels. Because of the narrower constriction, F_1 is relatively low in frequency. The frequency of F_2 varies with place of articulation, and is therefore relatively high (about 2400 Hz) for **y**, midrange for **l** and **r** (about 1200 Hz), and low for **w** (about 600 Hz). The semivowels **l** and **r** are distinguished chiefly by their F_3 frequencies, which range from 2400 to 3500 Hz for **l**, and from 1200 to 2400 Hz for **r** (Borden and Harris, 1980).

Nasals. As is the case with vowels and semivowels, the nasals **m, n** and **ng** are both voiced and resonant. However, the resonating vowel tract consists of the pharynx, the occluded oral cavity, and the nasal cavities. Thus, the oral cavity now acts essentially as a side-branch resonator, because sound is radiated from the nostrils instead of from the lips.

The most important acoustic result of the resonating nasal cavities is the presence of a peak in the spectrum of the nasal consonants corresponding to the resonant frequency of the vocal tract at about 300 Hz. This spectral prominence is known as "nasal murmur," and is a powerful perceptual cue for nasality.

Differences in place of production are signaled primarily by the frequency of the antiresonance of the oral cavity, which is now acting as a side-branch resonator. The antiresonance frequency depends on the place at which the oral cavity is occluded, and occurs at about 800 Hz for the bilabial **m,** at 1500 to 2000 Hz for the alveolar **n,** and at about 5000 Hz for the velar **ng** (Pickett, 1980).

Fricatives. The fricatives **f, v, th, s, z, sh, zh,** and **h** are produced by forcing the breath stream through an extremely narrow constriction in the vocal tract. The acoustical result is a fairly broad, flat-spectrum noise that serves as the only sound source for the unvoiced fricatives.

The noise source spectrum is shaped mainly by the resonances of the vocal tract anterior to the place of constriction. The fricatives characterized by the lowest resonant frequencies, and therefore the lowest-frequency noise spectrum, will be those produced with the constriction located at the most posterior points in the vocal tract. The fricative **h,** for which the noise source is at the glottis, is characterized by a spectral maximum at about 1000 Hz. As the point of constriction moves anteriorly, the resonant frequency increases to about 3000 Hz for **sh,** 4000 Hz for **s,** 5000 Hz for **th,** and 4500 to 7000 Hz for **f** (Pickett, 1980).

The noise spectrum of a voiced fricative is shaped in the same way as is the spectrum of its unvoiced counterpart. For a voiced fricative, the laryngeal sound source is activated, and the output spectrum is essentially the product of both laryngeal and noise sources, and of the vocal tract filtering that is applied to both.

Stops. The stop consonants **p, b, t, d, k,** and **g** are the most complex of all phonemes, both in an articulatory and in an acoustic sense. For a stop, the vocal tract is completely occluded at some point; during this phase, pressure builds up behind the occlusion due to the continuing expiratory breath stream. When the occlusion is released abruptly, a transient noise burst occurs, after which voicing begins for the following phoneme.

For voiced stops, voicing may simply continue through the occlusion phase, the burst, and the movement into the following phoneme, or voicing may begin up to 20 msec or so after the burst occurs. The interval between the onset of the burst and the onset of voicing is known as "voice onset time" (VOT); voiced stops are characterized by short VOT, the exact length of which is somewhat dependent on the place of articulation.

In an unvoiced stop, the VOT is longer—not less than 25 milliseconds for a bilabial. The interval between burst and onset of voicing is usually occupied by aspiration noise produced by air rushing through the trachea and vocal tract prior to the closing of the vocal folds for voice production. Thus, the voicing feature of a stop consonant is not simply signaled by the presence or absence of the laryngeal sound source, as it is for fricatives. Instead, it is the timing relations between noise production and initiation of voicing—and the complex acoustical results of these relationships—that determine the voicing characteristics of stops.

As is the case for fricatives, the spectra of the noise portions of stop consonants are the result of resonant shaping of the noise source by the vocal tract anterior to the place of noise production. Velar stops **k** and **g** are produced with a relatively large cavity anterior to the place of occlusion, and are thus characterized by noise burst maxima in the 2000-Hz region. The alveolars **t** and **d** have burst maxima above 2000 Hz. For bilabials **b** and **p,** in which there is essentially no anterior cavity, the burst spectrum is fairly diffuse, extending upward from 1500 Hz (Pickett, 1980).

Other Characteristics. There are many other acoustic characteristics of individual phonemes that may figure importantly in speech perception. Their characteristics may change substantially when they are uttered in the context of other phonemes in a syllable, word, or phrase. Important information pertaining to the identity of one phoneme may even be contained in other phonemes in the utterance. For example, the length of a vowel preceding a stop consonant may carry most of the voicing information for that consonant; a longer-duration vowel leads to the perception of a voiced stop, while a short-duration vowel indicates a following unvoiced stop (Raphael, 1972).

Changes in vocal tract resonances occur as the tract moves between consonant and vowel positions. These movements result in formant *transitions* that carry a great deal of information about the identity of both vowels and consonants. Formant transition rate functions as a cue for manner differences, with fast transitions signaling stop consonants, slower transitions signaling semivowels, and very slow transitions signaling diphthongs. Slowing the consonant-vowel transition rate in the syllable **be-** (as in bed), for example, leads to the perception of **we-,** while an even greater decrease in transition rate produces the two-vowel combination **oo-e-.** Because the second formant is closely associated with place of articulation of both vowels and consonants, it is not surprising that the frequency characteristics of the F_2 transitions between consonants and vowels are important indicators of the place characteristics of both.

The acoustic parameters of individual phonemes do not constitute all the phonemic information to be found in the speech signal. Even so, it would be helpful to have a general idea of where those acoustic characteristics of individual phonemes are to be found in the speech spectrum. Figure 2.2 represents a rough demarcation of the frequency ranges in which speech information pertaining to consonant voicing, manner, and place is to be found. Voicing information extends from low frequencies where energy corresponding to the vocal fundamental frequency is to be found, upwards to relatively high frequencies, reflecting the ability of the upper-frequency harmonics of the fundamental to signal the presence of voicing.

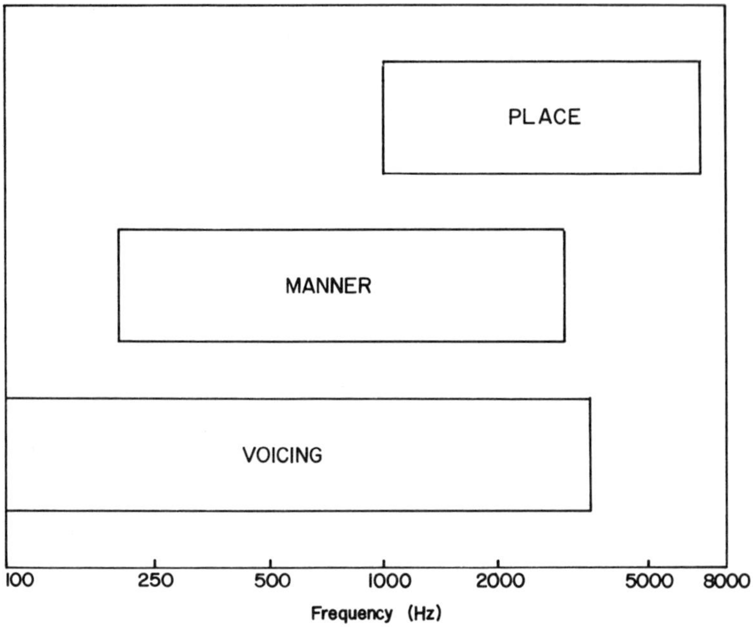

Figure 2.2. Frequency ranges of consonant place, manner, and voicing information.

Manner information is widely distributed across the spectrum, because acoustic cues for manner consist mostly of the timing of speech events. For instance, the difference in transition rate among stops, semivowels, and diphthongs cues a manner difference among those phoneme classes, and is essentially a temporal one.

Unlike manner and voicing information, place information is confined to a relatively narrow frequency range around 2000 Hz. The noise associated with stops and fricatives, the second formant, and the F_2 transitions lie in this area. All of these serve as cues for place of articulation of consonants and/or vowels.

Given this division of phoneme information into spectral areas, the shape of the long-term spectrum depicted in Figure 2.1 becomes more informative. Clearly, the high-energy, low-frequency portion of the spectrum contains information about consonant voicing and manner, in addition to vowel first formant energy. The low-energy, high-frequency portion of the spectrum contains some consonant manner and voicing information and almost all consonant place information, in addition to the upper formants of the vowels.

Knowledge of the speech spectrum described above can be used to predict the effects of a given hearing loss on phoneme recognition. Hearing loss in different frequency ranges will affect speech perception in different ways, and the speech perception deficit should vary in kind as well as in severity among hearing impaired individuals. This variation is the result of the interaction of the unique characteristics of an individual's hearing loss with the unique acoustic characteristics of speech.

Phonemic Perception by Hearing-Impaired Listeners

The perception of speech is a human process, and is therefore subject to the full spectrum of variables that influence human behavior. The source of some of the most significant of these variables is the way in which speech perception is usually assessed, both clinically and experimentally. There are at least three components of any assessment procedure.

1. The Speech Stimuli

The investigator has a choice of many different types of speech materials. The most widely used are lists of monosyllabic words, but nonsense syllables, multisyllabic words, sentences, and even continuous discourse are also used.

2. Auditory Presentation of the Speech Stimuli

Speech stimuli can be presented to listeners via loudspeaker, earphone, insert receiver, and other devices. They can be presented at various intensity levels, and they can be distorted in many different ways. Two forms of distortion that are commonly used are filtering and masking with either noise or speech.

3. Evaluation of Responses

After auditory presentation of each stimulus, the listener must indicate in some way what was actually heard. Usually, this is done by repeating the stimulus, writing it down on an answer sheet, or answering questions about its message content. Once the responses have been recorded, either a *quantative* or a *qualitative* method may be used to evaluate them, depending on the nature of the speech stimuli and on the information that the assessment task was designed to obtain. The use of a quantitative method entails counting the number or percent of the stimuli to which the listener responded correctly. The information obtained with this method pertains to the *extent* or *severity* of the subject's speech perception problem. Qualitative assessment methods involve the analysis of the erroneous responses made by the subject, as opposed to simply counting them. The use of these methods can yield information about the *nature* of the speech perception process and the problems experienced.

To examine the ways in which hearing loss affects the perception of the information-bearing acoustic parameters of the speech signal, it is first necessary to eliminate or control those nonacoustic variables that can affect subjects' performance on speech recognition tasks. The choice of speech stimuli is crucial, and for this purpose is limited to two types:

1. Meaningful Words in a Closed-set Response Format. Restricting the subject's response options to four or five items effectively brings linguistic variables under experimental control. That is, the vocabulary size of the subject ceases to be a factor in how the subject will respond, because the working vocabularies of all subjects will consist of only the four or five possible responses for each stimulus item. Perception of single phonemes can be tested in this way if all response alternatives differ in terms of only one sound. To investigate perception of the initial consonant in the word "bill," for example, response alternatives could be limited to the words "bill," "pill," "till," and "fill."

2. Nonsense Syllables. The use of nonmeaningful speech stimuli eliminates the possible contribution of contextual or other linguistic variables to subjects' responses. If the amount of acoustic information (i.e., number of phonemes) is held constant, then subjects could presumably base their responses only on the perceived phonetic characteristic of the stimuli.

In addition to careful selection of materials, a qualitative method of response analysis may be employed. The way in which phoneme recognition data are most commonly analyzed is to first cast the data into a confusion matrix. In this way, responses are compared to the stimuli that elicited those responses. Response data can then be further analyzed to determine what type of recognition errors were made and whether those error types form some sort of pattern. Figure 2.3 depicts a

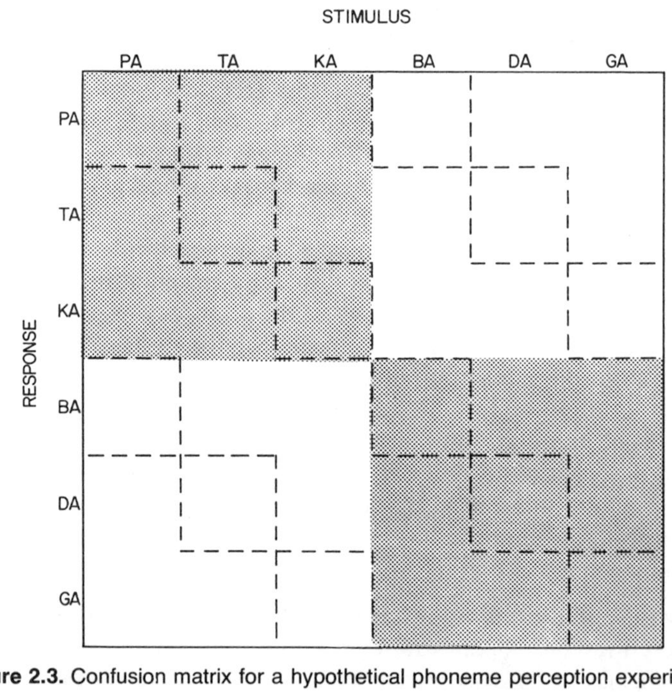

Figure 2.3. Confusion matrix for a hypothetical phoneme perception experiment.

confusion matrix for a hypothetical experiment in which the stimuli were the nonsense syllables "pa," "ta," "ka," "ba," "da," and "ga." Correct responses would be represented by entries along the main diagonal. Responses that were correct in terms of the voicing feature would be those entries inside the two shaded areas, while responses correct in terms of place would be confined to entries within the dashed boxes. Phoneme confusion matrices can be analyzed in this way for information regarding the number of phoneme errors and the type of subphonemic feature errors.

There have been many investigations of the phoneme confusions made by hearing impaired subjects for nonsense and closed-set materials. Although much of the data are contradictory, certain trends do emerge from these studies, and they are described below.

Meaningful Words. A number of investigators have employed consonant-vowel-consonant (CVC) words as stimuli for testing perception of single phonemes by hearing impaired listeners. Recall that phoneme perception information is obtained by providing the subject with a finite number of response words (usually four) that differ only in terms of the single phoneme being tested. When this approach is used, a consistent pattern of results usually emerges.

First, hearing-impaired subjects make few errors in vowel perception (Owens, Talbott, and Schubert, 1968; Owens, Benedict, and Schubert, 1971). When errors do occur, they tend to be on front vowels, which are characterized by higher-frequency second formants. In this case, subjects typically confuse the stimulus vowel with another vowel having a similar first formant frequency (Pickett, Martin, Johnson, Smith, Daniel, Willis, and Otis, 1972).

The error rate for consonants is much higher than that for vowels, and tends to be highest for consonants in word-final position (Owens and Schubert, 1968; Pickett et al., 1972; Sher and Owens, 1974; Owens, 1978). The overwhelming majority of consonant errors made by hearing impaired subjects involves the subphonemic feature *place* of articulation (Owens and Schubert, 1968; Owens, Benedict and Schubert, 1972; Pickett et al., 1972; Byers, 1973; Sher and Owens, 1974; Owens, 1978). *Manner* of articulation is perceived somewhat better, although errors on this feature do occur. It is noteworthy that errors involving the perception of nasality, or nasal manner of production, seldom occur (Owens and Schubert, 1968; Byers, 1973). Finally, the *voicing* feature is usually perceived accurately (Owens and Schubert, 1968; Pickett et al., 1972; Byers, 1973).

Relatively few investigations have explored the relation of audiometric configuration to phoneme perception. Owens and his coworkers (1972) did observe that the probability of error for stimulus phonemes **s, sh, ch, j, t, th** increased with increasing hearing loss in high frequencies. By the same token, some investigators have reported that these same phonemes are likely to be perceived erroneously both by subjects with high-frequency sensorineural hearing loss and by normally hearing subjects listening to CVC speech stimuli distorted by low-pass filtering (Owens et al., 1972; Sher and Owens, 1974). However, in no case has it been shown that phoneme error *type* is related to audiometric configuration. That is, the phonemes on which hearing-impaired subjects are likely to make errors are to some extent predictable on the basis of the configuration of hearing loss. On the other hand, the type of errors they make on those phonemes, or the subphonemic features that they perceive incorrectly, apparently are not predictable on the same basis.

Nonsense Syllables. When the speech stimuli are consonant-vowel (CV) or vowel-consonant (VC) nonsense syllables, and subjects have a larger number of response alternatives among which to choose, information obtained about phoneme perception is somewhat different. Again, very few errors are made on vowels, at least by subjects who have hearing loss only at frequencies above 1000 Hz (Lawrence and Byers, 1969).

In contrast to the meaningful-word data, consonants in nonsense syllable-initial position tend to be in error more often that those in final position (Bilger and Wang, 1976; Wang, Reed, and Bilger, 1978). In addition, the type of phoneme errors made by hearing-impaired subjects on these materials does appear to be related to audiometric configuration. Persons with flat or rising losses (better thresholds at high frequencies) (see Figure 2.4) make errors involving *nasality*. Features of *sibilance*

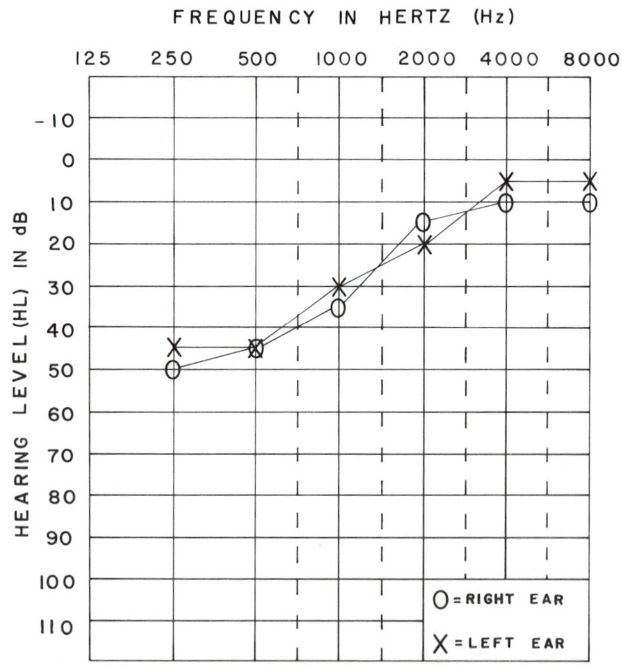

Figure 2.4. Audiogram depicting a rising hearing loss configuration.

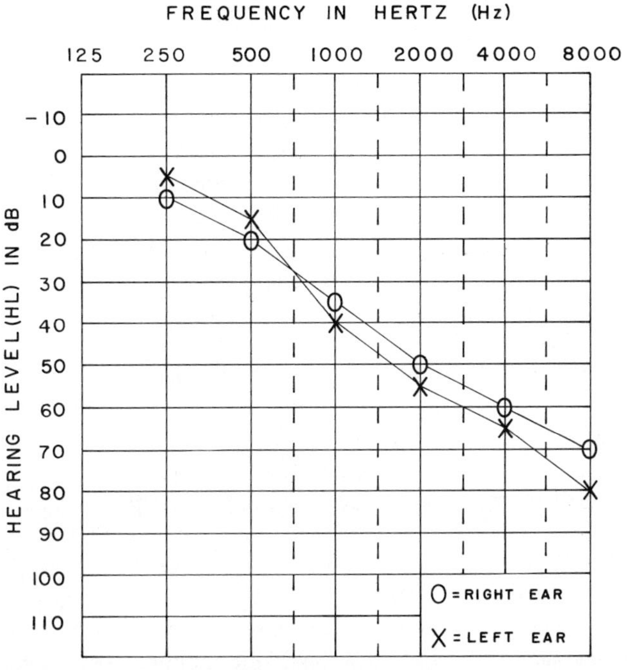

Figure 2.5. Audiogram depicting a sloping hearing loss configuration.

(presence of high-frequency consonant noise), *duration* and *voicing* are perceived correctly, while *place* is perceived somewhat more poorly (Reed, 1975; Bilger and Wang, 1976).

For persons with sloping high-frequency losses as depicted in Figure 2.5, *nasality* and *voicing* appear to be easy to perceive. Sibilance, on the other hand, is perceived poorly or not at all (Bilger and Wang, 1976). There is conflicting evidence on the perception of *place* of consonant articulation: Reed's (1975) subjects did not perceive it well, while subjects in the Bilger and Wang study (1976) performed better on this feature.

In a later study, Wang, Reed, and Bilger (1978) demonstrated that these same phoneme error patterns were characteristic of normal-hearing subjects listening to filtered nonsense syllables. Specifically, subjects listening to high-pass filtered syllables made errors similar to those made by subjects with flat or rising sensorineural losses. Low-pass filtering produced errors similar to those made by subjects with high-frequency sensorineural loss.

Another important finding of these studies was that phoneme error rate and phoneme error type did not seem to be related. Bilger and Wang (1976) showed that two subjects who performed at the same level in terms of percent of correct responses did not necessarily show similar types of errors. This clearly demonstrated that the speech perception information obtainable through the use of quantitative scoring methods is very different from that obtainable by qualitative, or error-analysis methods.

The meaningful-word data and the nonsense-syllable data differ in three major ways: (1) error rate on initial versus final consonants, (2) the proportion of *place* errors made relative to other types of errors, and (3) the relation of error type to configuration of hearing loss. These differences probably result from the combined effects of speech material, talker, response set, and subject training differences between the two types of studies, and provide ample evidence that even the most rigorously controlled speech perception studies are not free from the effects of all factors other than the acoustic characteristics of the stimuli.

Predicting Phoneme Perception. In retrospect, the data just reviewed on phoneme perception by hearing-impaired subjects would have been almost entirely predictable on the basis of the frequency location of information in the speech signal. Vowels are the most intense phonemes, and energy in the first formant region accounts for much of the energy in the long-term speech spectrum. It is therefore not surprising that vowels are perceived more accurately than consonants by hearing-impaired listeners, because vowel energy would likely remain audible even if some consonant energy were rendered inaudible by hearing loss.

Errors on front vowels may occur most often because front vowels have higher-frequency second formants. Because the amplitude of vowel formants decreases as their frequency increases, the F_2 energy in front vowels is also lower in amplitude than is F_2 energy in back vowels. Hearing-impaired persons are likely to have abnormal auditory thresholds at high frequencies. This characteristic of hearing loss, combined with the acoustic structure of front vowels, results in a reduction in the audibility of F_2 energy in front vowels. The lower-frequency, higher-intensity first formant remains audible and becomes the only information on which the listener can base vowel judgments. Thus, vowels that share F_1 frequency characteristcs may be confused with each other.

The consonant errors reported also make sense in terms of the frequencies associated with speech information. Persons with hearing loss at high frequencies have little difficulty perceiving low-frequency voicing information. The low-frequency nasal murmur, which is a powerful cue for nasal manner information, is also usable. This is reflected in the low incidence of phoneme errors involving nasality. Other types of manner information, however, extend to higher frequencies, and are thus more likely to be perceived inaccurately. The most disruptive effects of high-frequency hearing loss could be expected to be exerted on speech information confined to the high frequencies. Place information fits this description well, and the meaningful-word phoneme confusion data show that place is the feature most likely to be in error in these listeners.

Increased difficulty with nasality cues experienced by persons with flat or rising losses may be a reflection of the attenuation of the nasal murmur by hearing loss in the low frequencies. It is reasonable to assume that speech information pertaining to manner and place will also be affected by the loss of hearing at higher frequencies. The voicing feature remains singularly resistant even to the effects of flat and rising losses, probably because voicing information is represented across much of the speech spectrum, as well as in temporal aspects of the speech signal.

In general, the nature of the phoneme perception disturbance caused by hearing loss appears to be determined by the frequency region in which the loss occurs. Speech sound information in a region of normal hearing can be expected to be perceived correctly, while information in the region of hearing loss will be reduced in effectiveness to some extent.

The selective misperception of speech information is demonstrated particularly well by people with normal hearing in low frequencies and hearing loss only at higher frequencies. They make good use of low-frequency vowel and consonant information, but are unable to perceive correctly the higher-frequency cues for place of consonant articulation and sibilance. It would be erroneous, however, to expect the same performance from persons who have high-frequency sloping losses but do *not* have normal hearing in low frequencies. Erber's work has shown that the low-frequency residual hearing of children with profound sensorineural hearing loss (the familiar "corner" audiograms shown in Figure 2.6) is not usable for perception

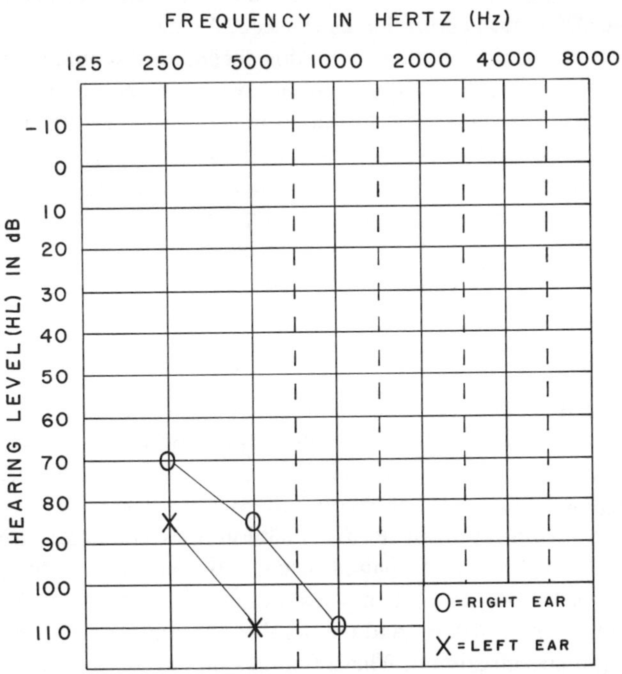

Figure 2.6. A "corner" audiogram in which hearing is limited to low frequencies.

of low-frequency speech information in the same way as is the low-frequency hearing of persons who have normal hearing in this region (Erber, 1979). Because these children's auditory thresholds may indicate vibrotactile instead of auditory sensitivity, or because their true auditory sensitivity may be restricted to an extremely narrow range of frequencies, they are apparently unable to make use of the spectral information contained in the low-frequency portion of the speech signal that may be detectable by them. For these children, the only speech information available auditorily is contained in the speech waveform envelope and consists mainly of the gross temporal aspects of speech such as vowel duration, vowel roughness, and syllabification.

The selective loss of speech sound information in the frequency region at which auditory thresholds are abnormal translates, for each hearing impaired individual, into a unique pattern of errors in the perception of phonemes and their subphonemic features. Because the same general pattern of errors may be elicited from a normally hearing listener by filtering the speech stimuli to simulate hearing loss, it has been convenient to think about hearing loss itself as a filter that simply attenuates speech information in the region of hearing loss. The appropriate goal of amplification, then, would be to return the hearing aid user's thresholds to normal by providing the appropriate amount of gain at frequencies at which hearing loss exists. This approach has been shown to be successful with persons have have fairly flat, moderate sensorineural hearing losses (Pascoe, 1975).

There are two major problems with this deceptively simple view of the hearing loss as a filter, the effects of which can be overcome by amplification at selected frequencies. First, the threshold of discomfort of the hearing-impaired listener may be equal to or even slightly lower than the normally hearing listener's threshold of discomfort. Because the hearing-impaired listener's sensitivity threshold in a region of hearing loss is higher than normal, the dynamic range of hearing, or range of intensities from detection threshold to threshold of discomfort, is smaller than it is for the normal listeners. Consequently, persons with severe hearing losses, and therefore small dynamic ranges, may not be able to tolerate the amount of amplification necessary to bring the speech signal to a suprathreshold level.

The other, more troublesome problem lies with the idea that hearing loss acts as a filter that simply attenuates the auditory signal differentially across frequencies. If this were truly the case, then we could expect the impaired auditory system to function normally once the appropriate frequencies of the signal were amplified to a suprathreshold level that was not uncomfortably loud. There is increasing evidence, however, that such a return of normal function does not occur. Results of recent studies indicate that hearing-impaired listeners perform more poorly than normals on auditory tasks involving frequency resolution (Wightman et al. 1977), frequency discrimination (Turner, 1979), and temporal resolution (Fitzgibbons, 1979) of suprathreshold non-speech stimuli. These findings are not restricted solely to frequencies at which a loss of sensitivity exists; Turner (1979) found that frequency discrimination by hearing impaired listeners may be poorer than normal even at frequencies where sensitivity thresholds are within normal limits. In light of these findings, it seems that hearing loss introduces much more complex signal distortions than simple filtering and attenuation.

Variability in Performance. The amount and type of speech sound information that is coded accurately by the peripheral auditory system varies greatly among hearing-impaired individuals. The nature of the acoustic speech information available to any given listener is related both to the configuration of hearing loss and to the way in which that configuration interacts with the distribution of phonetic information within the speech signal itself. While this interaction may involve simple attenuation of speech information, it is clear that sensorineural hearing loss introduces other types of signal distortions that are only beginning to be understood. Understanding of the spoken message is not entirely limited by the ability of a listener to recognize individual phonemes. Assuming that the phoneme perception ability of a hearing-impaired listener reflects the perceptual limits imposed by hearing loss, how does the hearing loss affect the ability of that listener to extract meaning from the speech signal?

Like anyone else, hearing-impaired listeners make use of a wide variety of both acoustic and linguistic cues in the process of speech perception. However, that process may differ in two important ways in the hearing-impaired population. First, the reduced amount of speech sound information to which the hearing-impaired listener has access may severely restrict the number of usable acoustic and linguistic cues. To the extent that phonetic information is preserved, the contextual information in speech will be used by hearing-impaired listeners in the same way as it is by normals. The same general rules apply: longer words may be more intelligible, as will be familiar words, words in sentences, and sentences about a known topic of conversation.

The second way in which the speech perception process may differ pertains to the way in which the available linguistic information may be used by a hearing-impaired listener. Many people who have hearing losses also have language problems that may be characterized by limited vocabularies and restricted knowledge of grammatical and phonological rules. For these individuals, linguistic information that is perceptible may still not be particularly useful. That is, the addition of linguistic context may do little to increase the intelligibility of speech for them.

As a group, hearing-impaired persons vary tremendously both in terms of the nature of their hearing losses and of their language sophistication. This being the case, we should expect that their performance on speech perception tasks would be highly variable. Indeed, the extreme variability among hearing-impaired listeners has been amply documented in the literature (Engelberg, 1968; Gengel, 1973). This variability does not appear to be appreciably reduced by grouping subjects according to audiometric configuration. Other factors, such as language competence, function to make hearing impaired people a highly divergent group. It is therefore crucial that no assumptions be made about the speech perception handicap of an individual hearing-impaired listener, even on the basis of audiometric data, until speech perception ability has been evaluated thoroughly. The exception to this rule occurs when attempting to predict how well a hearing-impaired infant will be able to use auditory information. Even then, prognosis should be made with extreme caution.

ASSESSMENT OF SPEECH PERCEPTION

There are many ways in which speech can be used as a stimulus for the clinical assessment of auditory function. In the measurement of auditory threshold for *detection* or *awareness* of speech, the audiologist is searching for the intensity level at which the presence of the speech signal can be just detected; the listener simply indicates whether or not a signal was heard, and makes no attempt to identify it. The intensity at which 50 percent of the speech stimuli (usually spondaic words) can be identified correctly by the listener is the speech *reception* threshold (SRT).

While determination of various speech thresholds is an important part of the audiological evaluation, the auditory communication ability of a client can be defined best by the ability to *recognize* speech stimuli presented at suprathreshold levels. This is the ability that is referred to throughout this chapter as "speech perception ability." Other terms often used to describe the same behavior are speech discrimination, word articulation, speech intelligibility, and speech recognition.

There are several reasons for assessing the speech perception abilities of hearing-impaired clients. Speech tests can be used to estimate the degree of communication difficulty a client is experiencing, to assess the effects of a hearing aid on speech perception, or to obtain information that may aid in determining the site of damage to the auditory system. Results of speech tests are essential to the design of an auditory and speech training program for any hearing-impaired individual and may be used periodically for assessing progress in such a program.

Although the evaluation of speech perception has several purposes, the assessment procedure itself is always the same and involves the selection of the speech stimuli, their auditory presentation, and analysis of the listener's responses. The examiner must first consider the kind of information that is needed, and then choose the combination of materials, presentation, response mode, and response analysis that will yield that information.

For purposes of remediation, there are two types of speech perception information to be obtained. The first type concerns what has been referred to as speech perception *impairment*. Specifically, we need to know which speech sounds and features are perceived accurately by the hearing-impaired individual and which are not. Second, we need to estimate the *handicap* imposed by hearing loss on the individual's ability to communicate effectively with others. The ways in which these two types of information may be obtained from adults and children will be reviewed briefly.

Assessment of Adults

Types of Speech Materials. To assess speech perception impairment materials must be chosen that allow the listener to respond on the basis of the acoustic structure of the speech stimuli only. Nonmeaningful speech stimuli or meaningful words in a closed-set response format may be used for this purpose. Nonsense syllables have been used primarily for experimental purposes; at present, standardized recorded versions of these materials are not generally available for clinical use. If speech perception handicap is to be measured, test materials should include meaningful words in an open set, sentences, or other stimuli that contain linguistic and contextual cues.

Materials Containing Minimal Linguistic Clues. Recorded versions of several closed-set meaningful-word lists are available. The most familiar set is the *Modified Rhyme Test,* developed by House and his co-workers (House, Williams, Necker, and Kryter, 1965) as a modification of Fairbanks' original rhyming word list (Fairbanks, 1958). For each stimulus word, there are six alternatives differing in either the initial or the final consonant. A more recent test is the *California Consonant Test* (*CCT*) (Owens and Schubert, 1977), which also assesses perception of initial and final consonants in meaningful words incorporating a four-alternative response set. Test items in the *CCT* were selected because of their difficulty for hearing-impaired listeners. The four response alternatives for each item test subphonemic feature contrasts on which hearing-impaired listeners are likely to err (manner and place features).

Another set of materials that may qualify as linguistically nonmeaningful is the *Synthetic Sentence Identification (SSI) Test* (Speaks and Jerger, 1965). These lists consist of 10 third-order approximations to real sentences. Each sentence contains seven words and is constructed so that any three contiguous words in the sentence are grammatically related, although the sentence may not be complete or have meaning. Two examples of synthetic sentences are: "Women view men with green paper should," and "Agree with him only to find out." The *SSI* is presented in a 10-sentence closed-response format. The listener identifies each spoken sentence as one of the 10 alternatives presented on an answer sheet or display panel.

Although all of these materials provide minimal linguistic cues to the listener, they are not equal in level of difficulty. The *CCT,* for example, is an extremely difficult test for hearing-impaired listeners, because the test items were chosen to reflect contrasts that are difficult for them to hear. On the other hand, the *SSI* is a very easy test when presented in quiet, because the stimulus items (sentences) are long and because the response format is closed-set. Degree of difficulty of test materials is important to the interpretation of test results.

Materials Containing Contextual Clues. Speech materials that contain linguistic and contextual clues are plentiful and in widespread use. The use of meaningful speech stimuli in an open-set response format always implies that both speech perception impairment and speech perception handicap are being evaluated, because the listener can make response decisions on the basis of the linguistic properties of the stimuli as well as their acoustic structure.

Lists of monosyllabic words that reflect the phonetic content of everyday spoken English are by far the most commonly used of these materials. The Harvard PAL PB-50 lists (Egan, 1948), the CID W-22 lists (Hirsh et al., 1952), and the Northwestern University Auditory Test No. 6 (Tillman and Carhart, 1966) are all familiar examples of monosyllabic word lists. Although monosyllables may appear to offer little in the way of linguistic clues, listeners are more likely to respond correctly to test items that are familiar words (Owens, 1961). For example, the Harvard PB-50 lists are more difficult for normally hearing listeners than the CID W-22 lists, which contain more familiar words. With hearing-impaired listeners, the familiarity of items is even more important. If they have reduced vocabularies, their performance on monosyllabic word lists may depend on test word familiarity to an even greater extent than it does for normally hearing listeners.

Sentence materials provide considerably more contextual clues than do monosyllabic words. The best known of these are the CID Everyday Sentences (Silverman and Hirsh, 1955), consisting of 10 lists, each of which contain 10 sentences of varying length. The listener repeats the entire sentence, although scoring is confined to the 50 "key words" in each list. Performance is determined by both the amount of acoustic information available and by the extent to which advantage can be taken of the linguistic information in the sentences.

A relatively new set of materials represents an attempt to quantify how well the listener can use contextual information. The *Speech Perception in Noise* (*SPIN*) *Test* (Kalikow, Stevens, and Elliott, 1977) consists of eight lists of 50 sentences each presented against a background of voice babble. The listener's task is to repeat the last word in each sentence. This word may be either a "high predictability" word or a "low predictability" word, depending on how much information about the identity of the word is contained in the rest of the sentence. For example, the word "*germs*" is considered to be low predictability in the context, "She should not have discussed the *germs*." It becomes a high-predictability word in the sentence, "Hospitals should be free of *germs*." Comparison of the number of low-predictability items versus the number of high-predictability items identified correctly can provide an index of the listener's ability to take advantage of the linguistic clues provided by the high-predictability sentences. The *SPIN* test provides a unique opportunity to obtain information about the speech communication handicap imposed by hearing loss.

Several sets of speech materials are used primarily as tests to determine rehabilitative needs or as auditory training materials. These include the Semi-Diagnostic Test Materials for Aural Rehabilitation (Hutton, Curry, and Armstrong, 1959), the Larsen Sound-Discrimination Lists (Larsen, 1963), and the Multiple-Choice Intelligibility Tests (Black, 1957). The Semi-Diagnostic Test was designed to assess auditory, visual, and combined auditory-visual reception.

This brief review of speech materials is by no means a complete description of all the stimuli that can be used for speech perception testing. There are many lists of nonsense syllables, monosyllabic and polysyllabic words, sentences, and even continuous discourse that have proved useful for this purpose. No matter which particular set of materials is used it is imperative that they be selected carefully and sensibly. The materials should be appropriate for the particular facet of speech perception ability about which information is desired. At the same time, materials should be neither too difficult nor too easy for the individual being tested.

Auditory Presentation of Speech Materials. Speech materials may be presented in live-voice or recorded form using many different types of equipment, depending on what is available at the testing site, and on the purpose of the testing. For example, a loudspeaker would be used for reproduction of the test stimuli during a hearing aid evaluation procedure, while earphones might be preferable for some other purpose. No matter what equipment is used, it is important that speech perception testing with adults be performed with recorded materials. This is imperative if test results are to be compared with test norms or with results obtained in another facility or at another time. It is also necessary if testing is to be done repeatedly, as might be the case in a hearing aid evaluation.

Given the same set of materials, listeners' test scores may vary substantially with different talkers. This variability may remain quite high even when the same set of materials is presented repeatedly, via live voice, by the same talker (Brandy, 1966). Test scores obtained from live-voice presentation of materials thus may reflect both the speech perception ability of the listener and the speaking characteristics of the tester, and it will be impossible to separate the effects of these two factors.

In most situations, there are two important decisions which must be made about auditory presentation of recorded speech materials. First, the tester must determine the intensity level, or levels, at which the stimuli are to be presented. Second, it must be decided whether to present the speech materials in quiet or in the presence of some form of competition.

Intensity Level. The selection of the intensity level, like other decisions about speech perception testing, will depend on the purpose for which testing is being performed. If this purpose is to estimate how well the listener perceives everyday spoken communication, then it is reasonable to present speech materials at a level similar to the average level of conversational speech. When measured 18 inches from the talker's lips, this level is approximately 74 dB SPL, a level that corresponds to 54 dB HL (ANSI, 1969) when presented via a Telephonics TDH-39 earphone. The average SPL of conversational speech at the greater distance of 1 meter from the talker's lips is approximately 60 to 65 dB. To simulate this more realistic situation, the clinician may wish to present materials at 40 to 45 dB HL (Bode, 1975; Hodgson, 1977). The equivalent sound-field presentation level will depend on the location of the subject in relation to the loudspeaker source (Dirks et al. 1972).

It is sometimes desirable to know the best performance of which a listener is capable with a certain set of speech materials. In this case, the level of the speech must be far enough above threshold to allow for maximum performance, but not so high as to cause discomfort or actual diminution of performance. Unfortunately, this optimal presentation level does not appear to be related in any simple fashion to the listener's audiogram or speech reception threshold (SRT). For example, presentation of speech materials at a level of 40 dB above the SRT, a level that is used commonly by audiologists, may produce maximum performance by one listener but not by another. Therefore, materials must be presented at more than one level to obtain a measurement of the listener's best performance. A useful rule of thumb has been suggested by Olsen and Matkin (1979): if possible, always present at least one list of materials at a hearing level above pure tone threshold for 2000 Hz. This makes sense in terms of what has already been discussed about the importance of the 2000-Hz region for consonant place information.

Testing in Noise. Speech perception testing may be done in a background of noise or speech competition for two reasons. First, this may make the speech materials more difficult to understand, and therefore more sensitive to the speech perception deficit experienced by a listener. Second, it may make the testing situation more realistic, considering the common occurrence of noisy backgrounds in everyday communication situations. Even mildly hearing-impaired listeners often complain that they have real difficulty understanding speech in a background of noise, although they may not experience any problem in quiet environments. Therefore, it is appropriate to present materials in some type of noise when the purpose of speech testing is to obtain an estimate of the extent of communication handicap resulting from hearing loss.

Background competition has also been used to make monosyllabic word lists more useful with listeners whose hearing losses are not severe. Carhart (1965) noted that only 39.4 percent of 170 hearing-impaired veterans scored poorer than 90 percent on the CID W-22 presented in quiet; this means that 60 percent of his listeners would not have been considered to have speech perception abilities out of the range of normal, on the basis of their performance on this test. These data exemplify a problem encountered in many clinics: patients often score high on the monosyllabic word lists, even though they complain of difficulties in understanding speech. Monosyllabic word lists presented in quiet may not differentiate between individuals who are communicatively handicapped by hearing loss and those who are not.

There is considerable evidence that presenting speech tests in noise reduces the performance of hearing-impaired listeners more than that of normally hearing listeners (Palva, 1955; Keith and Talis, 1972; Shapiro, Melnick, and Ver Muelen,

1972). Given two individuals who both score 94 percent on the CID W-22 in quiet, for example, the addition of noise might produce a different score for the person with an impairment of speech perception than for the one with normal hearing.

A more sensitive test of speech perception would make it unnecessary to increase the sensitivity of monosyllabic word lists by adding background noise. The *California Consonant Test* appears to be one such test. Persons with high-frequency hearing losses, who typically score high on monosyllable tests, do not perform well on the *CCT* (Owens and Schubert, 1977). For these individuals, administration of the *CCT* in quiet might serve the same purpose as administration of the CID W-22 in noise, providing that the goal is to separate the performance of a hearing impaired listener from that of normally hearing listeners.

In summary, the intensity level of stimulus presentation and the presence or absence of background noise or speech can be manipulated in various ways. To estimate degree of communication handicap, it is appropriate to present speech materials at an average conversational level, in the presence of a noise or speech background. Other clinical or rehabilitative goals may indicate presentation at several different intensities, in quiet or in noise.

Analysis of Responses. For tests that employ open-set format, the listener may respond either verbally by repeating the stimulus item or by writing the item on an answer sheet. The verbal response mode is faster but introduces the extraneous variable of the tester's judgment of the listener's spoken response. This is especially critical when the person being tested has a speech production disorder, as is frequently the case with hearing-impaired persons. In such instances an incorrect response may reflect either a true perceptual error or a speech production error. The write-down response mode must then be used, even though it is considerably more time consuming. The written mode also requires that the listener be literate and that some provision be made for dealing with spelling errors. For closed-set tests, the listener usually checks or circles one of the alternatives listed on an answer sheet. These tests are valid only if the person being tested is able to read the test items accurately.

Once the responses are obtained, they may be scored by quantitative or qualitative methods. The quantitative method simply involves counting the percentage of stimulus items that were responded to correctly. These items may be single words, "key" words in sentences, or entire sentences.

A qualitative method involves the recording and subsequent analysis of the listener's error responses. Some materials, such as the *Modified Rhyme Test* and the *California Consonant Test,* were designed to be scored in this way. Error responses can be scrutinized for patterns of phoneme errors and phoneme error types using a confusion matrix such as that described earlier. It is more difficult to perform error analysis on responses to other speech tests, such as monosyllabic word lists because these lists were not designed specifically to test phoneme perception.

Quantitative scoring methods yield measures that may be used to describe an individual's test performance in relation to test norms, or in documenting changes in performance with different levels of noise, different stimulus presentation levels, or different hearing aids. The accurate description of speech perception impairment requires a qualitative analysis of response. Because the percentage of test items repeated correctly and the types of phoneme perception errors made are not necessarily related, measures of both types of performance are necessary for the accurate description of an individual's speech perception ability.

Choosing Combinations of Tests. The possible combinations of speech materials, presentation of materials, and response analysis are seemingly endless. The choice of tests should depend on careful consideration of the individual to be tested and the information needed to plan habilitation. For example, phoneme perception should be tested only if the client possesses enough residual hearing for perception of at least some of the phonetic information in the speech signal. This is unlikely to be the case for people with ''corner'' audiograms.

When testing of phoneme perception is appropriate, the speech materials should be of the type designed for that purpose, the *MRT,* the *CCT,* or another closed-set of words or syllables designed to test perception of subphonemic feature contrasts. The materials should be presented in quiet, at a level at which the listener can perform best. Because this level is not always easy to predict, it might be preferable to administer the test at more than one level. The listener should be familiar with all response alternatives and be able to read them. Error responses should be analyzed for phonemes and subphonemic features perceived incorrectly.

For the purpose of estimating communication handicap, an entirely different combination would be appropriate. Materials should be meaningful and incorporate some of the linguistic context encountered in everyday speech. Sentence lists, including the SPIN test, would be appropriate, although monosyllabic word lists also have been used for this purpose. Speech should be presented at a level similar to that of conversational speech, in a noise or speech background. Response mode can be verbal or written, according to the abilities of the listener, and a performance-level (percent-correct) measure should be calculated.

Other clinical purposes, such as hearing aid trials, site-of-lesion testing, or evaluation of progress in rehabilitation demand that clinicians use other combinations of materials, presentation, and response analysis, keeping in mind the effects of these variables on speech perception.

Interpreting Results. There is much to be gained from a carefully designed assessment of speech perception, but there are limitations on the ways in which results may be interpreted. First, it has not been demonstrated satisfactorily that an individual's performance on speech tests is well correlated with actual communicative efficiency. Results may indicate only a slight communication handicap for a person who actually is experiencing considerable difficulty, or vice-versa.

A second factor that limits interpretation of speech test results is their variability. Suppose a hearing-impaired person scores 50 percent, 60 percent, and 65 percent on three 50-word lists of the W-22 presented at 30, 40, and 50 dB HL, respectively. Do the differences among scores really indicate performance differences at the various intensity levels, or do they represent variations that simply occur by chance? Traditionally, clinicians have accepted differences greater than ±8 to 10 percent as indicative of significant differences. However, a recent publication by Thornton and Raffin (1978) showed that the 95 percent critical differences for scores on the CID W-22 lists varied as a function of the magnitude of the obtained score and the number of items presented (see Table 2.2). For example, the 95 percent critical difference range around a score of 50 percent for a 50-word list of CID W-22 extends from 32 to 68 percent; this indicates that 95 times out of a hundred, a score outside this range will be significantly different from that score of 50 percent. Returning to our hypothetical three scores of 50 percent, 60 percent, and 65 percent, it is apparent that all three lie inside the 95 percent critical difference range; therefore, none of these scores is significantly different from any other. From the data of Thornton and Raffin, it seems that the 8 to 10 percent rule would be appropriate only for W-22 scores less than 2 percent or greater than 98 percent. Critical difference ranges are larger for midrange scores, necessitating a much greater range between scores before they could be considered to be truly different.

The Thornton and Raffin data should prove useful in interpreting results obtained using the word lists presented in quiet. Unfortunately, no comparable index is available for use with word lists presented in noise. Until such time as more test-retest data are available for these other uses, interpretation of performance-level scores, and of differences among them should be undertaken very carefully.

Table 2.2 Lower and Upper Limits of the 95 Percent Critical Differences for Percentage Scores

Percent Score	n = *50*	n = *25*	n = *10*	*Percent Score*	n = *100*
0	0–4	0–8	0–20	50	37–63
2	0–10			51	38–64
4	0–14	0–20		52	39–65
6	2–18			53	40–68
8	2–22	0–28		54	41–67
10	2–24		0–50	55	42–68
12	4–26	4–32		56	43–69
14	4–30			57	44–70
16	6–32	4–40		58	45–71
18	6–34			59	46–72
20	8–36	4–44	0–60	60	47–73

(continued)

Table 2.2—*continued*

Percent Score	n = *50*	n = *25*	n = *10*	*Percent Score*	n = *100*
22	8–40			61	43–74
24	10–42	8–48		62	49–74
26	12–44			63	50–75
28	14–46	8–52		64	51–76
30	14–48		10–70	65	52–77
32	16–50	12–56		66	53–78
34	18–52			67	54–79
36	20–54	16–60		68	55–80
38	22–56			69	56–81
40	22–58	16–64	10–80	70	57–81
42	24–60			71	58–82
44	26–62	20–68		72	59–83
46	28–64			73	60–84
48	30–66	24–72		74	61–85
50	32–68		10–90	75	63–86
52	34–70	28–76		76	64–86
54	36–72			77	65–87
56	38–74	32–80		78	66–88
58	40–76			79	67–89
60	42–78	36–84	20–90	80	68–89
62	44–78			81	69–90
64	46–80	40–84		82	71–91
66	48–82			83	72–92
68	50–84	44–88		84	73–92
70	52–86		30–90	85	74–93
72	54–86	48–92		86	75–94
74	56–88			87	77–94
76	58–90	52–92		88	78–95
78	60–92			89	79–96
80	64–92	56–96	40–100	90	82–96
82	66–94			91	82–97
84	68–94	60–96		92	83–98
86	70–96			93	85–98
88	74–96	68–96		94	86–99
90	76–98		50–100	95	88–99
92	78–98	72–100		96	89–99
94	82–98			97	91–100
96	86–100	80–100		98	92–100
98	90–100			99	94–100
100	96–100	80–100		100	97–100

Adapted from A. Thornton and M. J. M. Raffin, Speech discrimination scores modeled as a binomial variable, *J. Speech Hear. Res.*, 21, 507–518, 1978.

Assessment of Children

The approach that is taken toward the assessment of speech perception abilities of hearing-impaired children is substantially different from that taken with adults. From an adult the clinician usually wants to obtain various measures of speech recognition. These typically include auditory threshold for speech recognition (SRT) and appropriate measures of the individual's ability to recognize speech at suprathreshold intensities. Very young or low-verbal children cannot be tested in this way, because they probably will be unable to respond to tests requiring them to recognize or identify sentences, words, syllables, or even phonemes. With these children the clinician typically uses speech stimuli to obtain a measure of auditory threshold for *detection* of speech, which requires only that the child give a behavioral response indicating that a stimulus was detected, regardless of its identity. The *Five-Sound Test* described by Ling (1976) is an example of the way in which speech detection can be used to predict speech perceptual abilities. This test consists of five isolated phonemes (**oo, a, ee, sh,** and **s**), which are spoken to the child at a normal conversational level. The child simply indicates whether or not each sound is heard. According to Ling, children with measurable hearing at frequencies up to 1000 Hz should be able to detect the three vowels; hearing through 2000 Hz should permit reception of the **sh;** and the **s** should be perceived if there is residual hearing at frequencies up to 4000 Hz.

Depending on the child, the clinician might also obtain measures of auditory discomfort threshold for speech, and of the child's ability to discriminate differences among various words or speech sounds, because neither of these measures requires that the child recognize or repeat the stimulus.

In many instances, it is possible to administer tests that require speech recognition ability of young children. Before this is attempted, it is critical that the clinician obtain some measure of receptive language age. Matkin (1977) stressed the importance of this step, and suggested that an appropriate language screening test or information obtained from parents and teachers be used. He also suggested that speech materials and testing procedures designed for use with adults be used only with children whose receptive language ages are above the 12-year level. The receptive vocabularies of children whose language ages are below this level will not contain many of the test words in the adult speech tests. Their scores on such tests are likely to reflect their lack of familiarity with the test items instead of their true speech perception abilities.

Special materials and procedures should be used for speech perception testing with children whose receptive language ages are between about 4 and 12 years. Children below this range may not be able to identify enough test words to make it feasible to administer speech tests that require recognition responses. Materials, auditory presentation of materials, and response analysis suitable for use with children with receptive language ages in the 4- to 12-year-old range will be considered in the following section.

Speech Materials. Familiarity of test items is the primary criterion when selecting speech materials for use with hearing-impaired children. Receptive vocabularies may be quite dissimilar even among children who are at the same receptive language age. For this reason, it is advisable for the clinician to ensure that the child knows all the words comprising the set of speech materials being considered. If there are words with which the child is unfamiliar, these should be omitted from the test or replaced by other items. Although this procedure is time consuming, it is the only way to ensure that the test results will indicate speech perception ability rather than vocabulary size and composition.

The same factors that influence the performance of adults on tests of speech perception are also operational with children. If phoneme perception is to be assessed, then the speech stimuli must be either nonsense syllables or meaningful items in a closed-set response format. This necessity severely limits the feasibility of performing such testing with children. First, there are no closed-set, meaningful-word materials available that are composed of words likely to be within children's vocabularies, and at the same time are designed to test specific phoneme contrasts. Second, many younger children may not be testable with nonsense syllable materials. Because of the speech production problems evidenced by hearing-impaired children, it is usually not advisable to require the child to respond by repeating the nonsense-syllable test items. This limits the options to a written response; the child typically circles or checks responses on an answer sheet. Thus, testing with nonsense syllables will require some reading skills on the part of the child to be tested.

With children who are able to respond reliably to the test items, the use of nonsense syllables can yield valuable information. Erber (1972) used stimuli composed of eight consonants, each in the bisyllabic context /a/ C (consonant) /a/ and required written responses. Results indicated that severely hearing-impaired children were able to perceive consonant voicing and nasality features fairly accurately when the stimuli were presented auditorily. Profoundly hearing-impaired children, by contrast, appeared unable to perceive any consonant phonetic information auditorily. This type of information would be useful in planning a program for a hearing-impaired child and should be obtained if the child's reading and language skills make it possible.

Even though profoundly hearing-impaired children may be unable to perceive phonetic information, information can be obtained about their ability to perceive other acoustic aspects of speech. Erber and Alencewicz (1976) devised an ingenious test for evaluating a child's ability to perceive stress patterns and syllable length of words; this information is contained in the low-frequency end of the speech spectrum and is sometimes available to children with low-frequency residual hearing. The *Children's Auditory Test* (*CAT*) consists of four nouns in each of the three stress categories of monosyllabic, trochaic, and spondaic. Response format is closed set; the child points to the picture corresponding to each stimulus item as it is presented auditorily. The clinician records the child's responses in a confusion matrix like the one depicted in Figure 2.7. The results then can be analyzed for number of test items correctly identified, which would correspond to entries on the main diagonal. In addition, responses can be analyzed for number of items correctly identified in terms of stress category; this corresponds to the number of entries inside those portions of the figure outlined in bold lines. Stimulus words can easily

STIMULUS

RESPONSE	Bed	Cat	Duck	Pig	Button	Chicken	Doctor	Turtle	Baseball	Birdhouse	Popcorn	Toothpaste
Bed												
Cat												
Duck												
Pig												
Button												
Chicken												
Doctor												
Turtle												
Baseball												
Birdhouse												
Popcorn												
Toothpaste												

Figure 2.7. Confusion matrix for the *Children's Auditory Test.* (Adapted from N. P. Erber and C. M. Alencewicz, Audiologic evaluation of deaf children, *J. Speech Hear. Disord.,* 41, 1976, 256-267.)

be changed to ensure the child's familiarity with all items, making this a useful and versatile test.

When a performance-level measure of speech perception is desired, a few appropriate sets of materials are available for use with children. Perhaps the most widely used materials are the PBK-50 word lists (Haskins, 1949). These phonetically balanced 50-word lists are made up of monosyllabic words that should be familiar to normally hearing children of kindergarten age. The response format is open set, so that the vocabulary of the child to be tested is an important factor. Matkin (1977) has cautioned that the PBK 50-word lists should be administered only to children whose receptive language ages are above 6 years.

With children whose receptive language ages are between 4 and 6, the *Word Intelligibility by Picture Identification* (*WIPI*) *Test* (Ross and Lerman, 1970) may be used. It consists of four lists of 25 monosyllabic words. Response format is closed-set; the child responds to each item by pointing to one of six alternative pictures.

If the vocabulary of the child to be tested is not sufficiently large to allow the use of either the PBK 50-word lists or the *WIPI,* some performance-level estimate of speech perception ability may still be obtained. The clinician may compose a list of words that are familiar to the child and use these for informal testing. Cramer and Erber (1974) recommend the use of a 10-word list of spondaic words selected on the basis of their familiarity to the child.

The speech materials available for testing children are much fewer and more limited than are those available for use with adults. Nevertheless, the resourceful clinician should strive to select or devise materials that are suitable for the child to be tested, in terms of both the purpose for which testing is to be performed and the language sophistication of the child.

Auditory Presentation of Speech Stimuli. Whether the person to be tested is an adult or a child, the same sources of error will be introduced into the test results if materials are presented via live voice. However, it may not be feasible to use recorded materials with children, who may require flexible timing between presentation of stimuli. In addition, the deletion and substitution of items necessary to ensure familiarity with all test stimuli is not possible with recorded materials. More often than not, speech perception testing of children will be done live voice, and test scores should be interpreted with caution.

The SPL at which stimuli are presented again will vary according to the purpose for testing. In some instances, it may be useful to present the test items at a conversational speech level in order to estimate the difficulty the child will have in conversational or classroom situations. Testing in a noise background will highlight further the speech perception problems the child may experience in those situations. Usually speech materials should be presented at a level where the child will perform best. As is the case with adults, this level is hard to predict. If time and the child's attention span permit, testing should be done at more than one SPL.

Analysis of Responses. Appropriate response modes for children are limited. The use of written responses is realistic only with children who have adequate reading and writing skills. Verbal responses are inappropriate when children have speech production disorders, as do many hearing-impaired children. The point-to-the-picture mode is the most useful, even though it may require the construction of picture materials if a test other than the *WIPI* is to be used.

Analysis of error responses can be performed when appropriate materials such as nonsense syllables or the *CAT* have been used. Other materials will require the calculation of a percent-correct score. Interpretation of these scores should be accompanied by considerable caution, for a number of reasons. First, children's word lists may contain relatively few items, as do the *WIPI* (25 words) and the 10-word spondee list suggested by Cramer and Erber (1974). This reduction in number of items serves to increase the test-retest variability over that expected with longer lists. Second, children's scores may improve over time as a function of their language growth, especially if the clinician has not checked each test word for familiarity. Third, performance levels may vary from test to test as a function of size of the response set. For example, chance performance on the *WIPI* will be 100 percent/6, or approximately 16 percent, because the child's responses are limited to six alternatives. By the same token, chance performance on a four-alternative response test would be about 25 percent. Clearly, a score of 25 percent on this test would not be directly comparable to a score of 25 percent on the *WIPI*. The final factor that limits interpretation of test results is live-voice presentation of materials and its attendant variability due to talker differences.

It is more difficult to test the speech perception ability of children than that of adults. The choice of materials is more limited, the testing is more time consuming, and the results are more likely to be affected by language factors. Nevertheless, assessment and monitoring of children's ability to perceive speech is an essential part of their management, and every effort should be made to obtain as complete a picture as possible of their ability to perceive speech auditorily.

TRAINING AUDITORY SKILLS

Once an estimate of the status of the speech perception ability of a client is obtained, rehabilitation plans can be made. For most hearing-impaired people, management will include some training aimed at improving speech reception through audition. Such training rarely constitutes the only treatment necessary; rather it should be an integral part of the total program for children and adults. Auditory training will be discussed here as a separate procedure, then referred to as a component of treatment programs to be described in succeeding discussions.

The basis of auditory management is development of the use of residual hearing to the fullest extent possible. Because the goals and procedures of auditory training are quite different for children and adults, they will be discussed separately.

Auditory Training For Children

The goal of auditory training is to enable hearing-impaired children to make maximum use of the acoustic speech signal by developing the auditory system to the fullest extent possible. Although there is some disagreement as to how this goal should be accomplished, two facts seem indisputable: (1) maximal use of residual hearing is beneficial to all hearing-impaired children, either as the primary means of reception or as a supplement to visual reception and (2) the use of appropriate amplification is basic to the process. To make auditory information an integral part of a child's experiences, parents, teachers, and clinicians must be alert to every possible event throughout the day that can be used to develop auditory skills. Calling the child's attention to sound sources, describing ongoing activities verbally, repeating the names of things and events, playing rhythmic games, reading aloud, and reciting and acting out nursery rhymes and songs are examples of common interactions between children and adults that foster auditory learning under ordinary circumstances and which can be used to develop auditory skills in hearing-impaired children. Auditory training should not be regarded as a special activity to be engaged in at specific times under certain circumstances. What is necessary is a consistent concern about the development of auditory perceptions under the most favorable circumstances, a commitment that can exist no matter which teaching methodology is employed. Realization of this goal requires consistent monitoring of amplification and the provision of auditory input that is *associated with interesting activities* and *that is provided consistently no matter what other stimuli are available at the time.*

Boothroyd (1967) defined auditory training as the provision of contrived experiences through which hearing-impaired children develop auditory skills that other children obtain naturally. Although special "contrived experiences" may be necessary to supplement any auditory training program, especially with children having limited residual hearing, teachers and clinicians must be careful not to interpret this to mean that periodic auditory training periods will be sufficient for the development of auditory skills.

A commitment to auditory training as an essential ingredient in habilitation stresses early detection of hearing impairment and the use of appropriate amplification as early in life as possible. If intervention occurs during the first months of life or soon after the onset of hearing loss, many of the consequences of sensory deprivation may be minimized. Early use of amplification should enable the child to make maximum use of the preschool years for language and speech development and to minimize problems accepting and adjusting to the hearing aid. Enrollment in a preschool program for hearing-impaired children should enhance all aspects of development and adjustment. If the child has sufficient residual hearing to make use of amplification for understanding some portion of speech, and if teachers and parents take overt steps to insure adequate auditory reception, growth of auditory skills can occur along with simultaneous reception of visual cues.

Auditory training should be suited to the individual needs of the child. Appropriate placement in a training program requires careful assessment of auditory, visual, combined auditory-visual, and language competencies. If auditory learning is to be a feature of the program, something more than passive use of speech, amplification, and hearing is required. Amplification appropriate to the child's needs must be selected, it must be adequately maintained, and practice using it in quiet and noisy environments must be provided. For optimal learning to take place, the acoustical environment in which the child functions must be monitored and controlled, and the teacher must use good speaking skills and be familiar with the use of amplification equipment. Periodic analysis of progress in auditory learning must take place. Auditory training should also include attempts to increase tolerance of loud sounds, localization of signals, and identification of nonspeech sounds, not as a precursor to speech perception, but as a means of increasing the usefulness of hearing in general.

As electronic hearing aid technology has improved, several different approaches to auditory training for children have developed. The differences among them reflect the effects of improved hearing aids and earlier identification and habilitation of hearing-impaired children.

The Carhart Approach. Carhart (1947) was one of the first audiologists to describe a systematic program of auditory training for children. He viewed the goals of auditory training as aiding in (1) developing a command of language, (2) developing speech, and (3) encouraging adjustment to the world of hearing people. His theory of auditory training comprises four major stages. The first stage is development of *awareness of sound*. The goal of this stage is for the child to recognize when a sound is present and to attend to it. The child should be surrounded with sounds that are related to daily activities and that are clearly audible. It is not clear from Carhart's writing whether amplification was advocated during this stage. Some clinicians do not utilize amplification at this point, preferring to wait until the child has developed awareness of sound and derived some meaning from the experience.

Carhart's second stage involves the development of *gross sound discrimination*. The child is trained to distinguish between highly dissimilar nonspeech sounds, such as bells, drums, cymbals, and whistles. In addition, animal sounds or other environmental noises are often employed. Training at this stage includes discrimination of several parameters of sound, such as intensity (loud versus soft), duration (long versus short), and frequency (high versus low pitch). Once the child can discriminate among highly dissimilar sounds, finer discriminations along each parameter are trained. For example, several bells with different frequency characteristics may be presented for discrimination.

The third stage involves development of *broad discriminations among simple speech patterns*. By now, according to Carhart, the child is aware that sounds differ and is ready to apply this knowledge to the understanding of speech. He recommended that the clinician begin by teaching the child to distinguish among vowels or familiar meaningful phrases that are sufficiently different to minimize confusion. "Show me the dog," and "Give me the baby," are examples of utterances that might be used.

The fourth stage involves the development of *fine discrimination of speech.* The child is taught to make all of the discriminations among speech sounds that are possible within the limits imposed by the hearing impairment. Ideally, the child should be trained to recognize subtle phonemic differences, learn a large vocabulary of spoken words, and be able to follow connected discourse.

Carhart did much to shape the philosophy and activities of auditory training for children. Some of his views are no longer shared by present authorities, but many clinicians and teachers of the hearing impaired continue to employ activities based upon the Carhart model. In the sense that Carhart described it, the first stage (awareness of sound) is of less concern today. Until the early 1960s children usually were not fitted with amplification before age 3 or 4, which meant the average child endured auditory deprivation for much longer than is common today. Helping a child adjust to hearing many new sounds at relatively high intensities requires careful management by appropriate professionals, but the task can be accomplished more quickly and naturally with a child under two years of age than with older children.

Serious questions have been raised about the second stage (gross discriminations of nonspeech sounds) as a necessary precursor for speech discrimination. Ling (1976) concluded that there are marked differences in the way speech and nonspeech sounds are processed and that no benefits to speech discrimination can be expected from training with nonverbal sounds. While training in the detection and identification of nonspeech sounds may be worthwhile for other reasons, present evidence indicates that it is not essential for auditory learning of language.

The Traditional Approach. Several authors (Hirsh, 1966; Ling, 1976) have described four levels of audition that contribute to the perception of conversational speech: detection, discrimination, identification, and comprehension. *Detection* requires only that the child be able to distinguish between the presence and absence of sound. *Discrimination* involves the differentiation of speech sounds (are they the same or different?). *Identification* requires the child to recognize the speech signal and to be able to identify it in some way, such as pointing to a picture, writing the word or syllable heard, or repeating the stimulus. The final level, *comprehension,* involves understanding of the message on a cognitive and linguistic basis. The child demonstrates comprehension by answering questions or performing appropriate tasks. Erber and Hirsh (1978) suggested an auditory training program in which increasingly complex speech stimuli are presented for processing through the four levels of audition. The resulting auditory skills matrix is illustrated in Table 2.3. Each child's auditory abilities are monitored closely and used to specify goals for future training. When possible, auditory perception develops from the ability to

Table 2.3 Auditory Skills Matrix for Hearing-impaired Children[a]

		Stimulus					
		Speech Elements	*Syllables*	*Words*	*Phrases*	*Sentences*	*Connected Discourse*
Response Task	Detection (presence/absence)						
	Discrimination (same/different)						
	Recognition (identification)						
	Comprehension (understanding)						

[a] From Hallowell Davis and S. Richard Silverman, *Hearing and Deafness,* 4th edition. Copyright 1947, © 1960, 1970 by Holt, Rinehart and Winston, Inc. Copyright © 1978 by Holt, Rinehart and Winston. Reprinted with permission by Holt, Rinehart and Winston.

detect the presence of isolated speech units to the comprehension of connected discourse.

The same set of auditory skills is involved in an individualized auditory training program designed to be self-administered by means of an audio-tape card system (Erber, 1976). *Detection* of speech stimuli is trained by having the child listen to a stack of cards, some of which contain recorded speech stimuli and some of which are blank, and sort them into YES and NO boxes for later tallying by the teacher or clinician. *Discrimination* tasks utilize cards that contain two speech stimuli. The child determines whether or not the stimuli on a single card are the SAME or DIFFERENT and sorts them accordingly. Further discrimination can be demonstrated by presenting three stimuli per card and requiring the child to designate which of the three stimuli is different. *Identification* tasks may involve placing each card in predetermined categories (male or female speaker, one or two syllables, rising or falling intonation pattern), labeling the card with the word or syllable heard, or some other response that indicates that identification has occurred. The final skill, *comprehension,* requires the child to demonstrate understanding of the message, by answering questions such as ''What is your name?'' or following directions such as ''Shut the door.''

Mastery of the lower levels of *detection* and *discrimination* is considered to be a prerequisite for successful performance at the higher levels of *identification* and *comprehension*. Children should progress through the four levels and the various stimulus complexities at their own rate and to the extent dictated by the status of their residual hearing. The child who cannot progress beyond sound detection of a variety of stimuli still will benefit from development of that skill.

Although the terms used to label the first two skill levels are similar to the stages proposed by Carhart there are fundamental differences.

The *detection* level in the matrix does not correspond to the *awareness stage* as proposed by Carhart, because it focuses on speech reception rather than awareness of sounds in general. In addition, there is no corollary in the Erber and Hirsh paradigm for the development of gross discriminations of nonspeech sounds as proposed by Carhart.

The Carhart and Erber and Hirsh models of auditory training represent structured approaches to the development of auditory skills. More global approaches are advocated by several educators (Wedenberg, 1967; Whetnall and Fry, 1964; Pollack, 1970; Griffiths, 1967).

The Acoupedic Method. Contending that the use of audition is hampered when attention is divided between two or more sensory inputs, Pollack (1970) proposed a unisensory approach toward education and habilitation of hearing-impaired children. Known as the *acoupedic* method, Pollack's procedures exclude the use of all visual cues, such as speechreading, during early training. Pollack does not consider the acoupedic method to be a form of auditory training and she distinguishes between the two by delineating the following principles of the acoupedic approach.

1. Hearing impairment must be detected early in life. Pollack does not suggest an age beyond which introduction of the acoupedic approach may not be feasible, but the procedures are designed for infants and toddlers.
2. Binaural hearing aids should be selected as soon as the hearing impairment is diagnosed. Exception to this rule may be made if there appears to be no residual hearing in one ear.
3. The child must be given the "fullest opportunity" to use residual hearing, so visual stimuli are not provided initially. Listening must be a continuous daily activity in order for an auditory feedback mechanism to develop.
4. Normal patterns of language are stimulated through the usual auditory channel, eliminating the need to present language visually.
5. A favorable attitude must be established for auditory learning. In short, the people who are involved must believe that the child can hear and learn to communicate normally.
6. Parents must become the primary teachers, assuming responsibility for providing intensive auditory stimulation more or less continuously.
7. A "special" educational environment must be avoided. The goal is for the

> child to be educated with normally hearing children, an accomplishment that cannot be achieved without the positive attitude described above.

The actual auditory training activities used by Pollack and others who advocate intensive auditory stimulation are similar to those described by Carhart and to the paradigm proposed by Erber and Hirsh, with some additions. Emphasis is placed on the development of an auditory feedback loop, which is demonstrated and refined by repeated imitation of auditory stimuli. Because the acoupedic method is intended to be introduced in infancy, its activities are based on normal interactions between babies and mothers, with emphasis on repeated auditory stimulation by the mother and imitation by the baby. Games involving the location of musical toys, repetition of the sounds made by animals or toys (airplanes, ambulances), and imitation of the inflectional patterns of nursery rhymes or baby games ("Peek-a-boo," "Where's Mommy? There she is," "Oh-oh, down it goes") are suggested.

Cognitive Auditory Approach. Grammatico (1975) proposed an auditory approach similar to that of Pollack's, in which auditory training is not viewed as an activity to be set apart from other educational procedures. Her approach stresses sound awareness, discrimination, localization, imitation of intonational patterns, and memory as the auditory skills to be developed. These skills are similar to those described by other authors, but the manner in which they are reinforced and the purpose given by Grammatico for their development are unique. She views audition as the basis for development of cognitive skills, and the materials and procedures employed are designed to foster thinking as well as listening skills. Children are encouraged to classify and group stimuli, to determine similarities and differences, and to generalize information from one situation to another. Insofar as traditional activities for identification, discrimination, and localization of sound can be used to enhance thinking skills, they are included in activities throughout the day. Visual stimuli are not emphasized and their use is mildly discouraged.

The success of unisensory approaches, such as the acoupedic and cognitive-auditory approaches described above, is predicated on very early identification, provision of amplification immediately on identification, extensive parental guidance, and exposure to normal language stimulation with primary emphasis on developing auditory skills through day-long attention to auditory input. The purpose, according to Pollack (1970), is to incorporate hearing into the personality of the child, so that special education is not necessary and audition serves as the primary sensory input for language learning and processing. This is a realistic goal for some, but not all, hearing impaired children.

The Verbotonal Approach. All of the auditory training approaches described thus far utilize conventional hearing aids or auditory training units that are designed to amplify maximally the frequencies at which the hearing loss is greatest. This type of selective amplification is the principle on which most commercial hearing aids are designed and selected, and traditional auditory training programs are based on knowledge of the effects of conventional amplification on the perception of acoustic speech information in various frequency regions. In contrast to the philosophies underlying the use of these hearing aids, a novel approach toward delivering amplified sound to hearing impaired listeners has been proposed, called the verbotonal method (Guberina, 1964). Developed by Peter Guberina, a Yugoslavian language teacher, the verbotonal method is designed to develop auditory perception and speech production through the use of special amplification equipment, tactual stimulation delivered by a bone conduction vibrator, and body movements calculated to produce varying degrees of muscular tension associated with the production of speech sounds.

The verbotonal method is based on the theory that amplification of the frequencies at which hearing impairment is greatest results in added distortion of auditory signals and should be avoided. Instead, Guberina advocates the use of a special auditory training unit (SUVAG II) composed of banks of filters that can deliver selected bands of frequencies from 20 to 20,000 Hz. Guberina hypothesized that each person has an "optimal band of frequencies" through which auditory information is least distorted; this frequency band usually corresponds to that frequency region in which hearing is best.

Instead of amplifying the areas of greatest loss, SUVAG II is adjusted to pass only the optimal field of hearing, determined for each child individually by presenting filtered and unfiltered nonsense syllables for detection or identification. Because most sensorineural hearing loss is greatest in the high frequencies, the verbotonal method stresses delivery of low-frequency amplification, auditorily through earphones and tactually through a small vibrator held in the hand. By having their attention called to low frequency, relatively undistorted energy, children are trained to perceive speech without amplification on the basis of low-frequency cues that have been present, but ignored prior to training.

In addition to the auditory and tactual stimulation, kinesthetic movements are associated with each speech sound and used by teacher and children during speech production. Movements of the limbs, hands, and body vary in tension and direction to reflect characteristics of individual phonemes that can be transferred to the articulators. The speech resulting from this training is claimed to be characterized by appropriate tension and duration as a result of practice of body movements and improved auditory perception.

In the early stages of verbotonal training, nonsense syllables or single words are used exclusively as auditory stimuli. Accurate imitation by the child, including normal vocal pitch, is the criterion for success. The speech stimuli are carefully selected to follow an orderly phonetic progression from low to high "tonality." An example of a syllable having low-pitch characteristics is **mu,** while **si** is a high-pitched syllable. The verbotonal method confines auditory training to perception and imitation of speech, represented by nonsense syllables, words, and sentences.

Perception is facilitated through modifications of one or more of the following parameters of speech: frequency, intensity, intonation, duration, rhythm, pause, and body tension during production.

Guberina (1964) advocates the verbotonal method for all ages and types of deafness, congenital or adventitious, regardless of the degree of hearing loss. Individual hearing aids are selected for children or adults only after the optimal field of hearing has been determined and speech perception training has been given.

Proponents claim that all aspects of language can be taught by the verbotonal method, that children will develop auditory skills sufficient for near-normal perception of speech, and that the speech produced by them will exhibit normal pitch, rhythm, and articulation. Data supporting these claims have not been published, at least not for children enrolled in verbotonal programs in English-speaking countries.

Auditory Training for Adults

Organized aural rehabilitation programs for adults were initiated in military hospitals during World War II and are available in speech and hearing centers in many communities. Unfortunately, they have not enjoyed the same degree of success among civilians as they have in military hospitals. In recent years there has been a rebirth of interest by audiologists in improving the quantity and quality of rehabilitation services offered to adults, spurred by increased awareness of the limitations of hearing aids and by more direct audiological involvement in hearing aid dispensing.

Auditory training is an essential ingredient of remediation of adults and includes procedures designed to familiarize them with the operation, care, benefits, and limitations of amplification and to teach them to take full advantage of the audible acoustic cues of speech. Aspects of this training can be accomplished during routine clinic appointments; others are best accomplished through special case management appointments on an individual or group basis. Recommendations for the development of such programs are found in Chapter 13.

The goals of auditory training are quite different for adults than for children. For children the task is a developmental one, learning to recognize and use acoustic cues for the first time. For adults the task is a remedial one, relearning to recognize familiar acoustic cues that have been rendered less usable by acquired hearing loss. The procedures advocated for adults are varied, but not to the same extent as those developed for children. Activities fall into two general categories those that stress drill on auditory or auditory-visual stimuli and those that focus on adjustment to the use of amplification. Most modern approaches combine the two in short-term programs for small groups. Typical examples are described below.

The Carhart Approach. Carhart (1947) proposed four stages of auditory training for adults incorporating the use of amplification whenever feasible. The first stage consists of development of an attitude of *critical listening,* regarded as essential because many adults become habitually inattentive after experiencing hearing loss. Family members of hearing impaired adults often believe they "can hear when they want to" and there is some evidence to support that belief. When it is necessary to attend closely in order to understand speech, many hearing-impaired adults report that listening is fatiguing and often not worth the effort. As a result they 'tune out," attending closely only when it seems important to them to do so and giving the impression of being selective in what they "choose" to listen to. To improve listening skills, Carhart recommended drills involving presentation of pairs of syllables to listeners, who must make a same-different judgment or repeat what is heard. Other activities involve the presentation of lists of words, such as those used in speech-perception testing, with the client repeating or writing what is heard. Drills can be repeated many times to "reawaken" and improve listening performance.

Carhart's second stage involves training in *precise and rapid recognition of phonetic elements*. The listening drills described above are repeated, but stimuli are presented only once, with emphasis on the development of accurate and quick identification.

The third stage involves *reestablishment of recognition of significant noises*. The purpose is to refamiliarize the client with common environmental noises which may not have been heard for some time or which sound very different when processed through a hearing aid.

The last stage is *training in auditory discriminations under adverse listening circumstances*. The purpose of this stage is to provide practice in listening under poor acoustic conditions simulating common communication situations, such as listening in noise, at low sensation levels, or to speech distorted through loudspeakers or over the telephone.

Carhart also developed a program for use in military hospitals, consisting of a series of group training sessions with three major goals: (1) to provide an optimal hearing aid for everyday use, (2) to make each patient familiar with hearing aid operation and care and to develop habits of efficient use, and (3) to promote psychological acceptance of amplification. The members of the group were given the opportunity to wear several appropriate hearing aids for at least a day, while participating in a variety of listening and counseling sessions. Practice in sound localization, speech discrimination, and listening under adverse circumstances was provided. The patients evaluated each hearing aid worn and participated in the final decision prior to obtaining a personal hearing aid. Lipreading instruction and speech conservation were also provided and were continued as long as necessary. DiCarlo (1948) described a similar program conducted in another military hospital.

National Technical Institute for the Deaf (NTID) Program. Sims (1978) described an auditory training program for severely and profoundly hearing impaired students attending NTID. Instruction in auditory training, speechreading, speech therapy, and manual communication are provided in curricular packages consisting of 20 hours of therapy. The auditory training program is designed to improve perception of phonemes and suprasegmental speech features such as intonation and stress. According to Sims, suprasegmental training is not popular with students in spite of demonstrations of the usefulness of these features in determining meaning. The auditory training program consists of self instruction based on the audio tape card system described earlier, including training in detection, discrimination, identification, and comprehension of various types of auditory stimuli.

Other Rehabilitation Programs. Johnson and Siegenthaler (1951) described a 20-session auditory training program for adults who have recently acquired hearing aids. Activities, including discussion sessions, are designed to (1) improve personal-social attitudes and relationships through a better understanding and acceptance of the hearing loss, (2) teach the care, operation, and limitations of hearing aids, (3) increase the individual's tolerance for amplified sound, (4) improve the ability to localize sound, and (5) improve perception of speech through specific listening activities with the hearing aid.

The verbotonal method, discussed before with reference to hearing-impaired children, has also been applied to the rehabilitation of adults (Santore, 1978).

REFERENCES

American National Standards Institute, *American National Standards Specifications for Audiometers,* ANSI, S3.6-1969. New York: American National Standards Institute, Inc., 1969.

Benson, R. and Hirsh, I., Some variables in audio spectrometry, *J. Acoust. Soc. Am.,* 25, 449-453, 1953.

Bilger, R. and Wang, M., Consonant confusions in patients with sensorineural hearing loss, *J. Speech Hearing Res.,* 19, 718-748, 1976.

Black, J., Multiple-choice intelligibility tests, *J. Speech Hearing Dis.,* 22, 213-236, 1957.

Bode, D., Speech signals and hearing aids. In M. Pollack (Ed.), *Amplification for the Hearing Impaired.* New York: Grune and Stratton, 1975.

Boothroyd, A., Discrimination by partially hearing children of frequency distorted speech, *Audiology,* 6, 136-145, 1967.

Borden, G. and Harris, K., *Speech Science Primer: Physiology, Acoustics, and Perception of Speech.* Baltimore: Williams and Wilkins Co., 1980.

Brandy, W., Reliability of voice tests of speech discrimination, *J. Speech Hearing Res.,* 9, 461-465, 1966.

Byers, V., Initial consonant intelligibility by hearing impaired children, *J. Speech Hearing Res.,* 16, 48-55, 1973.

Carhart, R., Auditory training. In H. Davis (Ed.), *Hearing and Deafness.* New York: Rinehart, Inc., 1947.

Carhart, R., Problems in the measurement of speech discrimination, *Arch. Otolaryngol.,* 82, 253-260, 1965.

Cramer, K. and Erber, N., A spondee recognition test for young hearing impaired children, *J. Speech Hearing Dis.*, 39, 304–311, 1974.

Dirks, D., Stream, R., and Wilson, R., Speech audiometry: Earphone and sound field, *J. Speech Hearing Dis.*, 37, 162–176, 1972.

Dunn, H. and White, S., Statistical measurements on conversational speech, *J. Acoust. Soc. Am.*, 11, 278–288, 1940.

Egan, J., Articulation testing methods, *Laryngoscope,* 48, 955–991, 1948.

Engelberg, M., Test-retest variability of speech discrimination testing, *Laryngoscope,* 78, 1582–1589, 1968.

Erber, N., Auditory, visual and auditory-visual recognition of consonants by children with normal and impaired hearing, *J. Speech Hearing Res.*, 15, 364–371, 1972.

Erber, N., The use of audiotape-cards in auditory training for hearing impaired children, *Volta Rev.*, 78, 209–218, 1976.

Erber, N., Speech perception by profoundly hearing-impaired children. *J. Speech Hearing Dis.*, 44, 255–270, 1979.

Erber, N. and Alencewicz, C., Audiologic evaluation of deaf children. *J. Speech Hearing Dis.*, 41, 256–267, 1976.

Erber, N. and Hirsh, I., Auditory training. In H. Davis and S. Silverman (Eds.), *Hearing and Deafness*. New York: Holt, Rinehart and Winston, 1978.

Fairbanks, G., Test of phonemic differentiation: The rhyme test, *J. Acoust. Soc. Am.*, 30, 596–600, 1958.

Fitzgibbons, P., Temporal resolution in normal and hearing impaired listeners, Ph.D. Dissertation, Northwestern University, 1979.

Flanagan, J., Some properties of the glottal sound source, *J. Speech Hearing Res.*, 1, 99–116, 1958.

Fletcher, S., Acoustic phonetics. In F. Berg and S. Fletcher (Eds.), *The Hard of Hearing Child: Clinical and Educational Management*. New York: Grune and Stratton, 1970.

Gengel, R., On the reliability of discrimination performance in persons with sensorineural hearing impairment using a closed-set test. *J. Aud. Res.*, 13, 97–100, 1973.

Gerber, S., The intelligibility of speech. In S. Gerber (Ed.), *Introductory Hearing Science: Physical and Psychological Concepts*. Philadelphia: W. B. Saunders, 1974.

Grammatico, L., The development of listening skills, *Volta Rev.*, 77, 303–308, 1975.

Griffiths, C., *Conquering Childhood Deafness*. New York: Exposition, 1967.

Guberina, P., Verbo-tonal method and its application to the deaf, *Proceedings of the International Congress of the Deaf.* Washington, D.C.: Gallaudet College, 1964.

Haskins, H., A phonetically balanced test of speech discrimination for children, Master's Thesis, Northwestern University, 1949.

Hirsh, I., Audition in relation to the perception of speech. In E. Carterette (Ed.), *Brain Function III: Speech, Language, and Comprehension*. Los Angeles: UCLA Press, 1966.

Hirsh, I., Davis, H., Silverman, S., Reynolds, E., Eldert, E., and Benson, R., Development of materials for speech audiometry, *J. Speech Hearing Dis.*, 17, 321–337, 1952.

Hodgson, W., Speech acoustics and intelligibility. In W. Hodgson and P. Skinner (Eds.), *Hearing Aid Assessment and Use in Audiologic Habilitation*. Baltimore: Williams and Wilkins Co., 1977.

House, S., Williams, C., Necker, H., and Kryter, K., Articulation testing methods: Consonantal differentiation in a closed-set response set, *J. Acoust. Soc. Am.*, 37, 158–166, 1965.

Hutton, C., Curry, E., and Armstrong, M., Semi-Diagnostic Test Materials for Aural Rehabilitation, *J. Speech Hearing Dis.*, 24, 319–329, 1959.

Johnson, A. and Siegenthaler, B., A clinical auditory training program, *J. Speech Hearing Dis.*, 16, 35–39, 1951.

Kalikow, D., Stevens, K., and Elliott, L., Development of a test of speech intelligibility in noise using sentence materials with controlled word predictability, *J. Acoust. Soc. Am.*, 61, 1337–1351, 1977.

Keith, R. and Talis, H., The effects of white noise on PB scores of normal and hearing-impaired listeners, *Audiology*, 11, 177–186, 1972.

Larsen, L., The Larsen Sound-Discrimination Lists. In H. Davis and S. Silverman (Eds.), *Hearing and Deafness*, 2nd edition. New York: Holt, Rinehart and Winston, Inc., 1963.

Lawrence, D. and Byers, V., Identification of voiceless fricatives by high frequency hearing impaired listeners, *J. Speech Hearing Res.*, 12, 426–434, 1969.

Ling, D., *Speech and the Hearing Impaired Child*. Washington, D.C.: A. G. Bell Association, 1976.

Matkin, N., Hearing aids for children. In W. Hodgson and P. Skinner (Eds.), *Hearing Aid Assessment and Use in Audiological Habilitation*. Baltimore: Williams and Wilkins Co., 1977.

Miller, G., Heise, G., and Lichten, W., The intelligibility of speech as a function of the context of the test materials, *J. Exp. Psychol.*, 41, 329–335, 1957.

Olsen, W. and Matkin, N., Speech audiometry. In W. Rintelmann (Ed.), *Hearing Assessment*. Baltimore: University Park Press, 1979.

Owens, E., Intelligibility of words varying in familiarity, *J. Speech Hearing Res.*, 4, 113–129, 1961.

Owens, E., Consonant errors and remediation in sensorineural hearing loss, *J. Speech Hearing Dis.*, 43, 331–347, 1978.

Owens, E. and Schubert, E., The development of constant items for speech discrimination testing, *J. Speech Hearing Res.*, 11, 656–667, 1968.

Owens, E. and Schubert, E., Development of the California Consonant Test, *J. Speech Hearing Res.*, 20, 463–474, 1977.

Owens, E., Benedict, M., and Schubert, E., Further investigation of vowel items in multiple-choice speech discrimination testing, *J. Speech Hearing Res.*, 14, 841–847, 1971.

Owens, E., Benedict, M., and Schubert, E., Consonant phonemic errors associated with pure-tone configurations and certain kinds of hearing impairment, *J. Speech Hearing Res.*, 15, 308–322, 1972.

Owens, E., Talbott, C., and Schubert, E., Vowel discrimination of hearing impaired listeners, *J. Speech Hearing Res.*, 11, 648–655, 1968.

Palva, T., Studies of hearing for pure tones and speech in noise, *Acta Otolaryngol.*, 45, 231–243, 1955.

Pollack, D., *Educational Audiology for the Limited Hearing Infant*. Springfield, IL: Charles C Thomas, 1970.

Pascoe, D., Frequency responses of hearing aids and their effects on the speech perception of hearing impaired subjects, *Ann. Otol. Rhinol. Laryngol.,* Supplement 23, 84, No. 5, 1975.

Peterson, G. and Barney, H., Control methods used in a study of the vowels, *J. Acoust. Soc. Am.,* 24, 175–184, 1952.

Pickett, J., *The Sounds of Speech Communication.* Baltimore: University Park Press, 1980.

Pickett, J., Martin, E., Johnson, D., Smith, S., Daniel, Z., Willis, D., and Otis, W., On patterns of speech feature reception by deaf listeners. In G. Fant (Ed.), *Speech Communication Ability and Profound Deafness.* Washington, D.C.: A. G. Bell Association, 1972.

Raphael, L., Preceding vowel duration as a cue to the perception of voicing of American English consonants in word-final position, *J. Acoust. Soc. Am.,* 51, 1296–1303, 1972.

Reed, C., Identification and discrimination of vowel-consonant syllables in listeners with sensorineural hearing loss, *J. Speech Hearing Res.,* 18, 773–794, 1975.

Ross, M. and Lerman, J., Picture identification test for hearing impaired children, *J. Speech Hearing Res.,* 13, 44–53, 1970.

Santore, F., The Verbotonal aural rehabilitation program with hearing impaired adults: A five year summary report, *J. Acad. Rehab. Audiol.,* XI, 33–44, 1978.

Shapiro, M., Melnick, W., and Ver Muelen, V., Effects of modulated noise on speech intelligibility of people with sensorineural hearing loss, *Ann. Otol. Rhinol. Laryngol.,* 81, 241–248, 1972.

Sher, A. and Owens, E., Consonant confusions associated with hearing loss above 2000 Hz, *J. Speech Hearing Res.,* 17, 669–681, 1974.

Silverman, S. and Hirsh, I., Problems related to the use of speech in clinical audiometry, *Ann. Otol. Rhinol. Laryngol.,* 64, 1234–1244, 1955.

Sims, D., Visual and auditory training for adults. In J. Katz (Ed.), *Handbook of Clinical Audiology,* 2nd edition. Baltimore: William and Wilkins Co., 1978.

Speaks, C. and Jerger, J., Method for measurement of speech identification, *J. Speech Hearing Res.,* 8, 185–194, 1965.

Thornton, A. and Raffin, M., Speech discrimination scores modeled as a binomial variable, *J. Speech Hearing Res.,* 21, 507–518, 1978.

Tillman, T. and Carhart, R., An expanded test for speech discrimination utilizing CNC monosyllabic words: Northwestern University Auditory Test No. 6, *USAF School of Aerospace Medicine Technical Report,* Brooks Air Force Base, TX, 1966.

Turner, C., Psychometric functions for frequency discrimination in normal and hearing impaired listeners, Master's Thesis, University of Minnesota, 1979.

Wang, M., Reed, C., and Bilger, R., A comparison of the effects of filtering and sensorineural hearing loss on patterns of consonant confusions, *J. Speech Hearing Res.,* 21, 5–36, 1978.

Wedenberg, E., Experience from thirty years, auditory training, *Volta Rev.,* 69, 588–594, 1967.

Whetnall, E. and Fry, D., *The Deaf Child.* Springfield, IL: Charles C Thomas, 1964.

Wightman, R., McGee, T., and Kramer, M., Factors influencing frequency selectivity in normal and hearing impaired listeners. In E. Evans and J. Wilson (Eds.), *Psychophysics and Physiology of Hearing.* New York: Academic Press, 1977.

CHAPTER 3

Visual Modes of Communication

When hearing is impaired, acts of oral communication often are accomplished under adverse conditions in which hearing alone is not sufficient for understanding. For most hearing-impaired people audition must be supplemented by visual information of some sort if speech is to be understood. Visual input may be provided in three major ways: through facial expression and gesture, through lipreading, and through manual communication. These cues are rarely used alone, but occur most often in combination with each other. The information obtained through lipreading and facial expression is available in most face-to-face conversations and in many public situations. Manual communication is used by fewer hearing impaired people, usually those with the most severe hearing losses.

The purpose of the following discussion is to describe these types of visual stimuli and to suggest ways of assessing and improving their use.

LIPREADING

Various terms have been used to describe the process by which the visual components of speech are used for comprehension of spoken messages. These include *lipreading*, *speechreading*, and *visual hearing*. Although the term lipreading is used most often, it is probably the least accurate way of expressing what is actually involved in the use of visual cues. The observation of lip movements is only one aspect of the process. Facial expressions, body posture, gestures, and environmental cues are also important. The sentence "Oh, my aching back." is difficult to lipread when spoken with a straight face and rigid body; it is immediately comprehended when spoken with a pained expression and one hand touching the back. If the speaker is also sitting in a hospital bed discussing a recent accident, the cues of lip movements, facial expression, body language, environmental cues, and context of the conversation all contribute to the accurate reception of the message by the listener.

Everyone lipreads under certain circumstances. If voice level of a lecturer suddenly drops, the microphone goes dead, or noise from some source invades the room, normally hearing listeners will automatically focus on the speaker, attending to the mouth shapes and movements that occur. Most of the research into the lipreading process has been accomplished on normal listeners, some of whom are excellent lipreaders. It is not unusual for hearing people to score *better* on a lipreading test than hearing-impaired people whose language skills are poor. Because many speech sounds and syllables are not visible on the lips, they must be predicted from the information that is available. This is accomplished most easily by people who know the rules of a language well. They don't have to see the "-ed" or the "to" in the sentence "Yesterday he walked to town" to know that they are present.

There is no question that lipreading is an important means of receiving language for hearing-impaired listeners. It is most useful when combined with auditory information. The acoustic cues of manner of articulation and voicing are most resistant to the effects of hearing loss; they are also the least visible features of speech. On the other hand, information about place of articulation is very difficult for hearing-impaired people to perceive auditorily but is the most visible aspect of speech. For example, the difference between *take* and *cake* is a place distinction. Most hearing-impaired people need visual cues to tell which of these words is spoken unless the context is clear. The combination of auditory information about manner and voicing and visual information about place of articulation allows more accurate reception of a message than either of these inputs alone.

Factors Influencing Visual Perception of Speech

Investigations into the lipreading process show extremely large variations in lipreading performance regardless of the population being tested, the nature of the task, or the circumstances under which lipreading occurs. There appear to be several relevant factors that act alone or in combination to influence lipreading performance. O'Neill and Oyer (1961) referred to these as the speaker-sender, the lipreader-receiver, the environment, and the stimulus. Jeffers and Barley (1971) discussed at length the visibility of speech as a primary factor in its reception. Early research into the lipreading process concentrated on the mental and personality characteristics of the lipreader as the primary determinant of lipreading performance. Unfortunately, in spite of many investigations, little is known about the relative contribution of these factors or ways in which lipreading performance can be enhanced. The following discussion represents a summary of some of what appear to be the most salient factors influencing the use of lipreading by hearing-impaired people.

Visibility of Speech Sounds. There are two major ways in which visibility influences the ability to distinguish speech sounds on the lips: the visibility of the articulators involved in their production and the degree to which the sounds can be distinguished from each other. Sounds that are produced near the front of the mouth with maximum lip, jaw, and tongue movements (**p, b, m, f, v, oo**) are more visible than those produced farther back in the mouth with little movement of the articulators (**k, g, h,** and **y**). Only a portion of the 30 to 40 phonemes of English are actually visible and distinguishable from each other; estimates range from 11 to 57 percent (Berger, 1972).

Under ordinary communication circumstances individual phonemes are distinguished from each other on the basis of acoustic cues, including those of manner, voicing, and place of articulation. Removal or reduction of acoustic information limits severely the phonemic features that are available for processing, leaving place cues as the primary criteria for discrimination. Unfortunately for the lipreader, there are a limited number of places of articulation and many of them look alike on the lips. For example, there are three bilabial consonants (**p, b, m**) that do not differ visually although they are easily distinguishable by audition. Phonemes that look alike (have similar place of articulation) are called *homophemes* and words that are indistinguishable visually are termed *homophenous* words. Groups of words like *bill, pill,* and *mill* or *ton, done,* and *none* are homophenous; they involve no articulator movements that can be differentiated on the basis of visual cues.

Phonemes can also be described in terms of visually contrasting groups called *visemes*. Investigation into observers' abilities to distinguish phonemes from each other has identified at least four major viseme groups for consonants and vowels and several subgroupings that are not as definite. Woodward and Barber (1960) identified four visually contrastive consonant groups as follows:

1. **p, b, m**
2. **f, v**
3. **w, r**
4. **th, t, d, n, l, s, z, sh, ch, j, y, k, g, ng, h**

Fisher (1968) suggested five viseme groups for consonants in initial and another five for those in final positions:

Initial Position	Final Position
1. **p, b, m, d**	1. **p, b**
2. **f, v**	2. **f, v**
3. **k, g**	3. **k, g, ng, m**
4. **w-, wh, r**	4. **sh, zh, j, ch**
5. **sh, t, n, l, s z, j, y-, h-**	5. **t, d, n, th, z s, r, l**

Binnie, Jackson, and Montgomery (1976) proposed a different set of ten consonant visemes:

1. **f, v**	6. **r**
2. **p, b, m**	7. **th**
3. **w**	8. **t, d, s, z**
4. **l, n**	9. **k, g**
5. **sh, zh**	10. **y**

Other authors (Berger, 1972; Walden, Prosek, and Worthington, 1974) have suggested further variations of these groupings. The differences reported probably result from procedural differences employed in the studies, such as stimulus material (CV syllables, monosyllabic words), response tasks (recognition versus discrimination), or speaker differences.

Vowel viseme groups have also been reported. Vowels differ from each other less than consonants in terms of place of articulation, and the differences that exist are often not obvious. Fisher (1963) proposed four vowel visemes:

1. **ee, -i-, oi, ur**
2. **a-e, -e-, -u-**
3. **-o-, -a-, ou**
4. **aw, o-e, oo**

In addition, Jackson, Montgomery, and Binnie (1976) identified five features of vowel production that are important to recognition. In order of their prominence they are:

1. Lip extension versus rounding (**ee** versus **oo**).
2. Vertical lip separation (**-i-** versus **ar**).
3. General size of mouth opening (**-e-** versus **-a-**).

4. Features unique to diphthongs.
   (a) Vertical movement from first to second nucleus (**a-e** versus **au**).
   (b) Size of opening of second nucleus (**i-e** versus **au**).

Fortunately, speech sounds are much easier to distinguish when contextual information is present, a situation that does not exist in most controlled studies of visibility. Therefore the limitations imposed by poor visibility and the similarity among sounds may be alleviated partially by the linguistic context in which they occur. Although the homophenous words like *pop, mop,* and *bob* cannot be distinguished in isolation, they are not likely to be confused in sentences such as "Did you bob for apples?" or "Give me the can of pop." Sentence familiarity (Lloyd and Price, 1971) and linguistic structure of sentences (Schwartz and Black, 1967) have been shown to influence lipreading performance, even when the target words to be perceived were the same.

The visual parameters of speech do not lend themselves to accurate perception by lipreading alone. Much of the variability in lipreading performance reported probably relates to how well individuals can combine linguistic knowledge with visual perception. Unfortunately, the precise relationship among visibility and other factors is poorly understood at present.

Rapidity of Speech. Not only is the hand quicker than the eye, there is evidence that the mouth is also. The average speaker produces about 15 speech sounds per second for an average duration per phoneme of 67 milliseconds. The briefest consonants (plosives) are about 30 milliseconds in duration, while the longest are about 300 milliseconds. If the movement of the articulators associated with these sounds is visible for approximately the same length of time, the lipreader would have to process short duration stimuli in rapid succession to correctly identify each sound. Because some of the sounds are obscure or homophenous, the lipreading task imposes severe limitations on the information processing capacity of the visual system. In spite of the availability of linguistic redundancy and environmental clues, lipreading for extended periods of time often produces fatigue. Assuming that brief unstressed phonemes will be reduced in visibility (e.g., **s**), the use of lipreading as a means of learning some of the simplest rules of language (how to form plurals or express possessives and verb tenses, for example) will be difficult.

Speaker Differences. Speakers who have mobile, expressive faces are easier to lipread than those who use little lip or jaw movements (Stone, 1957). Precise articulation, such as that which contributes to auditory intelligibility, seems to result in visual intelligibility as well (O'Neill, 1951). The natural use of gestures enhances lipreading, but inappropriate or random gestures serve only as visual distractions (Berger, Martin, and Sakoff, 1970; Popelka and Berger, 1971).

The familiarity of the speaker also contributes to lipreading success. Deaf children have been shown to lipread their teachers more accurately than other adults

(Day, Fusfeld, and Pintner, 1928). People who rely on lipreading to communicate often report having to become familiar with a speaker before lipreading is possible.

Lipreaders vary in their reactions to the presence of beards and mustaches, with some viewing them as obstructions to lipreading and others considering them as "frames for the mouth." There is general agreement that people who speak while eating, chewing gum, or holding cigarettes or pipes in the mouth are difficult to lipread.

The rate of speaking is the most common speaker characteristic mentioned by lipreaders, who complain that rapid speech is very difficult to comprehend. Experimental investigations of this observation have resulted in conflicting data. Mulligan (1954) and Frisina and Bernero (1958) found that lipreading performance improved when filmed lipreading tests were slowed down from a normal rate of 24 frames per second. Byers and Lieberman (1959) and Black, O'Reilly, and Peck (1963) found no improvement in lipreading under the same conditions. These findings are difficult to relate to the daily experiences of lipreaders for several reasons. First, the rate of speaking on the films was slightly slower than normal to begin with so no measure of the attempts to lipread rapid speech were obtained. Second, speech was slowed by reducing the rate at which the film was projected, an artificial way of "slowing down" speech. The natural way to reduce the rate of speech is to increase the number and length of the pauses that occur during speech production. The relative duration and rate of phonemes and syllables remains normal; only the overall rate is reduced. When speakers produce rapid, normal and slow rates of speech naturally, significant differences in lipreading performance occur, with scores being best for the slow, but not distorted, rate (Rios-Escalera and Davis, 1977).

Environmental Factors. Factors such as distance and lighting affect lipreading performance in predictable ways. Lipreading is possible at distances up to about 24 feet, but it is easier at distances representative of typical conversational situations (5 to 10 feet), with 5 feet being optimal (Berger, 1972; Erber, 1971). The amount of light available is less critical than its location, except in cases of actual darkness or visual defects experienced by the lipreader. The light source should never be behind the speaker, since looking toward the speaker (into the light) causes constriction of the pupils and reduced visual acuity. The speaker's face may become a silhouette, the features dim and imprecise. Lipreading under such circumstances is very difficult. Otherwise, lighting factors are not critical as long as the speaker's face can be seen clearly.

Characteristics of the Lipreader. Lipreaders show great variability in performance and much effort has been directed toward determining what makes a successful lipreader. Early research efforts were based on the hypothesis that good lipreaders probably exhibited mental abilities or personality characteristics that differed from those of poor lipreaders. Reviews of the extensive research into the psychological traits associated with lipreading skills have been provided by O'Neill and Oyer

(1961), Berger (1972), Jeffers and Barley (1971), and Oyer and Frankmann (1975). Most investigations have resulted in negative findings. Neither intelligence nor personality variables, such as introspection or motivation, appear to correlate highly with lipreading ability. The ability to synthesize material appears to be mildly helpful, and the willingness to take a chance has been suggested as a significant variable. In general, there do not appear to be personality traits that are associated with the ability to lipread well.

There is some evidence that females lipread better than males, at least on sentence tasks (Taaffe, 1957; Wynn, 1964; Lesner, 1979). Hearing-impaired people do not appear to lipread better than those who hear normally. In addition, the severity and duration of the hearing loss are not directly related to lipreading ability. There is a tendency, however, for people with less severe hearing losses to be better lipreaders than those with profound hearing losses. This fact may simply reflect the linguistic advantages enjoyed by normally hearing people.

Because lipreading makes use of visual input, it seems obvious that the visual acuity of the lipreader would be an important factor in lipreading performance. Studies of the relationship between the ability to distinguish fine details (as usually measured by a Snellen chart using letters of the alphabet) and lipreading performance have resulted in conflicting opinions as to the importance of visual acuity to lipreading. Goetzinger (1964) and Evans (1960) reported no significant correlation between visual acuity and lipreading performance, while Lovering (1969), Hardick, Oyer, and Irion (1970), Glaser (1972) and Romano and Berlow (1974) reported opposite conclusions. For example, Lovering's subjects obtained lipreading scores of 20 percent at 20/100 and 80 percent at 20/20. Shepard, DeLavergne, Frueh, and Clobridge (1977) reported a correlation of −.90 between neural firing time in the visual system and performance on a lipreading test. These findings suggest that lipreading performance is strongly related to the rate of transmission of coded visual information through the neural system. The question is an important one. Both hearing and visual acuity deteriorate with age, resulting in a large population of people with reduced auditory input who need to use visual cues to supplement auditory ones, but whose visual acuity is also diminished. In the case of children, educators and health professionals believe that those with visual acuity less than 20/40 are at risk educationally. The combination of reduced vision and hearing is likely to interact in such a way as to seriously hinder educational achievement.

Studies of the effects of age on lipreading ability illustrate the complex interaction of variables that affect lipreading and the impossibility of predicting performance from one characteristic. Normal and hearing-impaired children appear to improve in the ability to lipread as they grow older, at least between the ages of 7 and 21 (Heider, 1947; Craig, 1964; Wynn, 1964; Evans, 1960, 1965). Conversely, young adults score higher on lipreading tasks than older people, with highest scores occurring prior to age 30 (Goetzinger, 1964; Farrimond, 1959; Pelsen and Prather, 1974). The development of linguistic and cognitive skills during childhood results in increased lipreading ability with age, up to a point, while the decrease in visual acuity that occurs as adults grow older results in decreased performance with age.

Attempts to isolate personal characteristics that contribute to lipreading performance have been largely unsuccessful and probably do not warrant further serious effort on the part of researchers. It is likely that almost any personal factor could be hypothesized as a contributor to lipreading performance. Two examples of research efforts will illustrate the infinite variety of factors that may be involved. First, recent studies of blinking rate reveal a direct relationship between this trait and lipreading ability, with poor lipreaders exhibiting more blinks per minute than good lipreaders. Interpretation of this finding is made difficult by the facts that (1) blinking rate increases with poor vision and (2) females blink fewer times per minute than males. Blinking rate may or may not be an important contributor to lipreading performance, but it *appears* to be on the basis of studies reported (Lesner, 1979). The second example involves extrasensory perception (ESP). One of the authors conducted a pilot study in which measures of ESP (using two standard sets of cards depicting geometric designs and words) and lipreading (using a sentence test) were obtained for a group of subjects who also differed in familiarity with the speaker. Results indicated a perfect correlation between lipreading ability and ESP. Furthermore, ESP scores were highest for the words on the cards that would have been most visible on the lips had they been spoken and significantly lower for the least visible words (king, sea). Instead of creating a desire in the experimenter to pursue this area of research, it demonstrated the elusive nature of the whole question of predicting lipreading performance on the basis of personal characteristics, many of which are probably beyond the control of the individual and therefore not easily modified through training.

Assessment of Lipreading Skills

In contrast to the tests that have been developed to assess auditory skills, available measures of lipreading ability have not been adequately validated nor are they used systematically throughout the professional community. Lipreading performance has been measured for research and clinical purposes using a variety of materials, ranging from nonsense syllables to short paragraphs. Some of the materials used, such as the CID Everyday Sentences, were designed for use as auditory, rather than visual, tests. The procedures used to administer lipreading tests are largely unstandardized. Some tests are presented on film; others are presented face to face. Frequently, the same materials are presented on film by one professional and live by another. Stimuli may be presented only once or two or more times, depending on the examiner's judgment. These factors probably contribute to the extreme variability in lipreading performance exhibited by both hearing and hearing-impaired individuals. They also complicate interpretation of test results and the exchange of information about a client from one class, school, or clinic to another.

Characteristics of Lipreading Tests. The most commonly used tests of lipreading are described in Table 3.1. All of these tests have one or more of the following deficiencies, which limit their usefulness as clinical tools.

1. The validity of the materials has not been satisfactorily demonstrated. A common method of establishing validity is to compare one test with another that is known or presumed to be a valid measure of the behavior being tested. Utley's test, *How Well Can You Read Lips?* (1945) was developed with considerable care and standardized on a large number of hearing-impaired people. It has been used often as the criterion against which the validity of other tests is evaluated. Unfortunately, the validity of the Utley test has been severely criticized. Heider (1947) suggested that roughly half of the items should be discarded because they are so difficult that they do not discriminate between levels of lipreading ability. DiCarlo and Kataja (1951) used the Utley test to evaluate performance of normally hearing people and hearing-impaired people divided into groups of good and poor lipreaders on the basis of ability to follow conversational speech by lipreading. The Utley test did not discriminate the normally hearing from the hearing-impaired group nor the good from the poor lipreaders. O'Neill and Stephens (1959) reported that teacher ratings of lipreading proficiency did not correlate significantly with Utley test results. Many of the other lipreading tests in use correlate with the Utley test, indicating that the same behavior is being assessed. The fact that test performance appears to be poorly related to the ability to comprehend conversations by lipreading may be interpreted in several ways. It is possible that these tests are not valid measures of the ability to lipread. Another interpretation is that the ability to lipread sentences is not related to the ability to lipread conversations. The third interpretation is that the tests are not sensitive enough to distinguish among varying degrees of lipreading skill except grossly.

2. Most lipreading tests are sufficiently difficult to discourage many subjects. Few subjects ever achieve a 100 percent correct score while 0 percent scores are not uncommon. It is unlikely that all 0 percent scores indicate an absence of lipreading ability. The normative data for the Utley sentence test was standardized on 761 hearing-impaired children and adults who used lipreading as an important aspect of speech reception. The range of scores among these hearing impaired subjects was from 0 to 84 with a mean performance of 33.6 items correct (27 percent of the 125 items on the test). The best lipreader only obtained 67 percent of the possible total.

3. Filmed tests are devoid of facial and gestural cues. Most of them were recorded many years ago and do not reflect contemporary dress or appearance. On the other hand, face-to-face testing introduces variability each time the stimulus materials are spoken.

4. Filmed and live presentations usually involve only one speaker. Because speakers are known to vary in their speaking ability, it may not be possible to generalize test results to other speakers or situations.

Table 3.1 Summary of Certain Characteristics of Several Lipreading Tests

Author	*Test Name*	*Type of Material*	*Equivalent Forms*	*Age or Language Competence Required*
Utley (1946)	How Well Do You Read Lips?	Words	2	Third-grade reading vocabulary.
		Sentences	2	Eight-year-olds in normative group. Most appropriate for adults.
		Conversational Dialogue	1 set of 6	
Barley (Jeffers and Barley, 1971)	Barley-CID[c]	Sentences	2	Based on CID Everyday Speech Sentences. Most appropriate for adults.
Taaffe (1957)	A Film Test of Lip Reading[a]	Sentences	2	Undetermined but all standardization accomplished with adults.
Craig (1964)	Craig Lipreading Inventory[c]	Words	2	Children—first through tenth grade.
		Sentences	2	
Costello (1957)	Costello Test of Speechreading[c]	Words	1	Kindergarten vocabulary
		Sentences	2	
Cavender (1949)	Cavender Test of Lipreading Ability[c]	Sentences	4	Vocabulary level—grades 1 to 3.

Mason (1943)	Visual Hearing Test	Nouns	2	Children.
Butt and Chreist (1968)	Butt Children's Speechreading Test	Questions or commands	1	Children down to 3 years. Comprehension indicated by motor action.
Myklebust and Neyhus (1970)	Diagnostic Test of Speechreading	Words	1	Vocabulary appropriate for deaf children aged 4 to 9.
		Phrases	1	
		Sentences	1	
Davis and Silverman (1978)	CID Everyday Speech Sentences	Sentences	10[b]	Developed for use with adults.
Hutton, Curry, and Armstrong (1959)	Semi-Diagnostic Test	Words	6	Vocabulary level—grades 1 to 4. Multiple-choice format so reading is required.
Binnie, Jackson, and Montgomery (1976)	Lipreading Screening Test	CV syllables	1	Has been used only with adults.

[a] Originally developed by Keaster at the University of Iowa. Also known as the John Tracy Clinic Test.
[b] It is not known whether the lists are equally difficult for lipreading or combined presentation.
[c] Forms of the test available in Jeffers and Barley, 1971.

5. Most lipreading tests have only one or two forms, rather than several lists equated for difficulty, visibility, familiarity, or other parameters.

6. Test materials are designed for reception by lipreading only. Materials designed to be presented through combined auditory and visual modes have not been developed and standardized, even though this condition is more representative of daily communication than visual reception alone and would allow better assessment of overall receptive proficiency.

Choosing a Test. At best, the available tests provide only general estimates of an individual's ability to lipread. The purpose of assessing lipreading skill and the limitations imposed by the age or linguistic competency of the client will determine the test to be chosen. For example, several of the tests shown in Table 3.1 use kindergarten and early elementary vocabulary. Their sentences represent simple structures. In some tests, such as the *Children's Speechreading Test* (see Appendix A), sentences consist primarily of frames for single vocabulary items (Show me the ______. Where is ______? Point to the ______.). Once the pointing response is established, it is not necessary for the child to understand the sentence frame to respond accurately, In contrast, the CID Everyday Sentences and the Utley test (shown in Appendix B) consist of sentences that vary in length and complexity; vocabulary level is not tightly controlled.

Response mode also varies among tests and can be used as a criterion for test selection. Most tests designed for children use a multiple-choice format, using either written key words or pictures depicting key words or sentence meaning. Tests for adults are open set tests, requiring repetition or writing responses.

Administration of Tests. The most common way to administer lipreading tests is face to face, with the examiner pronouncing the materials either in the same room without voice or with voice from a different room with the client viewing the examiner through a window. This common procedure does not allow the use of auditory information during testing. Although there are instances in which pure measures of visual reception of speech may be useful, people do not ordinarily lipread in the absence of auditory input, however slight or distorted. If lipreading is measured without sound, the test should be repeated with auditory information available. Comparison of the two scores may be used to estimate the usefulness of amplification, the need for lipreading or auditory training, and the efficacy of past training in one modality or the other. Although lipreading tests have not been designed for combined presentation, their questionable validity makes it doubtful that auditory-visual presentation will compromise their usefulness.

Because words and sentences are rarely spoken in exactly the same way across repetitions, live presentation of lipreading tests introduces the variable of consistency of production. Face-to-face presentations should never be used for research purposes or when close comparisons among lipreaders are important. When testing children, however, it is often necessary to present materials live to help maintain interest in the task and to ensure that the child is observing closely when stimulus items are presented. Many clinicians make their own videotape recordings of materials, thereby avoiding use of outdated filmed materials while controlling for consistency of presentation. Videotaped presentations also allow the examiner to control the amount of auditory information provided during testing by increasing and decreasing volume as desired.

The effects of three-dimensional (face-to-face) versus two-dimensional (filmed) presentations on lipreading performance are questionable. Differences reported between performance on live and filmed presentations of lipreading materials (Jeffers and Barley, 1971; Berger, 1972) are probably due as much to speaker differences as to basic effects of three- versus two-dimensional viewing.

Regardless of the presentation mode employed, materials to be lipread should be presented under optimal viewing conditions. Lighting should be on the speaker's face, viewing should be straight on or at a slight angle (45 degrees or less), and distance between lipreader and speaker should be from 5 to 10 feet.

Lipreading Training

Training in the ability to read lips constituted the earliest form of rehabilitation for hearing-impaired children and adults. As long ago as the 1600s educational procedures for hearing-impaired children were based on teaching students to recognize speech and to produce it on the basis of visual cues. Because the cues available for lipreading were used as a basis for producing speech, early methods of lipreading instruction tended to stress analysis of articulatory movements whether or not the lipreader had a good knowledge of language. Although lipreading instruction began as an educational procedure used in classes or schools for deaf children, the most detailed descriptions of instructional methods were published by teachers of adults (Nitchie, 1912; Bruhn, 1915, 1927, 1947; Kinzie and Kinzie, 1931, 1936; Bunger, 1932).

From about 1870 to 1940 lipreading classes were popular in most cities. Several different lipreading "methods" were developed, based on philosophical issues of the time, such as whether lipreading constituted a visual or a psychological process. Although lipreading instruction is still available in some speech and hearing centers, its relative contribution to rehabilitation has decreased greatly. No new methods have been developed since the mid-1930s, and schools devoted to lipreading instruction have disappeared. A combination of circumstances has contributed to the decline in the teaching of lipreading as a rehabilitative tool. Most influential has been the availability of hearing aids and their improved fidelity, which have increased the contribution made by audition to speech perception, thus reducing the degree to which lipreading is used by many hearing-impaired listeners. In addition, the importance of linguistic competency to the lipreading process is now recognized.

The ability of many normally hearing people to lipread and the wide variability among inexperienced and experienced lipreaders make it obvious that many people "learn" to lipread without formal instruction, while others do not use visual cues effectively even after instruction and practice.

For some reason, however, the notion persists that lipreading is the primary rehabilitative procedure, especially for adults. Most adults are referred to speech and hearing centers either by others or as self-referrals for lipreading instruction, rather than for auditory training. Several examples will illustrate the variability among hearing-impaired adults regarding their need for lipreading instruction.

> The first example is a 33-year-old woman who referred herself for lipreading lessons. She had been hearing impaired since early childhood but believed her hearing loss was worsening and wanted to improve her lipreading skills in case she lost her hearing altogether. She had used binaural hearing aids for several years. Informal and formal measures of lipreading revealed her to be an excellent lipreader, whose scores were around 80 percent without auditory cues and 100 percent when minimal auditory cues were provided. Nevertheless, she considered herself a mediocre lipreader. The treatment program designed for her involved analysis of her communication problems, identification of ways of managing situations to enhance her considerable ability to lipread, and practicing lipreading under extremely adverse conditions such as the absence of auditory information, poor viewing angles, and amid visual and auditory distractions. This was not lipreading instruction in the strictest sense; lipreading lessons did not appear to be appropriate for her needs.

> The second client was a 64-year-old man who was referred for lipreading instruction by a physician about three months after suddenly suffering a severe bilateral hearing loss. His ability to communicate was severely impaired; auditory discrimination was 20 percent; lipreading performance was 30 percent without auditory information, but 70 percent when amplification was provided. Although he had been referred for lipreading training and had not considered the use of amplification, the treatment program consisted of selection of a hearing aid combined with brief training in its use and the use of simultaneous visual and auditory information available in common communicative situations. Lipreading lessons were not provided because his ability to use combined visual and auditory information improved rapidly. He became a confident communicator who exhibited no need for extended therapy.

> The third example is a 46-year-old man who suffered a profound bilateral hearing loss in his early twenties. He had never used a hearing aid and was reported to be a poor lipreader and a social isolate. Referred by a vocational rehabilitation counselor for lipreading instruction, he was tested and found to have 0 percent auditory discrimination and a lipreading score of 0 percent on a sentence test. Attempts to communicate with him were frustrating for everyone concerned. This man had undergone lipreading instruction in the past, with no apparent success. He was enrolled again for lipreading lessons, which had little effect on his communication skills. A hearing aid was selected and combined visual and auditory training was provided. His communication skills improved almost immediately, as evidenced by a sharply improved ability to follow

conversations, including shifts in topics. Improvement in isolated lipreading or auditory skills could not be demonstrated. Lipreading lessons were terminated and treatment concentrated on the analysis and manipulation of communicative situations to maximize his ability to communicate effectively.

None of these individuals required lipreading lessons, per se, but each of them depended heavily on lipreading in order to communicate. For each, the use of amplification was more important to improved speech reception than was lipreading instruction. Although they exhibited varying skill in lipreading, their abilities did not appear to be related to the amount of lipreading instruction or practice they had experienced. The poorest lipreader had been dependent on lipreading as a means of communication for more than 20 years. The man whose hearing loss was only of a few month's duration was already a good user of visual skills when they were combined with minimal auditory information.

Most hearing-impaired individuals make good use of visual information with or without training. The patient most likely to benefit from lipreading lessons is one who experiences a sudden hearing loss, resulting in a severely disrupted ability to communicate. This is frightening and depressing, and immediate treatment is important to the person's adjustment to the hearing loss. Analysis of the visual information available in speech and training in its use may be the most helpful treatment that can be provided, especially if it is combined with efforts to enhance the use of whatever residual hearing remains. In some cases, severe problems tolerating loud sound may preclude the use of amplification; in those cases, lipreading will be the primary means of speech reception and every effort should be made to enhance its use.

Approaches Toward Teaching Lipreading. In the early 1900s several methods for teaching lipreading were developed and used widely with adults and children (Nitchie, 1912, 1950; Bruhn, 1927, 1947; Bunger, 1932). These methods differed from each other primarily in the way in which speech sounds were introduced and the emphasis placed on their recognition as the basis for perception of speech. These

Table 3.2 Classification of Consonants Used to Introduce Articulatory Position and Movement in the Nitchie Method of Lipreading

Sounds Formed and Revealed by the Lips	*Formed by the Tongue, Revealed by the Lips*	*Formed and Revealed by the Tongue*	*Revealed by Context*
p, b, m	**r**	**th**	**y-**
f, v	**s, z**	**l**	**k, g**
wh, w-	**sh, zh, ch, j**	**t, d, n**	**h-**

Nitchie, 1912.

same distinctions characterize modern approaches toward the teaching of lipreading, even though specific methods are rarely identified by name any more.

There are two major approaches toward the teaching of lipreading. The first, often called an *analytic* approach, involves making the lipreader familiar with the phonemes of English, how they look on the lips, and the movements associated with their production. Speech sounds are classified according to certain criteria which vary with different proponents. Tables 3.2 and 3.3 show two systems of classifying consonants; the viseme groups described earlier represent other classification systems. Analytic lipreading lessons involve the following types of activities:

1. Speech sounds are introduced and classified. Their production is demonstrated in isolation and in syllables.
2. Lipreaders practice identifying phonemes, usually in CV, VC, or CVC contexts. In the beginning lessons are built around one or two phonemes from different viseme groups. The target phonemes are easily distinguished from each other, and they are combined with a variety of vowels to encourage recognition of the sound in various contexts. Feedback is given often to help the lipreader monitor performance.
3. When the lipreader can recognize most consonants and vowels consistently, drills involving a variety of phonemes presented at increasing rates are accomplished.
4. Practice in lipreading words, phrases, sentences, and longer messages constitutes the final step in analytic training.

The analytic approach has as a major goal improvement of visual perceptual skills. Speech involves rapid movements of the articulators, which must be recognized, classified, and used to make decisions about the message received. Proponents of phoneme and syllable drill believe that visual perception can be improved through practice with materials that progress from highly visible stimuli, spoken slowly and in relative isolation, to visually obscure, rapid stimuli that require well-developed visual skills.

The second approach to lipreading is called *synthetic*. It involves less drill than the analytic approach, concentrating instead on perception of the meaning of an

Table 3.3 Classification of Consonants According to the Mueller-Walle Method of Lipreading

Class I: Produced with the Cavity of the Mouth Closed	*Class II: Produced with the Cavity of the Mouth Open*
f, v, s, z, m, p, b, w-, wh, sh, ch, th	**k, g, d, t, h-, l, n, r**

From Bruhn, 1947.

utterance rather than its phonemic components. (Of course, the final goal of any lipreading training is the effective use of visual cues to obtain meaning from speech.) To achieve this goal, synthetic teaching strategies involve training the lipreader to anticipate information (based on context, situation, and linguistic rules) and thereby process it more rapidly and successfully. The ability to "fill in" information that is missing because of poor visibility or the rapidity of the signal is a linguistic rather than a visual skill. It is this view of the lipreading process that differentiates synthetic from analytic training. Synthetic lipreading lessons usually involve the following types of activities:

1. The visibility limitations associated with speech are discussed and demonstrated. The effects of rate, distance, and phonemic content on recognition of speech are described along with the necessity to supplement the available visual cues with information based on linguistic context and situational data.
2. Lipreaders are given situations and asked to predict the utterances that would occur naturally during them. Stimuli may include pictures depicting interesting situations (such as old *Saturday Evening Post* covers or other illustrations by artists like Norman Rockwell), cartoons, descriptions of everyday activities (shopping, going to the movies), and familiar stories.
3. Stimuli like that described above are presented along with appropriate spoken utterances. The lipreaders attempt to understand the content, rather than specific elements of the utterances. Situations may be role played by group members while other lipreaders attempt to follow the meaning of what is said.
4. As the lipreaders become more confident, short paragraph-long stories or jokes are told, and the lipreaders attempt to understand the most salient pieces of information that will allow them to follow the events accurately.

Synthetic approaches usually do not involve syllable drill or practice unless the lipreaders simply cannot process longer speech units, an unusual occurrence.

Developing Lipreading Lessons. Regardless of the approach taken toward teaching lipreading, several general principles should be used as guidelines for developing lessons. The materials and stimuli used should be relevant to the communicative needs of the lipreader. A 10-year-old child needs to be able to recognize the words used by classroom teachers and peers; lipreading instruction could be concentrated on new vocabulary from curriculum materials, the latest slang expressions, the names of popular movies, songs, performers, and school activities. A secretary, physician, or salesman would benefit most from assistance in recognizing words, phrases, and questions related to their respective jobs and their environments. Lists of such materials can be provided by clients. Lipreading lessons should not revolve around a topic chosen at random by the clinician.

Because people seeking lipreading training are hearing impaired, visual aids should always be used to introduce the topics to be discussed and to explain the rules of the activities to follow. This will avoid confusion and encourage relaxation, a necessary state for easy lipreading. If the lesson is introduced adequately, the lipreader develops a preparatory set for what is to follow that contributes to early success.

The spoken materials involved should be presented in a logical manner, so that context can be used as an aid to understanding. Unexpected shifts in topics should be avoided. Lessons should begin with easy materials and progress toward more difficult stimuli and more difficult viewing conditions. Distance and viewing angle can be changed as the lipreaders become more relaxed and confident. The effects of these factors should be discussed.

Combined Auditory-Visual Training. Although there may be times when training in the use of visual cues alone will be beneficial, the major contribution of lipreading to communication lies in its use as an adjunct to audition. Lipreading is most helpful in distinguishing the place of articulation, enabling differentiation between words like *tin, pin, sin, fin,* and *thin* when they cannot be distinguished on the basis of acoustic cues alone. The simultaneous presentation of auditory and visual information is the most natural and beneficial way to encourage improvements in communication. This type of training can be accomplished with videotaped materials ranging from nonsense syllables to stories. Presentation by videotape allows easy manipulation of the volume of the auditory signal and distance and viewing angle for the visual signal. Different speakers can be used within a single lesson to demonstrate the effects of different speaking rates, styles, accents, and other characteristics on reception of similar material.

If desired, the auditory signal can be degraded by the addition of noise or by filtering so that greater reliance on visual information occurs. This technique was described by Montgomery (1977).

Benefits of Lipreading Training. The contribution of lipreading to communication by hearing-impaired people is obvious and real. Unfortunately, little is known about how lipreading skills are developed or what factors contribute most to the process. There are virtually no data available that document the benefits of lipreading training. Anecdotal reports from clients are almost always positive, however. Clients express belief that their lipreading skills are improved through training, no matter how brief. It is possible that the changes they perceive are too subtle to be detected by the lipreading tests currently in use, or that the perceived improvement is related to greater confidence in their communicative abilities. The most logical explanation for the consistent belief that lipreading skills are improved through training lies in the relationship between lipreading and the use of audition. Many clients seek rehabilitation who are poor users of amplification. In addition they need assistance in analyzing their communicative needs. As a result, their attempts to lipread are hampered by poor auditory perception and the failure to manipulate the environment to aid communication. When these factors are addressed and improvements made, the use of visual cues is enhanced and the ability to lipread appears to have improved.

MANUAL COMMUNICATION

For some hearing-impaired people, use of lipreading as the only visual input is not sufficient for easy communication. This is especially true if acoustic cues are not audible or if visual problems interfere with fine visual discriminations. These people require less ambiguity than that involved in lipreading; for them non-oral forms of communication may be necessary for language reception and expression.

Types of Manual Communication

The term *manual communication* refers to several types of messages produced by the hands, arms, face and body, and received by the eyes (Mayberry, 1978). The major forms of manual communication are *gestures, fingerspelling,* and *sign.* Gestures are used widely by most people as natural adjuncts to speech or in place of it under special circumstances when speech is not appropriate (in church or at a distance). Fingerspelling and sign are used primarily by persons who have been deaf since early in life. Among deaf adults sign is the dominant form of communication, used alone or in combination with speech, lipreading, and hearing (Schein, 1978). Gestures and signs are commonly used by deaf children among themselves, regardless of the communication modes they are expected to use with teachers or others (Moores, 1978).

As is the case with spoken forms of language, manual forms undergo constant change and evaluation. Contrary to popular belief, there is no international manual language. The communication systems described as follows are representative of those used in this country.

Fingerspelling. In the United States the manual alphabet is produced with one hand; in some countries, such as England, both hands are used. Figure 3.1 shows the manual alphabet used in this country. Fingerspelling provides a visual representation of spoken language. Words are spelled in the air, usually at shoulder level and slightly to the right of the body. Since the hands generally do not move as rapidly as the articulators, it is difficult to fingerspell at a normal speaking rate, although some fingerspellers are able to spell words and speak fluently at the same time. One method of teaching deaf children, the Rochester method, consists of simultaneous fingerspelling of each word that is spoken.

The manual alphabet is easy to learn and produce. Most people can learn to spell words accurately and rapidly in a short time. Reading fingerspelling is a more

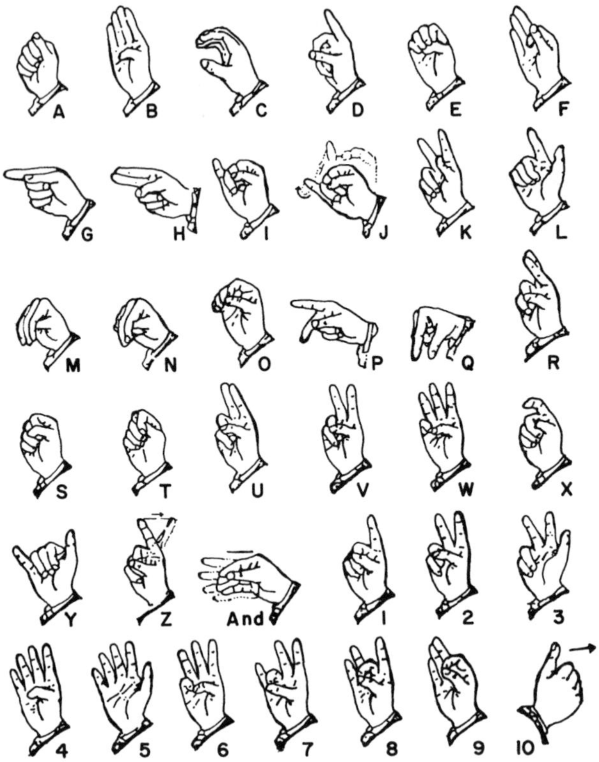

Figure 3.1. Manual alphabet.

difficult task and requires much practice. Many of the letters are visually similar and difficult to distinguish when produced rapidly. For example, the letters, **e, o, a, s, t, m,** and **n** all resemble a closed fist, and the observer must learn to note minor differences in the hand configurations.

Except for children and teachers in programs using the Rochester method, most people use fingerspelling only as an adjunct to sign. English words or concepts for which there are no established signs, technical terms, and proper names are fingerspelled. It is also used to clarify misunderstandings among people who use different signs for the same message.

Sign. The last 10 years have brought widespread acceptance of sign as a means of communication. Deaf persons have always signed, either as a result of being exposed to a formal sign system or being forced to invent one to meet their needs (Moores, 1978). Until recently, however, sign was not well accepted by the public, professionals serving the deaf, or parents of deaf children. The controversy surrounding its use with deaf children has raged for hundreds of years and is discussed in Chapter 10.

Mayberry (1978) described two major types of sign: sign *languages,* which are independent of spoken language, and sign *systems,* which are derived from oral languages. *American Sign Lanugage* (*ASL or Ameslan*), the sign used by most deaf adults, represents the former category. Recent research into its structure indicates that it is a separate language having its own lexicon and grammar, both independent of spoken English (Wilbur, 1976). Several recently developed sign systems fall into the latter category, consisting of signs representing English words and structure. These systems are used primarily in educational programs for deaf children. Sign in general may be more acceptable to hearing people now because of its resemblance to English; on the other hand, the development of the new systems may be an outgrowth of increased acceptability. The reasons for it probably cannot be determined, but the new popularity of sign has increased communication between deaf and hearing people, which, in turn, has resulted in increased understanding of the impact of deafness on communication and the feelings of deaf people regarding their unique language mode.

Signs are produced by one or both hands at various places on or near the upper body and head. Each sign has three major elements: the shape of the hand(s), their position relative to the body and each other, and the movement involved. Variation in any of the three may change the meaning of the sign. For example, the *ASL* sign for *blind* is made by bent, clawlike index and middle fingers brought to the eyes. The same hand shape and movement at the throat means *stuck,* or, interestingly, *pregnant*.

Some signs are iconic; they resemble their referents so closely that their meaning can be determined by someone with no knowledge of sign. An example is the sign for *me,* made by touching the chest with the index finger. The sign for *baby* is made by cradling the arms at the chest and rocking them gently from side to side. The sign for *drive* is produced with both hands holding an imaginary steering wheel and turning it slightly once or twice. Most signs are not iconic, however, and their meaning cannot be determined without knowledge of sign. Signs for many "words" are the same in several or all of the sign systems in current use; others vary widely. Descriptions of the most commonly used forms of sign follow.

American Sign Language (ASL). *ASL* is based on French sign language and was brought to America in 1816 by Thomas Gallaudet and Laurent Clerc, founders of the American School for the Deaf. Because its structure and vocabulary are not those of English, it has often been described by hearing people as an incomplete language or a poor representation of English. The nature of *ASL* can best be illustrated by describing a few of its characteristics that differ from spoken English. First, *ASL* signs do not represent words, although some signs may be accurately translated into English words (book, school, drink, work). Others do not have

English equivalents, such as the sign for *to-fall-in-love*. A single sign may represent several English words related to a central concept. For example, an index finger brought from the signer's chin forward a few inches may mean any present tense form of the verb *to be* (is, am, are, be), *indeed, yes, sure, certain,* or *true*. All these words represent a state of existence. The sign described above for *drive* is another example; it is also used to represent *car*. Conversely, a single English word may be represented by several different signs, depending on its meaning in context. For example, signs for the word *right* are produced differently when the word conveys the meaning of direction (turn right), accuracy (that's right), and acquiesence (all right).

Second, although *ASL* contains no specific signs for many pronouns, modifiers, articles and other function words, they are accurately conveyed by shifts in body position, the direction in which signs are made, pointing, and facial expressions. Objects or people to be referred to are named, assigned a position in space near the signer, then referred to by eye or head movements or slight body shifts.

Third, stress is conveyed by slowing down or speeding up the movement of signs or producing them with sharp emphasis. Rate may also change meaning; speeding up the sign for *month* produces *rent*.

Finally, repetition may alter a single sign by making it plural (house, houses), or changing its meaning (*again* repeated two or three times becomes *often*).

Hearing people must learn *ASL* as a foreign language. The task is complicated because it cannot be written. Pictures or drawings make it possible to learn *ASL* signs relatively easily, but the syntax must be observed and practiced extensively with other *ASL* signers. Examples of the differences between *ASL* and English syntax are shown in Table 3.4. These sentences illustrate the complexities of shifting from one language to the other.

ASL is not directly related to English, and it is impossible to speak English and sign *ASL* at the same time. Users of *ASL* either do not speak while signing, or they

Table 3.4 Examples of Utterances as They Are Expressed in Spoken English and *ASL*

English	*ASL*
1. She has already told me she wants to go back next year.	1. Finish say next year want again go there.
2. I was tired when I got home last night.	2. Yesterday night arrive home tired.
3. I have been to Chicago many times.	3. Finish touch Chicago many time.
4. I was surprised at how many questions they asked me.	4. Me surprise many many questions, question, question they question me.
5. I haven't eaten yet.	5. Eat late, me.

produce *ASL* signs in English word order, a combination referred to as *ASL-English pidgen* (Mayberry, 1978). The ability to do this requires a knowledge of English. For most *ASL* signers, English is a second language, and their ability to shift from one language to the other varies considerably. Attempts by hearing people to impose English structure and literal interpretation on *ASL* often results in cross communication and misunderstanding.

Bellugi and Fischer (1972) have shown that a given message can be communicated as rapidly in *ASL* as in spoken English, even though hand movements are slower than speech. As a means of communicating it is quick, colorful, and effective. It does not have the precision necessary for representing technical material, analyzing philosophical discussions, or teaching abstract subject matter, however. Recognizing this, several authors have devised new systems of sign that attempt to represent spoken and written English, referred to as "contrived" or "artificial" sign systems. It may be more accurate to refer to them as translations of English into manual form. Mayberry (1978) has labeled them "manual English systems."

Manual English Systems. Several attempts to represent English in manual form have been made. The impetus for them has been the need for a way to stimulate deaf children with English in a nonambiguous, meaningful form. Educators reasoned that, if deaf children could *see* English similar to the way in which hearing children *hear* it, learning would occur naturally through repeated exposure.

The first attempt to develop a manual English system was made by David Anthony and a group of his associates. The system was called *Seeing Essential English* (SEE_1). Two other systems were spawned from SEE_1: *Signing Exact English* (SEE_2) and *Linguistics of Visual English* (*LOVE*). An independent effort by researchers at Gallaudet College to produce a sign system for kindergarten children resulted in the development of *Signed English*. Three of these systems are described briefly as follows.

1. *Seeing Essential English* (SEE_1). Initially, Anthony and his associates (1971) sought to combine *ASL* and English, using a "one-word, one-sign" philosophy. Each sign represented a single word in English, based on the pronunciation, spelling, and meaning of the word. If two of these three characteristics were the same for words used in different contexts, the sign representing them was the same. The earlier example of *right* can be used to demonstrate this rule. Because the word *right* is spelled the same and sounds the same in all the contexts described earlier, a single *ASL* sign was chosen to represent the word. Thus, the directionality sign for right is used in SEE_1 whenever the word *right* is signed, regardless of its meaning within a given context. The one word, one sign rule also precludes use of a single sign for *car* and *drive,* or for *is, am, are, true,* and *sure* because these words are spelled and pronounced differently. Each of these words is represented by a different sign in SEE_1. New signs were devised for word endings, such as *-ing, -s, -ed, -ly, -ment, -tion, -ity, -ist,* and *-ous*. Articles, pronouns, infinitives, and other words for which *ASL* has no designations were assigned formal signs. Many *ASL* signs for words like *happy, understand,* and *balance* were carried over into *SEE_1*.

As *SEE_1* developed, Anthony and his associates began to disagree regarding the extent to which *ASL* vocabulary should be used and the way in which signs were assigned to words. By 1976, Anthony had shifted to a morpheme-based sign system. He defined morphemes to include suffixes, prefixes, and roots of words. Words like *balance* were represented by two signs: *bal(l)* + *ance*. *Accompany* was signed *a* + *come* + *pan* + *y*. *Happy* became *hap(p)* + *y* and *understand* became *un* + *der* + *stand*. The semantic base for words and their signs was discarded in favor of a syllabic orientation. Long before the syllable-based signs became dominant in *SEE_1*, some of Anthony's associates defected and founded other sign systems.

2. *Signing Exact English SEE_2)*. *SEE_2* is almost identical to the early *SEE_1*. It was renamed by Gustason, Pfetzinger, and Azwolkow (1972) and represented an attempt to prevent further artificial breakdown of words and signs. The one-word, one-sign rule was maintained and numerous word endings were used. When first published the only difference between *SEE_1* and *SEE_2* was the manner in which they were represented in print. Instead of the elaborate written code used by Anthony, signs were represented in the *SEE_2* dictionary as drawings. At present, there is little resemblance between the two systems.

3. *Signed English*. Sometimes referred to as Gallaudet Signed English, this system was devised by Bornstein (1974) and others at Gallaudet College for use with preschool deaf children. Most of the vocabulary comes from *ASL;* the most common word endings (-ing, -s, -ed, -en, -ly, -y, -'s, -er, -est, -or) are also signed along with pronouns, auxiliary verbs, and articles not used in *ASL*. There are a number of colorful materials available in Signed English. The *Signed English Dictionary* (Bornstein, Hamilton, Saulinier, and Roy, 1975) contains about 1500 signs, depicted by colored drawings and written descriptions. Children's books are available, written in sign and words; these include books of nursery rhymes and children's stories, such as *Little Red Riding Hood*.

The manual English systems have several features in common:

1. Signs represent English words.
2. Signs are produced in English word order.
3. Some manual representation of common word endings is included.
4. Synonyms or words constituting classes or families of related words are formed by the use of similar hand positions and movements, but different hand shapes. For example, signs for *class, group, family,* and *organization* are made by bringing the two hands apart and together again as they describe an imaginary circle in front of the body. Different hand shapes representing letters of the manual alphabet are used for each word: C, G. F, and O, respectively.
5. Relatively little fingerspelling is used; pronouns, infinitives, prepositions, modal verbs, articles, and other function words are usually signed instead of spelled.

Cued Speech. This system of hand signals is not usually considered a form of manual communication. It is designed to be used as an adjunct to lipreading, and the cues have no intrinsic meaning of their own. The system consists of 32 cues that are combinations of eight hand shapes and four placement positions near the head and neck. A single cue (hand shape plus position) cannot be interpreted in the absence of the lip movements associated with it. Cued speech is described in detail in Chapter 10.

Assessment of Manual Communication Skills

The ability to use manual communication for receiving and expressing messages is not usually evaluated. One reason for this may be that traditionally it has not been considered an acceptable form of communication to be encouraged or taught. Gochnour (1973) suggested that assessment of deaf persons without the use of manual communication would result in underestimation of their ability to use language. She suggested ways of including the use of manual communication during language assessment procedures but no mention is made of evaluating the hearing-impaired person's own reception and production of sign.

Evaluation of the ability to produce or read sign and fingerspelling independent of language status is rare. Unlike the articulation of speech, the accuracy of production of signs does not have established norms. Variations in production occur; which ones of them are normal and which are deviant have not been ascertained. Wilbur (1976) described the "phonology" of sign, in which certain features of production were described, but stated that further research is necessary before a standard description of the physical characteristics of sign will be available. Schlesinger and Meadow (1972) described the development of expressive sign in young children, indicating that early attempts to produce sign were often distorted and sometimes unintelligible. Gradual approximations to the adult form of sign occurred.

If interested in the accuracy of production of signs, clinicians may analyze them according to hand shape, place of production, and movement, describing any variations from the accepted forms. Because of the wide differences of production that are typical among signers, it is unwise to label slight deviations in production as incorrect, especially when the person being evaluated is a native signer and the observer is not.

Assessment of sign reception and production is useful in planning new habilitative programs or when considering modifications of existing programs. It is most often used by postsecondary programs for deaf students, such as Gallaudet College and NTID. Gallaudet is the only liberal arts college for the deaf in the world; NTID is the only four-year technical training center for the deaf currently in existence. Instructors at both of these institutions use simultaneous communication in the classroom to enhance comprehension by the deaf students. Students from all types of educational programs attend these colleges; they exhibit widely varying manual or simultaneous communication skills. To assess these skills, NTID personnel administer videotaped communication tests, including signed and fingerspelled presentations of the CID Everyday Sentences. Results are used to help students decide whether or not to enroll in communication skills training (auditory training, lipreading, sign language, and fingerspelling). Often, their attempts to communicate with their classmates are instrumental in their seeking ways to improve their communication skills.

Teaching Manual Communication Skills

Because most hearing-impaired people who use manual communication learn it from each other, it is seldom taught in the traditional sense. Children attending educational programs for the deaf learn sign from their classmates and dorm neighbors whether or not it is used in the classroom by teachers or children. Deaf adults who were not exposed to sign in childhood learn it easily when they come in contact with other deaf people, socially or at work. Signing appears to be an easy skill to master if sufficient practice occurs.

Because of the increased acceptance of sign that has occurred in the last few years, classes in manual communication are available in most communities. Because of the dynamic nature of sign, it is seldom learned sufficiently from books alone. Instruction by an accomplished signer or regular interaction with people who use sign to communicate are the best ways to learn it well enough to use it in communication.

Occasionally the decision is made to introduce sign to a child or an adult in a therapy or tutoring situation. This is usally accomplished by simply signing what is spoken during sessions, but it may involve actual teaching of individual signs. There are not well-established methods of accomplishing this. It makes sense, however, to introduce signs that will be useful immediately, used often, and thereby reinforced quickly.

REFERENCES

Anthony, D. and Associates, *Seeing Essential English Manual.* Anaheim, CA: Anaheim Union High School District, 1971.

Bellugi, V. and Fischer, A., A comparison of sign language and spoken language, *Cognition,* 1, 173-200, 1972.

Berger, K., *Speechreading Principles and Methods.* Baltimore: National Educational Press, 1972.

Berger, K., Martin, J., and Sakoff, R., The effect of visual distractions on speechreading performance, *Teach. Deaf,* 68, 384-387, 1970.

Binnie, C., Jackson, P., and Montgomery, A., Visual intelligibility of consonants: A lipreading screening test with implications for aural rehabilitation, *J. Speech Hearing Dis.,* 41, 530-539, 1976.

Black, J., O'Reilly, P., and Peck, L., Self administered training in lipreading, *J. Speech Hearing Dis.,* 28, 183–186, 1963.
Bornstein, H., Signed English: A manual approach to English language development, J. Speech Hearing Dis., 39, 330–343, 1974.
Bornstein, H., Hamilton, K., Saulinier, K., and Roy, H., *The Signed English Dictionary for Preschool and Elementary Levels.* Washington, D.C.: Gallaudet College, 1975.
Bruhn, M., *The Meuller-Walle Method of Lip-Reading for the Deaf.* Lynn, MA: The Nichols Press, 1915.
Bruhn, M., *Elementary Lessons in Lipreading: The Mueller-Walle Method.* Lynn, MA: The Nichols Press, 1927.
Bruhn, M., *The Mueller-Walle Method of Lipreading for the Hard of Hearing.* Boston: Leavis, 1947.
Bunger, A., *Speechreading—Jena Method.* Danville, IL: Interstate, 1932.
Butt, D. and Chreist, F., A speechreading test for young children, *Volta Rev.,* 70, 225–244, 1968.
Byers, V. and Lieberman, L., Lipreading performance and the rate of the speaker, *J. Speech Hearing Res.,* 2, 271–276, 1959.
Cavender, B., The construction and investigation of a test of lipreading ability and a study of factors assumed to affect the results, Master's Thesis, Indiana University, 1949.
Costello, M., A study of speechreading as a developing language process in deaf and in hard of hearing children, Ph.D. Dissertation, Northwestern University, 1957.
Craig, W., Effects of pre-school training on the development of reading and lipreading skills of deaf children, *Amer. Ann. Deaf,* 109, 280–296, 1964.
Davis, H. and Silverman, S. (Eds.), *Hearing and Deafness,* 4th edition. New York: Holt, Rinehart and Winston, 1978.
Day, H., Fusfeld, I., and Pintner, R., *A Survey of American Schools for the Deaf 1927–1952.* Washington, D.C.: National Research Council, 1928.
DiCarlo, L. and Kataja, R., An analysis of the Utley lipreading test, *J. Speech Hearing Dis.,* 16, 226–240, 1951.
Erber, N., Effects of distance on visual reception of speech, *J. Speech Hearing Res.,* 14, 848–857, 1971.
Evans, L., Factors related to listening and lipreading, *Teach. Deaf,* 58, 417–423, 1960.
Evans, L., Psychological factors related to lipreading, *Teach. Deaf,* 63, 131–136, 1965.
Farrimond, T., Age differences in the ability to use visual cues in auditory communication, *Language and Speech,* 2, 179–192, 1959.
Fisher, C., Confusions within six types of phonemes in an oral-visual system of communication, Ph.D. Dissertation, The Ohio State University, 1963.
Fisher, C., Confusions among visually perceived consonants, *J. Speech Hearing Res.,* 11, 796–804, 1968.
Frisina, D. and Bernero, R., A profile of the hearing and speech of Gallaudet College students, *Volta Rev.,* 60, 316–321, 1958.
Glaser, R., The relationship of speechreading performance to altered visual acuity, Master's Thesis, Kent State University, 1972.
Gochnour, E., Evaluating the communication skills of the adult deaf, *Asha,* 15, 687–691, 1973.

Goetzinger, C., A study of monocular versus binocular vision in lipreading, *Proceedings of the International Congress on Education of the Deaf and the Forty-First Meeting of the Convention of American Instructors of the Deaf.* Washington, D.C.: United States Government Printing Office Document No. 106, 1964.

Gustason, G., Pfetzinger, D., and Azwolkow, E., *Signing Exact English*. Rossmoor, CA: Modern Signs Press, 1972.

Hardick, E., Oyer, H., and Irion, P., Lipreading performance as related to measurements of vision, *J. Speech Hearing Res.,* 13, 92–100, 1970.

Heider, G., The Utley lipreading test, *Volta Rev.,* 49, 457–458, 1947.

Hutton, C., Curry, E., and Armstrong, M., Semi-diagnostic test materials for aural rehabilitation, *J. Speech Hearing Dis.,* 24, 319–329, 1959.

Jackson, P., Montgomery, A., and Binnie, C., Perceptual dimensions underlying vowel lipreading performance, *J. Speech Hearing Res.,* 19, 796–812, 1976.

Jeffers, J. and Barley, M., *Speechreading (Lipreading)*. Springfield, IL: Charles C Thomas, 1971.

Kinzie, C. and Kinzie, R., *Lipreading for the Deafened Adult*. Philadelphia: John C. Winston, 1931.

Kinzie, C. and Kinzie, R., *Lipreading for Children*. Washington, D.C.: Volta Bureau, 1936.

Lesner, S., An investigation of involuntary eyeblinks during lipreading, Ph.D. Dissertation, The Ohio State University, 1979.

Lloyd, L. and Price, J., Sentence familiarity as a factor in visual speech reception (lipreading) of deaf college students, *J. Speech Hearing Res.,* 14, 291–294, 1971.

Lovering, L., Lipreading performance as a function of visual acuity, Ph.D. Dissertation, Michigan State University, 1969.

Mason, M., A cinematographic technique for testing visual speech comprehension, *J. Speech Hearing Dis.,* 8, 271–278, 1943.

Mayberry, R., Manual communication. In H. Davis and S. Silverman (Eds.), *Hearing and Deafness*. New York: Holt, Rinehart and Winston, 1978.

Montgomery, A., Assessment of a new auditory visual integration technique. Paper presented at the Annual Convention of The American Speech and Hearing Association, Chicago, 1977.

Moores, D., *Educating the Deaf: Psychology, Principles and Practices*. Boston: Houghton Mifflin, 1978.

Mulligan, M., Variables in the reception of visual speech from motion pictures, Master's Thesis, The Ohio State University, 1954.

Myklebust, H. and Neyhus, A., *A Diagnostic Test of Speechreading*. New York: Grune and Stratton, 1970.

Nitchie, E., *Lipreading: Principles and Practice*. New York: F. A. Stokes, 1912.

Nitchie, E., *New Lessons in Lipreading*. Philadelphia: J. B. Lippincott, 1950.

O'Neill, J., An exploratory investigation of lipreading ability among normal hearing students, *Speech Monographs,* 18, 309–311, 1951.

O'Neill, J. and Oyer, H., *Visual Communication for the Hard of Hearing*. Englewood Cliffs, NJ: Prentice-Hall, 1961.

O'Neill, J. and Stephens, M., Relationships among three filmed lipreading tests, *J. Speech Hearing Res.,* 2, 61–65, 1959.

Oyer, H. and Frankmann, J., *The Aural Rehabilitation Process*. New York: Holt, Rinehart and Winston, 1975.
Pelson, R. and Prather, W., Effects of visual message related cues, age, and hearing impairment on speechreading performance, *J. Speech Hearing Res.*, 17, 518-525, 1974.
Popelka, G. and Berger, K., Gestures and speech reception, *Amer. Ann. Deaf,* 116, 434-436, 1971.
Rios-Escalera, A. and Davis, J., An investigation of lipreading performance as a function of speaking rate. In K. Berger (Ed.), *Research Studies in Speechreading*. Kent, OH: Herald Publishing House, 1977.
Romano, P. and Berlow, W., Vision requirements for lipreading, *Amer. Ann. Deaf,* 119, 383-386, 1974.
Schein, J., The deaf community. In H. Davis and S. Silverman (Eds.), *Hearing and Deafness*. New York: Holt, Rinehart and Winston, 1978.
Schlesinger, H. and Meadow, K., *Sound and Sign: Childhood Deafness and Mental Health*. Berkeley: University of California Press, 1972.
Schwartz, J. and Black, J., Some effects of sentence structures on speechreading, *Central States Speech J.,* 18, 86-90, 1967.
Shepard, D., DeLavergne, R., Frueh, F., and Clobridge, C., Visual-neural correlates of speechreading ability in normal-hearing adults, *J. Speech Hearing Res.*, 20, 752-765, 1977.
Taaffe, G., A film test of lipreading. *John Tracy Clinic Research Papers,* No. 2, (November) 1957.
Utley, J., Development and standardization of a motion picture achievement test of lipreading ability, Ph.D. Dissertation, Northwestern University, 1945.
Utley, J., A test of lipreading ability, *J. Speech Hearing Dis.,* 11, 109-116, 1946.
Walden, B., Prosek, R., and Worthington, D., Predicting audio-visual consonant recognition performance of hearing impaired adults, *J. Speech Hearing Res.,* 17, 270-278, 1974.
Wilbur, R., The linguistics of manual systems. In L. Lloyd (Ed.), *Communication Assessment and Intervention Strategies*. Baltimore: University Park Press, 1976.
Woodward, M. and Barber, C., Phoneme perception in lipreading, *J. Speech Hearing Res.,* 3, 212-222, 1960.
Wynn, M., Norms for a film presentation of the semi-diagnostic test in aural rehabilitation, Master's Thesis, Michigan State University, 1964.

APPENDIX A
Children's Speechreading Test[1]

TEST B

For children 3 years of age or older. The following toys and materials are required.

1. Toys, durable, realistically colored, and in correct proportion: 3-inch baby doll, 1-inch baby doll, doll bed, table, and chair, doll shoe, car, airplane, bus, train, gun, top, toy

[1]From Butt and Chreist, 1968. Reprinted with permission from *Volta Rev.,* 70, 225-244.

wrist watch, button, bell, cellophane wrapped candy, toy cup, fork, and spoon, child's toothbrush, 1-inch rubber ball, ½-inch rubber ball, cow, chicken, pig, horse, fish.

2. Blocks: five 1-inch counting blocks of uniform color.
3. Color chips: 1-inch colored paper squares: yellow, blue, black, white, red, and brown.
4. Ten picture cards 8½ inches × 11 inches that can be constructed from colored pictures in children's books or magazines. Each picture must be realistic and easily recognized by a child:

   Card (a) baby, kitten, flower.
   (b) Mother, father, boy, girl.
   (c) Bird, dog, hammer, spoon.
   (d) Television set, motor boat, house, bed.
   (e) Girl putting on her shoes; boy eating at the table; girl or boy swimming.
   (f) Child playing with a ball; child taking a bath; girl jumping rope.
   (g) Child in bed; child reading a book; child playing with blocks.
   (h) Apple, water faucet and glass of water, pie, butter.
   (i) An orange; milk carton and glass of milk; loaf of bread and a piece of bread; a vegetable.
   (j) Banana, cookies, cooked meat, soup.

5. Paper dolls with clothes. Boy and girl dolls should be mounted on separate 8½ inch × 11 inch cards, and the clothing should be cut so it can easily be placed in position: two dolls with pants, shirt, dress, pajamas, hats, and shoes.

Part I. Identification of Objects

Place objects in random order on the table. Encourage child to watch your face while you name the object three times, then allow child to indicate the correct object. Replace object after each task. It is helpful to keep each set of objects in a separate box.

Present: fish, shoe, ball, train

_____ **1.** Show me the fish. _____ **2.** Show me the ball.
_____ **3.** Show me the shoe.

Present: top, airplane, baby, gun

_____ **4.** Show me the airplane. _____ **5.** Show me the top.
_____ **6.** Show me the gun.

Present: chair, toothbrush, button

_____ **7.** Show me the chair. _____ **8.** Show me the button.
_____ **9.** Show me the toothbrush.

Present: fork, table, car, bus

_____ **10.** Show me the table. _____ **11.** Show me the car.
_____ **12.** Show me the bus.

Present: candy, watch, bell, hat

_____ **13.** Show me the bell. _____ **14.** Show me the candy.
_____ **15.** Show me the watch.

Part II. Numbers

Place five blocks on the table. Demonstrate the first task by saying, "four," and scooping four blocks toward you. Replace the blocks, repeat the word "four" and indicate for the child to push the correct number toward you.

______ **16.** one ______ **17.** three ______ **18.** two

Part III. Picture Identification

Present Test Card (a) and say,

______ **19.** See baby? Where is baby? ______ **20.** Where is the flower?

Present: Test Card (b)

______ **21.** Where is mother? ______ **22.** Where is father? (or daddy)

______ **23.** Where's the boy?

Present: Test Card (c)

______ **24.** Point to the bird. ______ **25.** Point to the dog.

______ **26.** Point to the hammer.

Present: Test Card (d)

______ **27.** Point to the TV (or television) ______ **28.** Point to the boat.

______ **29.** Point to the home. (or house)

Part IV. Color Identification

Place color squares on table three at a time. Say the name of one color and reach your hand out to receive it. Change color cards for each item.

Present: blue, yellow, and white. ______ **30.** blue

Present: black, white, and brown. ______ **31.** white

Present: yellow, red, and brown. ______ **32.** brown

Part V. Actions. Present Test Card (e)

______ **33.** Who put on her shoes?

______ **34.** Who eats her supper? (or dinner)

Present Test Card (f)

______ **35.** Which one plays ball? ______ **36.** Which one takes a bath?

Present Test Card (g)

______ **37.** Who goes to bed?
Who sleeps in bed?

______ **38.** Who reads a book?

Part VI. Foods

Present Test Card (h) to child. Allow him or her to examine it and proceed.

______ **39.** Show me the apple.
______ **40.** Where is the water?
______ **41.** Point to the pie.

Continue with Card (i)

______ **42.** Show me the orange.
______ **43.** Where is the milk?
______ **44.** Where is the bread?

Card (j)

______ **45.** Show me the banana.
______ **46.** Where are the cookies?
______ **47.** Show me the meat.

Part VII. Descriptive Words

Place on the table a large ball and a small ball, a 3-inch baby doll and a 1-inch baby doll.

______ **50.** Where is your mouth?
______ **51.** Where are your eyes?
______ **52.** Where is your nose?
______ **53.** Show me your teeth.
______ **54.** Show me your arm.
______ **55.** Where are your feet?

Part IX. Animal Names

Place the animals on the table in random order. Include chicken, pig, sheep, cow, horse. Replace after each item.

______ **56.** Give me the cow.
______ **57.** Give me the horse.
______ **58.** Give me the pig.
______ **59.** Give me the chicken.

Part X. Clothing

Place on the table a paper doll mounted on 8½ inch × 11 inch card. Use a boy or a girl doll according to the sex of the child. Place the doll's clothes beside test card. Demonstrate the first item. "Put on his (her) pajamas." Replace each piece before proceeding with the next item.

Part XI. Simple Directions

Place these objects on the table: chair, bed, baby, cup, table.

______ **64.** Put the baby to bed. Put her to bed. Go to bed, baby.
______ **65.** Put the spoon in the cup. Put it in the cup.
______ **66.** Put the fork on the table. Put it on the table.

Part XII. Activities

Stand up and gesture for the child to stand. Say, "Stand up." "Do what I do." "Can you hop?" Hop and encourage the child to perform this action as a demonstration. Avoid gesturing with the actual test items to follow.

_______ **67.** Can you jump? Jump.
_______ **68.** Can you walk? Walk. Walk to the door.
_______ **69.** Open the door. Go open the door. Open it.
_______ **70.** Come here. Come.

Scoring. Each correct response receives one point. Total possible score is 70. All items should be administered. Results with 124 hearing-impaired children from 3 to 8 years of age were:

Age	Mean	Standard Deviation
3	28	24
4	26	19
5	35	20
6	39	22
7	40	19
8	52	16

APPENDIX B
How Well Can You Read Lips?[1]

PRACTICE SENTENCES

1. Good morning.
2. Thank you.
3. Hello.
4. How are you?
5. Goodbye.

TEST FORM A

1. All right.
2. Where have you been?
3. I have forgotten.
4. I have nothing.
5. That is right.
6. Look you.

[1]From Utley, 1946. Reprinted with permission.

7. How have you been?
8. I don't know if I can.
9. How tall are you?
10. It is awfully cold.
11. My folks are home.
12. How much was it?
13. Good night.
14. Where are you going?
15. Excuse me.
16. Did you have a good time?
17. What did you want?
18. How much do you weigh?
19. I cannot stand him.
20. She was home last week.
21. Keep your eye on the ball.
22. I cannot remember.
23. Of course.
24. I flew to Washington.
25. You look well.
26. The train runs every hour.
27. You had better go slow.
28. It says that in the book.
29. We got home at six o'clock.
30. We drove to the country.
31. How much rain fell?

TEST FORM B

1. What happened?
2. It is all over.
3. How old are you?
4. What did you say?
5. O.K.
6. No.
7. That is pretty.
8. Pardon me.
9. Did you like it?
10. Good afternoon.
11. I cannot help it.
12. I will see you tomorrow.
13. You are welcome.
14. You are all dressed up.
15. What is your number?
16. I know.
17. It is cold today.
18. I am hungry.
19. I had rather go now.
20. What is your address?
21. What does the paper say about the weather?
22. It is around four o'clock.
23. Do you understand?
24. They went way around the world.
25. The office opens at nine o'clock.
26. None of them is here.
27. Take two cups of coffee.
28. Come again.
29. The thermometer says twenty above.
30. It is your turn.
31. It is hard to keep up with the new books.

Scoring. One point for each correct word. Maximum score is 125. Results with filmed version administered to 761 hearing-impaired subjects from 8 years of age to adults were:

	Form A	**Form B**
Range	0–84	0–89
Mean	33.6	33.8
Standard Deviation	16.4	17.5

APPENDIX C
A Film Test of Lipreading[1]

FORM A

1. How are you?
2. Do you have a piece of paper?
3. What hours do you work?
4. Do you have a pencil?
5. Do you like to go to the movies?
6. How far is it to the post office?
7. How much time have you?
8. How far is it from here to Chicago?
9. Where do you work?
10. Did you enjoy the baseball game?
11. The train leaves at five o'clock.
12. Do you have an umbrella?
13. What is your favorite television program?
14. This is a cold day.
15. Have you any children?
16. How much snow did we have last night?
17. Did you finish high school?
18. Do you have chains on your car?
19. Have you ever lived in the West?
20. I'm going south for my vacation.
21. How many miles did you drive your Ford?
22. Did you get my letter?
23. What does the paper say about the weather?
24. I think it is going to snow.
25. The bank closes at two-thirty.
26. The snow is five inches deep.
27. Isn't this a beautiful day?
28. It was a perfect day for a football game.
29. You had a long distance call while you were gone.
30. It rained most of the night.

FORM B

1. What time is it?
2. Do you have a dog?
3. What time did you have breakfast this morning?
4. Do you have a new car?
5. What kind of a dog do you have?

[1]From Taaffe, 1957. Reprinted with permission.

6. Have you read the newspaper this morning?
7. Where is your home?
8. How are your family?
9. Are you going home for vacation?
10. Do you like to shop?
11. Do you think it will rain this afternoon?
12. Would you like to go to the show with us?
13. What is your occupation?
14. Do you like to watch television?
15. What are your hobbies?
16. What kind of a car do you drive?
17. What day of the week is this?
18. Do you drink your coffee black?
19. My watch is slow.
20. Have you any brothers or sisters?
21. The wind is blowing from the northeast.
22. My watch doesn't keep good time.
23. What shall we do tonight?
24. Did you drive or come by train?
25. Can you have lunch with me Friday?
26. I have an appointment at three o'clock.
27. Are your parents living?
28. I'll meet you at three o'clock.
29. You could drop me a postcard to let me know.
30. Do they allow children in that building?

Scoring. One point for each correct word. Maximum score is 188. Results with filmed version administered to normally hearing college students were:

	Form A		*Form B*	
	Male	*Female*	*Male*	*Female*
Mean	84.7	102.0	94.9	109.8
Standard deviation	33.2	32.8	34.2	29.4

CHAPTER 4

Amplification

For most hearing-impaired people the selection and use of appropriate amplification is the most important component of successful habilitation. Except in rare cases the use of audition is essential to the development of the best possible communication skills, and amplification is essential to the maximal use of audition.

The most commonly used forms of amplification are hearing aids and auditory training units, both of which will be discussed here.

PURPOSES OF AMPLIFICATION

The purpose of any kind of amplification is to make speech louder; this is accomplished by increasing the amplitude of the frequencies that make up speech sounds so that they are audible to the listener. Most hearing aids are designed to amplify the frequencies that are important to the perception of consonants, which also tend to be the frequencies at which sensorineural hearing loss is greatest (above 1000 Hz). This approach toward the use of amplification has not moved much beyond the concept of hearing loss as a frequency filter, even though the filter theory is an inadequate explanation of the communication difficulties imposed by sensorineural hearing loss. Within these limitations the objective of hearing aid use is to improve the intelligibility of speech by making it loud enough to be heard.

Who Can Use Hearing Aids?

Any hearing-impaired person who has difficulty communicating in common situations should consider using a hearing aid. The effects of reduced hearing on ease of communication can be illustrated by examining the relationship between the intensity of a signal and its perceived loudness. The average SPL of conversational speech measured 1 meter from the source is between 60 to 70 dB; this level corresponds to an audiometric attenuator dial reading of 40 to 50 dB HL, a scale that relates hearing level to the average threshold of normal hearing. The relationship of intensity to loudness is such that a 10 dB decrease in intensity results in a halving of the sensation of loudness. Table 4.1 indicates the relation between changes in intensity and the resulting perceptions of loudness by a listener.

This relationship between intensity and loudness means that people with a mild hearing loss of 30 dB HL, for example, will hear speech only one-fourth as loudly as normally hearing listeners. Under these circumstances listening is a difficult and tiring task. The less intense speech sounds are inaudible and any noise interferes seriously with speech perception. The most helpful thing that can be done for someone who hears speech one-fourth as loudly as others it to make that speech louder, more audible, and, possibly, more intelligible. For people with mild hearing losses using a hearing aid may make the difference between tense, strained listening and easy communication.

For people who cannot hear conversational speech (those who have hearing losses greater than 50 dB HL), a hearing aid is even more essential to communication, because it allows the user to go from zero intelligibility to some degree of speech perception, an improvement whose importance cannot be overemphasized. It may make the difference between understanding little of what is said and understanding most of what is said through a combination of auditory and visual perception.

For persons with profound hearing impairment, the purpose of amplification is to make available some amount of auditory information that may be useful for making decisions about speech that is heard and seen and to monitor the speech that

Table 4.1 The Effects of Changes in Intensity on the Perception of Loudness by Listeners

dB HL	*Loudness Perceived*
50 dB	Normal loudness for speech
40 dB	Speech sounds ½ as loud as normal
30 dB	Speech sounds ¼ as loud as normal
20 dB	Speech sounds ⅛ as loud as normal

is produced. For a very few, amplification does not appear useful at all, but these people are rare. Selection of amplification for these people is a complex and time-consuming task, but the results are worth the effort if their perception of speech can be enhanced.

When listening conditions are less than optimal, the usefulness of hearing aids may increase. People who can hear fairly well unaided in a one-to-one conversation may have great difficulty understanding speech from a distance of 10 feet or when mild noise is present. Using a hearing aid may be all that is required to overcome the effects of distance and mild interference on communication. Under more severe background noise conditions, however, a hearing aid may produce little or no benefit.

Limitations of Hearing Aids

Unfortunately, as helpful as amplification is to hearing-impaired listeners, it cannot and does not restore hearing to normal. In the case of conductive hearing loss, little distortion of the auditory signal occurs as a result of the hearing loss itself, making amplification of speech an effective way of overcoming the most important effect of the hearing loss—reduced sensitivity to sound. Because the frequency response of hearing aids is limited, however, amplified sound does not have the same fidelity as that received by a normal ear.

People with sensorineural hearing loss experience distortion because of the damage sustained by the sound receptors located in the cochlea or the nerve fibers involved in neural transmission from the cochlea to higher auditory centers. Because amplified speech is subject to the same frequency and timing distortions as unamplified speech, the use of a hearing aid does not result in normal speech perception. Nevertheless, being able to *hear* speech more easily, even if it is not perfectly clear, contributes significantly to communication.

ELECTROACOUSTIC CHARACTERISTICS OF HEARING AIDS

The functioning properties of hearing aids can be described in terms of certain electroacoustic characteristics that must be monitored carefully if hearing aids are to achieve their intended purposes. Hearing aids are subject to damage and malfunctioning parts just as are other electronic devices. Because hearing aids are worn daily, they are affected by several sources of stress, including moisture (from perspiration or weather conditions), accidents (being dropped or banged around during physical activity) and other incidents which they are not designed to withstand (being chewed on by dogs, for example, a surprisingly common occurrence). An understanding of the normal characteristics of a given hearing aid is necessary for adequate monitoring of how well it is functioning.

Gain

Gain is the preferred term for what is colloquially called volume. It refers to the amount of amplification (stated in decibels) that is added to the input signal by the hearing aid. Each hearing aid is designed to provide a range of amplification from some minimum to some maximum increment. Hearing aids are described as having mild (approximately 25 to 40 dB), moderate (approximately 40 to 55 dB), or high (more than 60 dB) gain. Within the range of a given aid, the amount of gain delivered at any moment is determined by the degree to which the gain control wheel is rotated.

The formula that describes the relation of gain to the function of the hearing aid is: input + gain = output. If a signal of 30 dB SPL impinges on the microphone of a hearing aid whose gain control is set to provide 40 dB of amplification, the output of the aid will be 70 dB SPL: input (30) = gain (40) = output (70). Input SPL and gain in dB are additive providing the frequency characteristics of the input are within the frequency range of the hearing aid and the maximum output of the hearing aid is not exceeded.

The amount of gain in dB provided by a given setting on a particular hearing aid is not always easy to determine. Few hearing aids have gain controls that are labeled; when provided the labels are meaningless for determining the amount of gain provided at that setting. The increase in output per degree of gain control rotation is called the *taper* of the control. Most of the gain of a hearing aid is associated with approximately the first half to two-thirds of the available rotation. This means that simply turning the aid on makes the minimal amount of gain available; as the gain control is rotated to the halfway mark the increase in gain is fairly rapid. Amount of gain per degree of rotation decreases as the control is turned beyond the one-half to two-thirds mark. Unfortunately, hearing aids differ widely in their taper rates. Figure 4.1 illustrates the taper of the gain control of an aid whose maximum gain is 45 dB. It shows that when the gain control is adjusted to 25 percent of its maximum rotation, the amount of gain delivered is 22 dB or almost half of the available gain; at 50 percent rotation the amount of gain is 29 dB; at 75 percent rotation, 35 dB is provided. If the same aid were equipped with a gain control labeled 1 to 5 at equal intervals, it is clear that the numbers could not be used to estimate gain unless the exact taper rate of that aid was known. For example, a setting of 4 (approximately the 75 percent mark and 35 dB) would not represent twice as much gain as a setting of 2 (approximately the 25 percent mark and 22 dB).

Determination of the amount of gain needed by a listener should be made before a hearing aid is selected. Most people do best when the needed gain can be provided in the middle third of the gain control rotation. If the appropriate gain occurs in the first third, the aid may be too loud for comfort; if it occurs in the final third, the aid may not provide adequate gain. An aid should never be operated habitually at full-gain setting because of the likelihood of distortion when the amplifier is being driven to its capacity.

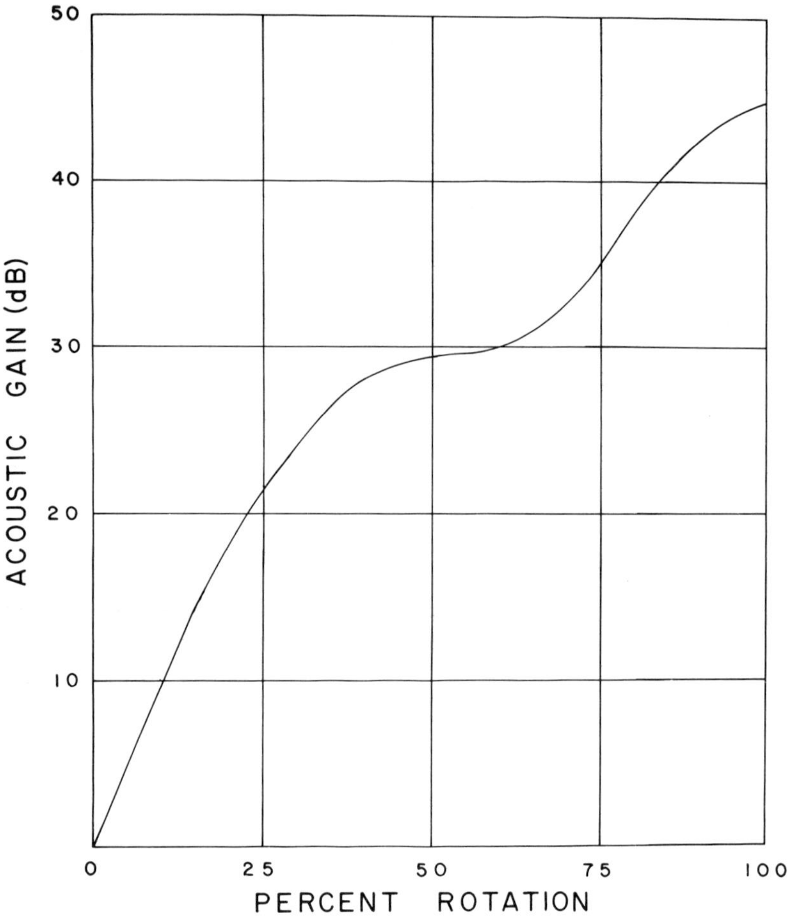

Figure 4.1. Gain control taper showing amount of gain as a function of percent rotation of gain control.

Saturation Sound Pressure Level (SSPL)—Maximum Power Output

Unless limited, the output of a hearing aid can be extremely loud if the input signal and the gain are both of high intensity. For example, if the input is a sound of 90 dB SPL (a loud shout), and the gain provided is 50 dB, the output could reach 140 dB SPL (the intensity level of a jet engine). It is necessary to avoid exposure to such intense sounds for two reasons: they may cause discomfort, especially to hearing-impaired listeners whose tolerance for loud sound is limited, and they may cause damage to residual hearing over time. Therefore, all hearing aids are equipped with output limiters. The highest output level delivered by a hearing aid is known as its *maximum power output* (MPO), which is operationally defined as a frequency response curve known as *$SSPL_{90}$* (saturation sound pressure level when the input signal is 90 dB) (ANSI 53.22, 1976). There are two basic ways of limiting the output of hearing aids: peak clipping and compression.

Peak Clipping. When an input signal becomes loud enough to exceed the SSPL of a hearing aid after it is amplified, the peaks of the waveform may be clipped symmetrically and prevented from being transmitted to the listener; only the middle portion of the sound wave is delivered at output. Figure 4.2 illustrates the effects of peak clipping on the output waveform. The gain of the hearing aid is not affected by peak clipping. The output is reduced, however, because only a portion of the input signal is transduced by the receiver. Input and gain are no longer additive because their combined value exceeds the allowable output of the aid. To illustrate, for an aid whose $SSPL_{90}$ is 132 dB and in which peak clipping is operating, input (90) + gain (50) = output (132). Peak clipping results in some distortion of the signal that may not be detrimental to normally hearing listeners but that may affect hearing-impaired listeners' perception of speech.

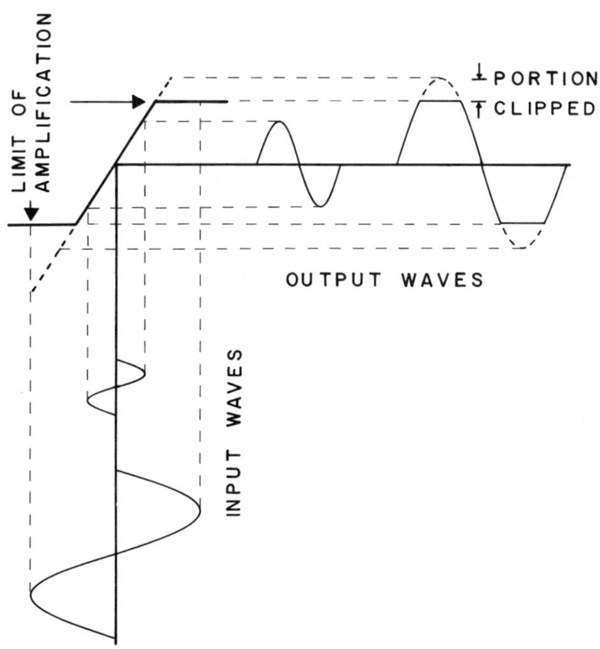

Figure 4.2. Diagram showing nonlinear distortion (peak clipping). The lower amplitude input signal is not distorted because it and the gain of the instrument are within the prescribed limits. The peaks of the higher amplitude input are clipped by the amount that combined gain and input amplitude exceed the limit. The clipped portion of the signal is shown as dashed lines.

Compression. Instead of eliminating the peaks of the amplified signal to limit output, compression amplification is designed to reduce the amount of gain applied to the input signal to achieve the same result. Usually referred to as automatic gain control (AGC) or automatic volume control (AVC), compression systems reduce the amount of gain the amplifier provides as input signals become more intense. The following example illustrates the principles involved. A hearing aid whose gain setting provides 50 dB of gain is exposed to a series of input signals ranging from 40 dB SPL to 90 dB SPL. If the $SSPL_{90}$ of that aid is 120 dB, the less intense signals will be subjected to 50 dB of gain as they are processed through the hearing aid. As the signal becomes more intense, however, the gain applied to it is reduced, limiting the output as it nears 120 dB SPL. The input-gain-output data might resemble the following:

Input	+	Gain	=	Output
40 dB	+	50 dB	=	90 dB SPL
50 dB	+	50 dB	=	100 dB SPL
60 dB	+	46 dB	=	106 dB SPL
70 dB	+	42 dB	=	112 dB SPL
80 dB	+	38 dB	=	118 dB SPL
90 dB	+	29 dB	=	119 dB SPL

Importance of SSPL in Hearing Aid Selection. The output of a hearing aid is an important consideration in its selection. If the SSPL exceeds the wearer's tolerance level, the aid will be uncomfortable and the person may not wear it regularly. Clients often turn down the gain of such aids in an effort to make their use more comfortable, but this is successful only if the aid is worn solely in quiet environments. Usually the hearing aid simply is not worn and the person complains that "sound is too loud." "the aid is noisy," "the aid makes me nervous," or "wearing it makes me tired." Whenever amplification is rejected by a client, the output of the aid should be measured and compared to the listener's tolerance levels for sound. If the output exceeds the listening level that is comfortable for the client, the audiologist should make recommendations concerning modifications of the hearing aid or replacing it with one that has a lower SSPL.

Frequency Response

The amount of gain provided by the hearing aid at different frequencies constitutes its frequency response. When approximately equal amplification for a broad band of frequencies occurs, the hearing aid is said to have a flat frequency response. When there is relatively more gain at high than at low frequencies, the aid is described as having a high-frequency emphasis (HFE). When the hearing aid frequency response includes frequencies below about 200 Hz or above 4000 Hz, the aid is said to have an extended low- or high-frequency response. The average hearing aid has a frequency response that extends from about 400 to 4500 Hz. Figure 4.3 shows a common hearing aid frequency response curve.

In comparison with amplification systems employed in broadcasting or stereo systems, hearing aids and auditory training units would be defined as low-fidelity systems. Not only do they employ greater amplification at some frequencies than at others, but the range of frequencies that are involved is restricted compared to high-fidelity recording and playback systems, many of which reproduce frequencies from 50 to 16,000 Hz.

Although some hearing-impaired individuals receive maximum benefit from amplification having a flat frequency response, the majority benefit most when they receive somewhat more amplification for high frequencies than for low frequencies. This results from both the nature of hearing impairment (the greatest hearing loss is usually in the high frequencies) and the importance of high-frequency information to speech perception. Many consonants are recognized on the basis of their high-frequency energy. This high-frequency acoustic energy, although essential for perception, is not very intense compared to the low-frequency energy associated with vowels, for example. If the hearing aid is to be maximally beneficial, it must make consonants more audible without interference from the more intense low-frequency components of speech. It is possible, for example, for amplified low frequencies associated with vowels to mask the high-frequency information associated with consonants. It is also common for relatively intense low-frequency sounds to trigger the output limiting device of an aid, causing peak clipping or reduced gain that prevents adequate amplification of high-frequency information. Finally, ambient environmental noise is usually composed of low-frequency energy; when it is amplified it is distracting and masks speech, interfering with speech perception. As a result of these factors, most hearing aids should have a smoothly rising frequency response curve.

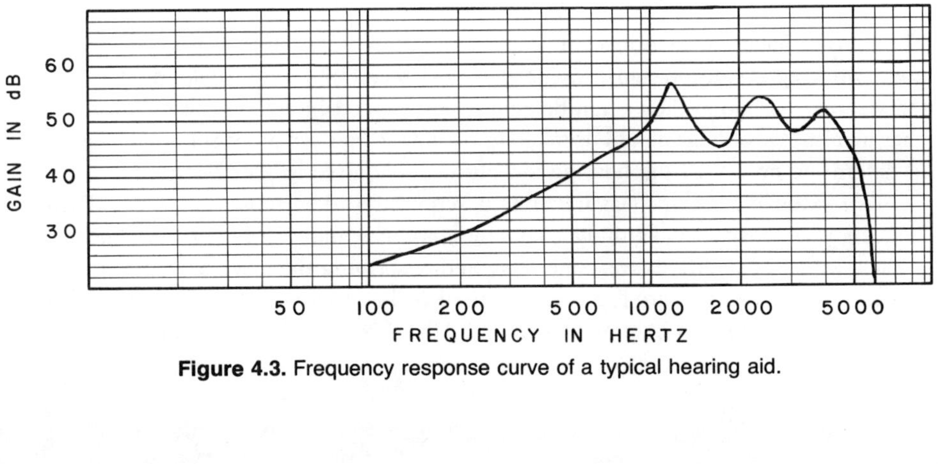

Figure 4.3. Frequency response curve of a typical hearing aid.

Distortion

Hearing aids are subject to several types of distortion that occurs when the input-output relationship of the system is not linear. The most common type of distortion is harmonic distortion; it is not likely to occur when each increase in input results in an equal increase in output. Because of the necessity to limit output, however, linear amplification over a broad intensity range is not possible. Nonlinearity of response occurs when the electronic system is forced to operate at or near its maximum limit. In a hearing aid the source of harmonic distortion may be the microphone, the amplifier, or the receiver, but the most common source is peak clipping of intense signals by the amplifier. Clipping changes the waveform; the clipped energy appears in the output signal as integral multiples of the fundamental frequency of the sound wave.

Harmonic distortion is less likely to occur in hearing aids whose output is controlled by compression rather than peak clipping. The extent to which harmonic distortion reduces the intelligibility of speech is unclear, but it is desirable to keep any source of distortion as low as possible to avoid adding to the listener's difficulties in perceiving speech. Generally, distortion should be kept below 10 percent.

Two other types of distortion are also associated with hearing aids: intermodulation distortion and transient distortion. Intermodulation distortion is related to harmonic distortion because it also results from amplifier nonlinearity. When two different sinusoid waveforms reach the microphone simultaneously, sum and difference tones will occur in addition to the harmonics. When harmonic distortion is present, intermodulation distortion is also probable.

Transient distortion occurs when there are resonant peaks in the frequency response curve. Impact or impulse noises trigger this type of distortion most easily, causing a "ringing" or an echo to occur. The ringing may persist, masking subsequent signals that reach the microphone. Besides being unpleasant to listen to, transient distortion may be detrimental to speech perception.

Measurement of Electroacoustic Characteristics

The performance of a hearing aid must be monitored carefully if it is to be kept in good working condition and provide the most beneficial amplification possible to the wearer. Although they often become sophisticated in behavioral monitoring of hearing aids, most hearing aid users do not have the equipment or training necessary to determine how well the hearing aid performs relative to its design.

An extensive set of measurements is required to determine how faithfully the frequency, intensity, and timing characteristics of sound are being reproduced by the hearing aid. Standards for measuring and describing the electroacoustic characteristics of hearing aids are regulated by the Food and Drug Administration (FDA); they are explained in a document known as the ANSI S3.22-1976 standard.

Several characteristics of hearing aids must be measured and reported by manufacturers, usually in a separate specification sheet for each model of hearing aid produced. Measurements are made using a special hearing aid test box that allows the response of the hearing aid to several input signals to be specified. Required measurements include the following:

1. The gain of a hearing aid is reported as an average of the amount of gain provided at the frequencies of 1000, 1600, and 2500 Hz when a 50 (for AGC aids) or 60 dB SPL input signal is presented. The gain control is set at full-on for this measure. Many of the other measures obtained are done at what is called the reference test position, a gain setting producing output 17 dB less than $SSPL_{90}$.
2. The $SSPL_{90}$ measurement is an output curve derived with the gain set full-on with 90 dB input into the aid. The average output at 1000, 1600, and 2500 Hz is calculated and referred to as the "high-frequency average" $SSPL_{90}$. The output curve will also yield the peak SPL and the frequency at which it occurs.
3. The frequency response of a hearing aid consists of a frequency by gain graph obtained for a wide frequency range (200–5000 Hz) under prescribed measurement conditions. An input level of 60 dB SPL is introduced to the aid with the gain in the reference test position.
4. Harmonic distortion is measured at 500, 800, and 1600 Hz with gain control and input levels varying depending on whether the aid incorporates peak clipping or some form of compression.

In addition to these basic measurements, ANSI S3.22-1976 requires that manufacturers report measures of automatic gain control characteristics, equivalent input noise level, induction coil gain, and battery current. Tolerance requirements for the parameters tested have been established to encourage quality control by manufacturers and to protect consumers.

The measurements described above should be made periodically by an audiologist as a part of a reevaluation of hearing or a rehabilitative program. If an aid does not meet the specifications established by its manufacturer, repairs are usually necessary. It is especially important to identify any problems that exist before the warranty expires so that expense to the user is minimized.

COMPONENTS OF HEARING AIDS

Hearing aids consist of the following main components: a microphone, an amplifier, a receiver, and a battery. In addition, all hearing aids contain one or more controls, including a gain (volume) control, on-off switch, tone control, telephone coil, and a control(s) for altering the amount of gain and output the hearing aid will produce.

Microphone

The microphone is a transducer; it converts energy from one form to another. In this case, the microphone converts acoustical to mechanical to electrical energy. The microphone contains a diaphragm that is sensitive to small changes in air pressure referred to as compressions and rarefactions. These compressions and rarefactions (acoustic energy) set the diaphragm into vibration (mechanical energy) and the small electric current thus generated (electrical energy) is conveyed to the amplifier. The most commonly used hearing aid transducer is the electret condenser microphone, which has broad and flat frequency response characteristics, is rugged and sensitive, is relatively immune to variations in humidity, and reduces the possibility of internal mechanical feedback that plagues many microphones.

The microphone is located within the plastic case of the hearing aid; its placement can be determined by a grilled opening in the case. This inlet may face toward the front, side, back, or top of the hearing aid, depending on its style.

Some hearing aids incorporate a modification known as a directional microphone, which produces a partial cancellation of acoustic energy at input. The purpose of the directional microphone is to reduce the effects of ambient noise on the reception of the desired signal. Such a hearing aid contains one microphone, but employs two sound inlets to the diaphragm. One of the inlets is in front of the diaphragm while the other is about one-half inch away on the other side of the diaphragm. Cancellation is accomplished by delaying sounds originating behind the hearing aid from reaching the diaphragm through the rear inlet by approximately the time it takes the same signal to travel forward, enter the front inlet, and reach the front side of the diaphragm. The two wave forms reach opposite sides of the diaphragm simultaneously (in phase), resulting in cancellation. Delaying the sound entering the rear inlet produces a reduction in the intensity of sounds originating behind the hearing aid through the frequency range of 200 to 2000 Hz (Olsen, 1977). Signals originating in front of the hearing aid are not canceled because they reach the diaphragm through the front inlet slightly before the same wave reaches the other side of the diaphragm through the rear inlet. Assuming that the hearing aid user is facing the preferred sound source, usually a speaker, any sound occurring behind the listener will be reduced in intensity and therefore less distracting. Research with this type of microphone reveals potential benefits when the aid is worn in a noisy environment (Nielsen, 1973; Lentz, 1972; Frank and Gooden, 1973). However, there is some indication that directional-microphone hearing aids are not preferred by all users (Causey, 1976), and that all directional-microphone hearing aids are not equally effective.

Amplifier

The weak electrical signal provided by the microphone is delivered to the amplifier. The function of the amplifier is to increase the voltage (amplitude of the signal) by an amount determined by the gain control setting and limited by the maximum power output of the hearing aid. The amplifier includes several amplification stages consisting of transistors and their associated circuitry arranged on a tiny printed circuit board. Each stage of amplification is capable of increasing the voltage by a fixed amount. If the hearing aid contains an automatic gain control (AGC), this circuit is also located in the amplifier. The amplifier cannot be seen by looking at the hearing aid, but it is represented on the case by the volume control dial.

Receiver

The electrical output of the amplifier travels by wire to the hearing aid receiver. The magnetic receiver performs the reverse function of the microphone: transducing electrical energy into mechanical energy, which generates acoustic energy. The receiver consists of a magnet and a metal diaphragm encased in a housing. As the current flow from the amplifier varies, the strength of the magnetic field does also, thereby increasing or decreasing attraction of the metal diaphragm. It is the to-and-fro movement of the diaphragm that recreates, with greater amplitude, the compressions and rarefactions of the input signal.

The output of the amplifier can be delivered to either an air conduction receiver or a bone conduction vibrator. Unless deformities of the pinna or ear canal make use of an earmold impossible or there is middle-ear pathology that precludes occluding the ear canal with an earmold, air conduction receivers are preferred. When these conditions exist, a bone conduction receiver may be substituted. Its function and placement are the same as for bone-conduction testing in audiometry. The bone-conduction vibrator is also a magnetic transducer, but is designed so that the case itself is set into vigorous vibration. This form of transduction is less efficient than that of the air-conduction receiver in that it requires a higher gain setting to reach threshold, sound quality is poor, and the effective frequency range is narrow. The bone-conduction receiver is recommended only as a last resort for those people who cannot use air-conduction receivers.

The receiver of a body type aid is a round ''button'' connected to the ear by a cord. The receiver of an ear-level hearing aid is contained within the case and cannot be seen.

Battery

Hearing aids are powered by small batteries that deliver voltage to the amplifier. The most commonly used batteries in modern hearing aids are either mercury cells that deliver 1.3 to 1.4 volts, or silver-oxide cells that deliver 1.4 to 1.5 volts. They are available in several sizes and shapes and are differentiated by model numbers. The manufacturer always specifies the battery number to be used in a given hearing aid as well as the type (mercury or silver-oxide). Hearing-aid batteries are manufactured by several companies, all of whom use the standardized numerical coding system. Therefore, batteries can be purchased on the basis of model number and type rather than by name of the manufacturer. They are sold in a variety of retail establishments and should be readily available at competitive prices. Inexpensive battery testers are also available for purposes of monitoring battery life. The life of a battery is estimated in hours and is dependent on the power of the hearing aid. Average battery life is approximately 200 hours, but powerful hearing aids consume more voltage per unit of time and therefore result in a shorter battery life. A few hearing aids allow a battery life of 600 hours. Because batteries are relatively expensive, battery life is taken into account during hearing aid selection procedures whenever possible.

Each hearing aid has a battery compartment designed to hold a specific battery size. A few aids employ rechargeable batteries that must be replaced less often than conventional batteries. Rechargeable batteries may last as long as a year, depending on the power of the hearing aid in which they are used.

Telecoil

Many modern hearing aids are equipped with a mechanism called a telecoil, by which direct input from a telephone receiver may be obtained. The telecoil is an induction coil consisting of tightly wound wire inside the hearing aid case. Current flow through the wire is induced when the hearing aid is placed in a magnetic field. This current flow is directed to the amplifier and processed in the same way as current flow from the microphone. The presence of a telecoil is indicated by a function switch located on the case of the hearing aid indicating microphone input only (M), telecoil input only (T), and, sometimes simultaneous microphone and telecoil input (M-T or B). When the switch is in the telecoil position the only signal amplified is that coming from the magnetic field of the telephone; if the switch is in the "both" setting the user will hear the amplified input to both microphone and telecoil. Use of the former setting may permit telephone reception in the presence of ambient acoustic noise, while the latter may be preferable in certain listening situations in a quiet environment.

The induction coils used in hearing aids are incompatible with newer telephone receivers. The new L-type magnetic telephone receiver does not develop a strong magnetic field. An adapter can be purchased to interface between the telephone receiver and the telecoil if the hearing-aid user must use the telecoil and this type of telephone. Many hearing-impaired people, however, report better telephone reception when the telephone receiver itself is equipped with a built-in amplifier.

Tone Control

Tone control adjustments are provided in some hearing aids to allow modifications in the frequency response characteristics of the hearing aid. The controls are usually labeled H (indicating high frequency), L (low frequency), and N (normal setting, usually a relatively flat frequency response), but sometimes numbers or the letters A, B, C, D are used.

Changes in tone control setting primarily alter the low-frequency response characteristics of the hearing aid. That is, a high-frequency emphasis setting usually means that amplification of low frequencies is reduced while high-frequency response remains unchanged. Low-frequency emphasis means that low-frequency tones are receiving more amplification relative to the high frequency emphasis setting. Some hearing aids contain a tone control accessible to the user, others have hidden or coded tone control adjustments that must be set by the dispenser, and still others have no provision for tone control adjustments of the amplifier.

On-Off Switch

Hearing aids usually have some provision for an on-off switch, but there is little uniformity relative to its type or location. It may be incorporated in the gain control, in the microphone-telephone switch, in the tone-setting switch, or as a part of the battery compartment door mechanism. If location is not obvious by inspection of the case, the owner's manual should be consulted to determine whether or not there is an on-off switch and where it is located. When the hearing aid is not in use the switch should be in the off position to conserve battery voltage.

The preceding discussion is designed to provide only a general orientation to the components of hearing aids and how they work. More detailed information about the working principles of hearing aid components may be found in Niemoller, Silverman, and Davis (1970), Bauer (1974), and Olsen (1977).

STYLES OF HEARING AIDS

Present-day hearing aids are available in four basic styles as shown in Figure 4.4. A fifth, experimental type of hearing aid prosthesis, the cochlear stimulator (Brackmann and House, 1976), must be implanted surgically and is not available to the public. Each style has distinct advantages and disadvantages that make it appropriate for certain types and degrees of hearing loss.

Body Hearing Aids

At one time all hearing aids were large units that were worn on the body; at present they account for no more than 4 percent of sales (Anonymous, 1978). Modern body-worn instruments are about half the size of a pack of cigarettes and small enough to be carried comfortably in a shirt pocket, in a special harness worn under or over clothing, or clipped to the clothing. The receiver, which is snapped into an earmold fitted to the ear, is connected to the body-worn unit by a thin cord. The case

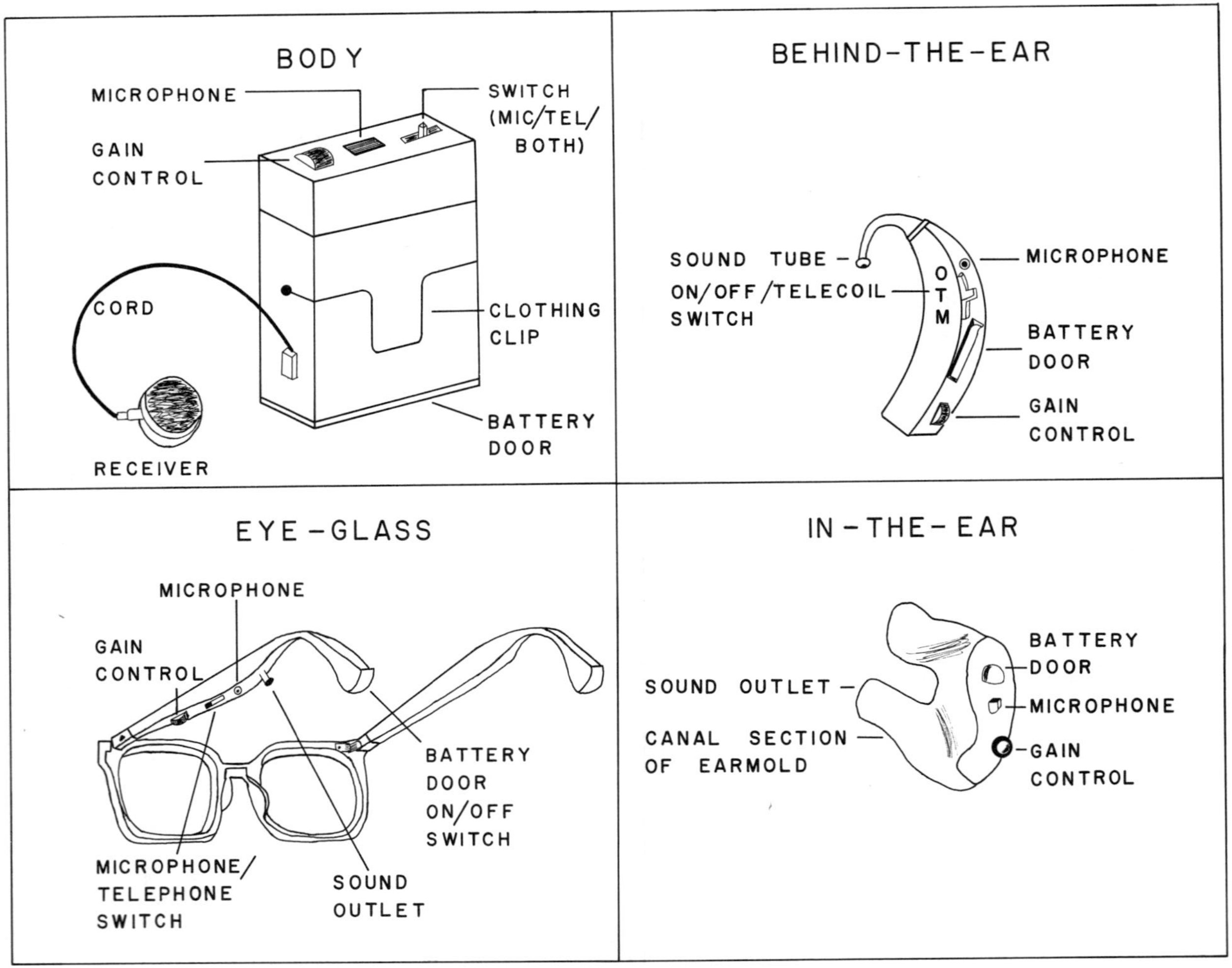

Figure 4.4. Four basic styles of modern hearing aids.

of the hearing aid contains the microphone, amplifier, battery, and controls (see Figure 4.4.).

Until the development of modern, miniaturized microphones, body aids provided higher gain and broader frequency responses than did the smaller, over-the-ear aids. They were required by people whose hearing losses were severe, regardless of age or preference. This is no longer true, but demand for the body-type of hearing aid remains because of the special needs of some severely hearing-impaired individuals, the multiply handicapped, very young children, and elderly people with poor hand-eye coordination, loss of finger sensitivity or impaired vision. Body aids have larger and more prominent operating controls and batteries that facilitate handling and encourage independent management. They also may be securely attached to the torso or clothing for protection from loss or damage. This type of aid also provides a mechanism for minimizing acoustic feedback because the distance from the microphone to the receiver is greater than for other types of aids, and it can be increased further by manipulating the placement of the aid on the body if necessary.

The fact that a body-worn aid can be placed under the clothing is an advantage when the wearer is a young child. This placement discourages removal of the aid or *ad hoc* adjustment of the controls. Generally speaking, the body aid is sturdier and more damage-resistant than smaller aids, making it a more ''childproof'' device. The disadvantages of this type of aid, however, outweigh advantages for most individuals. The noise produced by clothing contacting the microphone opening is often distracting and the aids lack cosmetic appeal. In addition, true binaural amplification is difficult to achieve even if two hearing aids are worn, because both microphones are located in approximately the same place, usually on the chest. Effects of head shadow and other factors that contribute to binaural processing of signals cannot be provided. Whenever possible other hearing aid styles should probably be used.

Behind-the-Ear Hearing Aids

The popularity of these head worn aids has steadily increased over the past 25 years until at present they represent more than 55 percent of the hearing aids sold (Anonymous, 1978). In the early years the amount of amplification that could be delivered by them was limited by the small amount of space available inside the case. With advances in microtechnology, including the development of microcircuitry and the incorporation of miniature electret microphones, over-the-ear hearing aids are now capable of delivering high gain across a wide range of frequencies. They can now be used by individuals with hearing impairments ranging from mild to severe.

All the essential components of the behind-the-ear aid are enclosed in a plastic case that rests on the top and back side of the pinna (see Figure 4.4). Amplified sound travels from the receiver through a plastic ear hook that passes over the top of the ear. Plastic tubing is connected to the ear hook and channels the sound into and through the earmold to the tympanic membrane.

This type of hearing aid, because it is worn at ear level, has several obvious advantages. Binaural arrangements for enhancing localization and improving speech intelligibility are possible, and noise produced by clothing and body movement are eliminated. Although the controls and batteries are smaller than body-worn instruments, they are readily managed by most people.

The major problem associated with the use of these head-worn instruments is acoustic feedback, the squeal that occurs when the sound amplified and delivered by the hearing aid receiver is picked up by the microphone. The distance between microphone and receiver is an important factor in the control of feedback, as is the seal at the ear provided by the earmold, a factor to be discussed later. Over-the-ear hearing aids are not large enough to allow much separation of microphone and receiver, so acoustic feedback is relatively common especially at higher gain setting. When the aid is worn within a confined space, such as that caused by wearing a hat, scarf, or coat with a high bulky collar, the probability of feedback increases.

Eyeglass-Type Over-the-Ear Hearing Aids

This style incorporates the electronic components of the over-the-ear hearing aid inside the plastic temple section of a pair of eyeglasses. Special hollowed-out bows are used that are wider and thicker than usual to accommodate the hearing aid components. When ear level hearing aids were first developed the eyeglass style was very popular; it now accounts for no more than 10 percent of sales, and a substantial proportion of these fittings are a special modification for unilateral hearing losses. In terms of electroacoustic characteristics and methods of ear coupling these hearing aids are similar to the self-contained over-the-ear hearing aids previously discussed.

The major advantages of this type of hearing aid are the same as those for the ear level aids. In addition, they can provide more variations in location of microphone placement. Some full-time users of eyeglasses prefer them because wearing two separate prosthetic devices is less comfortable, but clinical experience indicates that the number of people who prefer eyeglass aids is relatively small.

There are several serious disadvantages to the incorporation of a standard hearing aid into an eyeglass frame. Removal of the glasses means removal of the hearing aid. Although the hearing aid may be turned off while the glasses are in place, the earmold(s) will dangle from the glasses temple bar if removed from the ear(s). Perhaps the most important disadvantage of the glasses-type hearing aid is the difficulty involved in keeping the frames adjusted so that they fit comfortably and properly on the bridge of the nose. Anyone who has worn glasses knows how often they must be adjusted; the fact that the bows contain electronic circuitry complicates fitting and adjusting. As a result, there are more maintenance problems involved with this type of hearing aid than any other.

In general, the disadvantages of eyeglass-type hearing aid outweigh the advantages except under unusual circumstances. Most people who wear eyeglasses can wear a separate ear-level hearing aid comfortably. The full-time benefits of amplification can be realized best if the hearing aid is independent of the glasses.

All-in-the-Ear Hearing Aids

This type of aid is the smallest currently available. All components of the system are located in the concha and the external ear canal of the wearer. The microphone-amplifier-receiver module may be connected to or be an integral part of the earmold. The microphone is located on the outside surface of the concha portion of the case and faces in the same direction as the opening of the auditory canal (see Figure 4.4). This arrangement takes advantage of the sound-focusing characteristics of the pinna and more closely simulates the function of the normal ear in terms of the head shadow effect.

Until recently these hearing aids were useful only to people with mild hearing losses, because more amplifier space than was available was required to achieve moderate gain. Internal mechanical feedback also was a common problem. Recent developments in microcircuitry and the application of the electret microphone have made it possible to produce higher-gain instruments with a reduction in the incidence of the internal form of feedback. As a result of these improvements, the popularity of all-in-the-ear aids is increasing rapidly (Griffing and Dahlberg, 1978). At present about 30 percent of hearing aid sales involve the all-in-the-ear aid.

The major advantages to this type of aid are the cosmetic aspects of its size and the location of its components when worn. Its major disadvantages are the somewhat limited gain available, the size of its controls, and the restrictions imposed by the semipermanent attachment of the hearing aid to the earmold. Obtaining and keeping a well-fitting earmold may be more difficult, especially for growing children. Setting the controls may be too difficult for some physically handicapped and elderly individuals. At present, these aids provide too little usable gain for people with severe or profound hearing losses.

Implantable Hearing Aids

The notion of restoring or improving hearing by implanting a device within the ear has intrigued researchers for decades. In recent years, two types of implantable devices have been developed and used on a limited, experimental basis. One type consists of placing a circuit in the middle ear or in a hollowed-out portion of the mastoid cavity (Vernon, Mahoney, and Schleuning, 1976). The output of the unit activates the stapes directly and the amplified sound proceeds through the usual auditory mechanism. The second type provides direct electrical stimulation to the VIIIth cranial nerve by implanting electrodes within the cochlea in close approximation to nerve fibers. The electrodes are connected through the round window to a miniature radio receiver button embedded in the skull behind the pinna. This button receives signals from a small antenna on the outside of the skin. The electrical energy delivered to the electrodes in the cochlea stimulates an electrical response in the nerve fiber. Normal nerve fibers are required for this transmission, even though there may be a profound sensory (cochlear) hearing loss. Implantations of this type have been done on humans who exhibited little or no functional residual hearing providing that evidence of a normal nerve could be demonstrated (Simmons, Mongeon, Lewis, and Huntington, 1964; Simmons, 1966; Michelson, 1971a; Michelson, 1971b; House and Urban, 1973). Studies of experimental patients indicate that some form of neural stimulation takes place but does not appear to be particularly useful in the reception of speech, probably because these early experiments involved single channel electrodes. As multichannel devices are perfected, it is possible that implanted hearing aids will become common. Much more research will be necessary to determine, among other things, whether or not the implant will cause damage or degeneration of the VIIIth cranial nerve.

EARMOLDS

An important determiner of successful hearing aid use is the earmold, a small plastic device that couples the hearing aid to the ear. Best results are obtained when a custom-fitted earmold is constructed from an impression made of the ear in which the hearing aid is worn. Earmold impressions are usually sent to a laboratory that specializes in making them, and they can be ordered in different colors, materials, and types. In addition, certain modifications in earmold construction can be made that will alter the nature of the sound delivered from the hearing aid to the ear.

Purposes of the Earmold

There are four primary purposes of the custom-fitted earmold.

1. To direct sound to the ear canal. Because the purpose of a hearing aid is to make sound louder and available to the listener for processing, it is important that the output of the aid be delivered to the ear as efficiently as possible. Unless the hearing aid receiver is coupled tightly to the ear, much of the amplified sound is dissipated before it reaches the hearing mechanism. A tightly fitting earmold reduces the amount of gain necessary to reach the listener's threshold, allowing effective use of amplification by persons with even severe and profound hearing losses.

2. To minimize the occurrence of acoustic feedback. This term refers to the squeal produced when the output of a hearing aid is picked up by the microphone. It occurs most often as a result of a poorly fitting earmold that allows amplified sound to leak from the ear and enter the microphone. Unless the earmold fits snugly, the gain of the hearing aid must be reduced to prevent feedback from occurring. This limits the usable gain of the aid. Furthermore, acoustic feedback can be distracting or painful to the hearing aid wearer and irritating to others in the environment.

The probability of feedback is related to the type of earmold worn and its condition. The type of earmold to be worn should be chosen carefully based on the individual hearing aid user's hearing loss and amplification needs. They must be replaced periodically if feedback is to be controlled adequately. Children often require frequent earmold fittings as the size of their ears increase.

3. To support the air-conduction receiver of a body-worn aid or to anchor the case of an ear-level aid to the head and to prevent damage to the hearing aid it is necessary to anchor it firmly to the ear; otherwise it may fall off. A well-fitted earmold provides a firm support for the aid or receiver button and minimizes unnecessary or irritating movement.

4. To maximize comfort. Unless the earmold fits properly, irritation of the ear canal may occur, making use of the hearing aid painful. A carefully fitted earmold will eliminate chafing and the necessity to adjust its position frequently, factors that determine comfort and ease of adjustment to the use of amplification.

Types of Earmolds

There are many types of earmolds in common use, but attempts to standardize earmold terminology have only recently been made. Nineteen earmold laboratories in the United States have formed the National Association of Earmold Laboratories (NAEL) in an attempt to reduce the proliferation of trade names used for various common earmold types (Nelson, 1978). The NAEL has identified the following standard types of earmolds: receiver, shell, half-shell, all-in-the-ear, skeleton, three-quarter skeleton, semiskeleton, canal, and canal lock (NAEL, 1970). Figure 4.5 shows these nine earmold types.

The major differences among earmold types fall into two categories: the length of the portion of the earmold that fits into the wearer's ear canal and the amount and shape of the body of the earmold that fits in the concha of the external ear. For example, the receiver-type mold usually has a relatively long canal portion and a large body. The long canal allows maximum delivery of low frequencies and the large body provides more support for the hearing aid receiver. The canal mold uses a relatively long canal, but no body at all.

A tenth type is the open or non-occluding mold, which differs from all the others in that the ear canal is not occluded, permitting normal entry of sound energy into the canal while providing delivery of amplified sound at the same time through tubing held in place by an extension of the earmold into the concha (the frame). It is

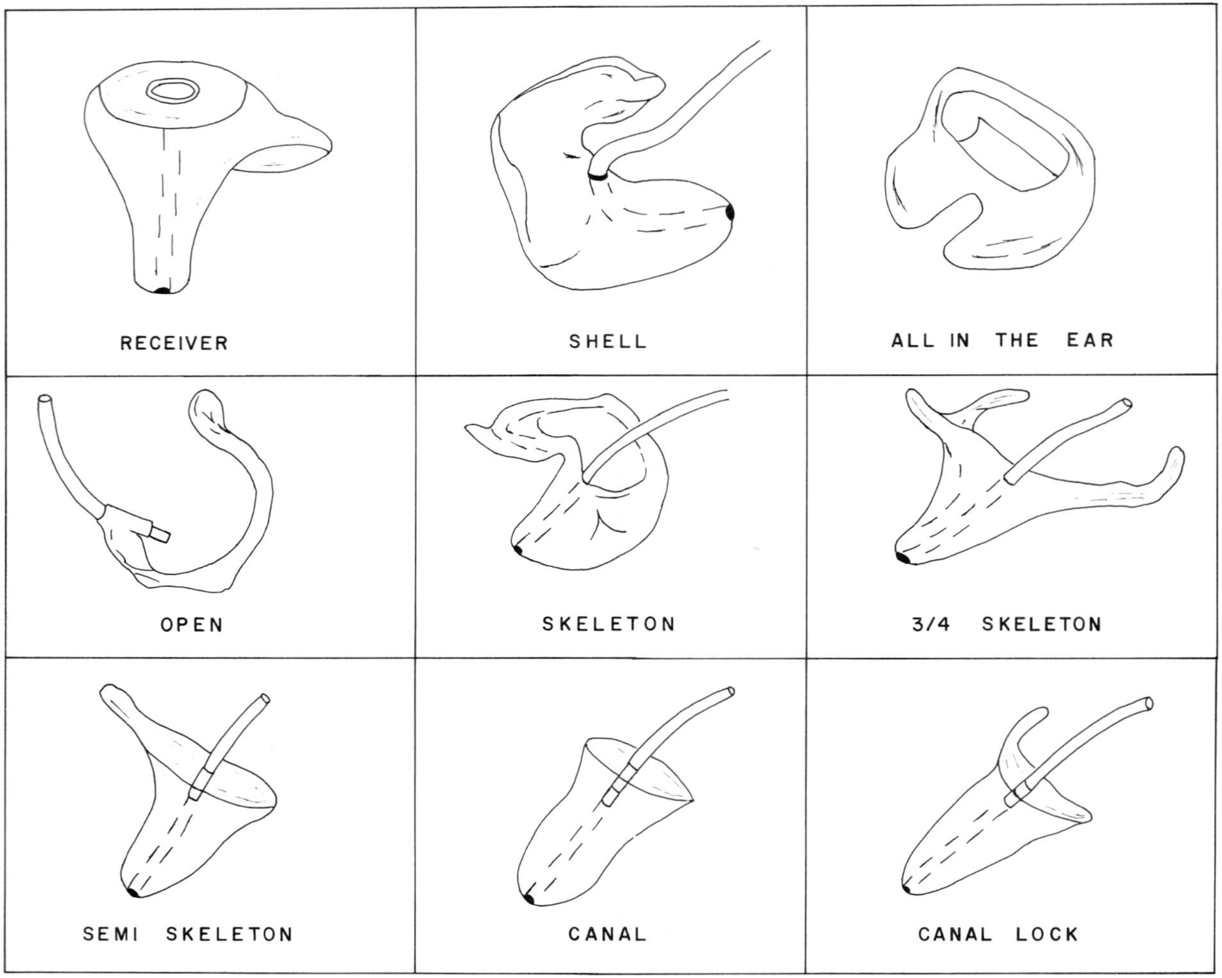

Figure 4.5. Basic earmold types. Skeleton, three-quarter skeleton, semiskeleton, canal, canal-lock, shell, half-shell, receiver, and all-in-the-ear molds are NAEL standard types. The half-shell is not pictured because its variation from the shell is slight. The open earmold has been added because of its increasingly frequent use since the NAEL standard was developed.

used when little amplification is desired and the probability of acoustic feedback is minimal.

The receiver mold is designed for use with a body-worn hearing aid. The receiver of the aid is snapped into a ring built into the earmold; the cord of the aid attaches the receiver to the body of the hearing aid. The all-in-the-ear mold is designed to hold an all-in-the-ear hearing aid and is usually attached semipermanently to it. The aid and mold fit snugly into the concha and ear canal. All the other earmold types are designed for use with ear-level hearing aids. They come with plastic tubing (as shown in Figure 4.5), which must be cut to fit the distance between the earmold and the sound tube of the hearing aid (also called an earhook) to which the plastic tubing must be attached. Tubing comes in several diameters, the dimensions of which affect the relative strength of the high frequencies that will be delivered to the ear.

Modifications of Earmolds

Hearing-impaired individuals may require minor modifications of the characteristics of a given hearing aid in order to use it most comfortably and effectively. Desired changes can often be accomplished by modifications of the earmold. For example, people who require less low-frequency energy than provided by a given hearing aid may benefit from use of a *vented* earmold, in which a small hole is drilled through the earmold. The size of the vent is one variable that determines the effect on the acoustical properties of the signal. A very small hole may not alter the signal, but it may provide relief from a sense of fullness in the ear reported by many users. Increasing the size of the vent will reduce low-frequency energy and shift the resonant peaks of the frequency response. The length of the vent and whether it intersects the sound channel also influence response (Hawkins, 1979).

Other ways of producing minor changes in frequency response include changing the diameter or length of the tubing, shortening or lengthening the canal portion of the earmold, or changing the internal cavity of a receiver-type mold. In addition to changing frequency response characteristics, these modifications also may have noticeable effects on speech intelligibility, quality judgments, listener preference, and comfort. Earmolds are an integral part of the amplification system and must be chosen and evaluated carefully. A more extensive discussion of earmold acoustics may be found in Studebaker and Zachman (1970), Lybarger (1972), Langford (1975), and Smith (1977).

USE OF HEARING AIDS

Successful use of a hearing aid depends on many factors that vary among individuals. There are three major factors, however, that appear to be important to all hearing-aid users. Consideration of these should always be included in the program of habilitation that is planned for individuals or groups of hearing-impaired clients.

Personal Adjustment

No matter how carefully a hearing aid is selected, its usefulness to the wearer will be limited unless there are reasonable expectations for its use and it is accepted for what it can provide. There are many reasons why hearing aids are rejected. Some of these pertain to the adequacy of the instrument, the purposes for which it is worn, and the attitudes toward hearing impairment held by the hearing-impaired person or other family members. These attitudes are discussed in subsequent chapters. Many hearing aids are rejected, however, because of unrealistic expectations concerning what the hearing aid can and cannot do to improve the reception of speech. A society that is accustomed to the use of eyeglasses that restore visual acuity to normal or near-normal levels is unlikely to expect less of a hearing aid. Unfortunately, hearing aids rarely equal eyeglasses in the degree to which they restore sensory function.

A hearing aid makes sound more intense. It may or may not make it clearer to the listener. Not only does an aid make the wanted signal (speech) more intense, it also amplifies unwanted ambient noise. If a hearing-impaired listener is not accustomed to hearing many sounds in the environment, their amplification often results in surprised irritation. The ability to attend to wanted sound in the presence of unwanted sound is reduced, and the degree to which unwanted sound exists almost everywhere usually has been forgotten. As a result, a period of adjustment to amplified sound is necessary for all but a handful of hearing-impaired listeners.

When assisting clients in adjusting to a hearing aid, it is important to stress the factors discussed below.

Fatigue. Many hearing-impaired individuals may have reduced tolerance thresholds for loud sounds, a condition that is known as recruitment and is associated with hearing loss of cochlear origin. Listening to amplified sound is tiring for these people, even when the hearing aid has been carefully selected so that its SSPL is lower than the individuals' tolerance level. These clients should be encouraged to wear the hearing aid for short periods of time at first, removing it when they become fatigued or nervous. The aid should be worn first in a quiet environment, so that unwanted sound is kept to a minimum. As tolerance for amplified sound is increased, the aid should be worn for longer periods of time and in more and varied environments.

The goal of this part of the adjustment program is to develop the ability to wear the aid regularly, preferably all day, with a minimum of gain control adjustments. Inexperienced hearing-aid users may adjust the gain setting of the aid frequently in an effort to avoid many sounds. If the aid has been carefully selected regarding its gain taper and SSPL, the client should be encouraged to find the most beneficial setting that will lead to casual, habitual use. This may take some time; it is important to respect the nervousness and fatigue that may result from initial hearing aid use; periods of rest and experimentation will usually result in eventual adjustment.

Situational Difficulty. Hearing-impaired people express remarkably similar descriptions of the situations in which listening is most difficult for them. These include listening from a distance, in the presence of noise of any kind, and when trying to converse with more than one or two other people. It is not necessary to remind them of these situations except with regard to hearing aid use. Clients seek out hearing aids because they have trouble communicating in these, and possibly other, situations. It is natural for them to assume that a hearing aid, designed to improve communication, will be beneficial to them when they need help the most. Otherwise why bother with one?

Although a hearing aid may eventually be quite helpful under adverse listening conditions, it may not be readily apparent in the beginning. Clients should be encouraged to use amplification under easy conditions first, gradually using it under more difficult ones. The worst thing a person can do is purchase a hearing aid, put it on, and wear it to a cocktail party or other noisy event. It is bound to be a disappointment at best and a catastrophe at worst. It is important to point out that the listening situations that are most difficult *without* a hearing aid are likely to be the most difficult *with* a hearing aid.

Steps in Hearing Aid Use. To minimize disappointment and fatigue, it may be helpful to suggest a sequence of situations for the user to move through relative to hearing aid use. The following list is an example of such a sequence; the time spent listening under each condition will vary according to individual needs and tolerance.

Condition 1: Listening in quiet
Situations: Quiet room at home
Quiet lawn or porch at home
Activities: Reading aloud (to become accustomed to the sound of one's own voice)
Conversing with one other person
Listening to a radio, TV, or music
Identifying outside sounds

Condition 2: Listening in controlled noise
Situations: A room at home, in which a noise source can be introduced at will. Examples: vacuum cleaner, radio, TV, refrigerator, fan
Activities: Conversing with one other person
Listening to a radio or TV

Condition 3: Listening under common noise conditions
Situations: Outside in traffic
Riding in a car
In small groups
In a theater or church
Activities: Conversing with individuals and small groups
Listening to a lecture or sermon
Listening to music
Identifying sound sources
Practicing changing position to enhance hearing

Condition 4: Listening under adverse noise conditions
Situations: Crowded rooms
Large meetings
Restaurants
In large conversational groups
Activities: Conversing with one or several people
Following an ongoing conversation

Monitoring and Troubleshooting Hearing Aids

A hearing aid is a delicate electronic instrument that is susceptible to unwanted changes in its sound-handling characteristics. Obvious malfunctions such as intermittent operation, a failure to amplify signals, or the presence of annoying internal noise are easily identified, but many subtle changes may occur without being recognized. It is essential for audiologists and clients to establish a monitoring schedule that includes daily listening checks by the client and periodic electroacoustic evaluation by the audiologist.

Daily monitoring is most important for hearing aids worn by young children. Children rarely report changes in hearing aid function unless they are gross, but their aids are more likely to develop problems because of the types of activities pursued by children. Investigations of the status of children's hearing aids by several investigators (Gaeth and Lounsbury, 1966; Zink, 1972; Porter, 1973; and Schell, 1976) have shown that approximately 50 percent of the hearing aids worn by children in educational settings are malfunctioning at any given time. Furthermore, many hearing aids that have been recently repaired fail to meet their original specifications (Zink, 1972; Warren and Kasten, 1976). If children are to receive the intended benefit from amplification, their hearing aids must be monitored daily by behavioral listening checks and periodically by electroacoustic analysis.

In the case of young children daily monitoring may be accomplished by parents, teachers, speech-language pathologists, or anyone else who comes in daily contact with the child. The presence of an audiologist in the school system can contribute greatly to the use of amplification within that setting. The audiologist will be responsible for electroacoustic analysis of hearing aids and for training other school personnel in their care and maintenance.

Daily Hearing Aid Check Procedures. The most common symptoms of hearing aid malfunction are no amplification, weak amplification, feedback, intermittent performance, scratchy sound, or fuzzy-distorted sound. These symptoms may have several different causes, which can be determined from systematic inspection and careful listening. Some malfunctions can be readily corrected while others require laboratory repair services. The following procedures should be completed daily by the hearing-aid user, parent, teacher, or clinician.

1. Make a careful visual inspection of the hearing aid and earmold.
   - **(a)** Are the switches in appropriate position for operation? This includes the on-off switch, the gain-control wheel, the tone-control switch (if available) and the microphone-telephone switch.
   - **(b)** Are the battery contacts clean and do they make contact with the battery? Is the battery inserted properly? Does the battery compartment door fit properly and securely? Does the battery have sufficient voltage to operate the instrument? (This requires use of battery tester or insertion of a battery of known voltage.)
   - **(c)** Is the earmold damaged? Is the channel through the earmold free of cerumen (ear wax) or foreign material? Are there any obvious cracks or holes in the tubing connecting the ear-level aid with the earmold? Is the ear hook snugly connected to the receiver outlet and is it structurally sound? If the aid is a body-type hearing aid, is the air conduction receiver-earmold coupling secure and tight?
   - **(d)** Are cord connections secure in body-type hearing aids? Is the insulation material on the cord intact? Is the air-conduction receiver cracked? Does the receiver rattle when lightly shaken?

2. Listen to the hearing aid. The following procedures can be accomplished by using an appropriately fitting earmold for body-type hearing aids or a hearing-aid stethoscope for head-worn units.
   - **(a)** Turn the hearing aid on and listen carefully as the gain control is rotated. Are there noticeable jumps in loudness? Is there a static-like noise while the wheel is rotated? Does the gain control wheel turn easily but not too loosely?
   - **(b)** Set the gain control at use level and listen to determine if speech sounds fuzzy or distorted. Listen for gross distortion of sounds including short duration (impulse) sounds. Gently shake the hearing aid to determine if movement produces noticeable variations in performance. Hold the hearing aid in different positions, upside down

or on its side, to determine if position has an effect on sound reproduction. Manipulate the switches on the hearing aid to determine if they are performing their function.

(c) Shake the cord (body-type aid) and gently manipulate it to see if this produces intermittent performance or static noise.

(d) If acoustic feedback is present its source may be determined by removing the hearing aid from the ear, turning the gain control full-on, and occluding the earmold channel with a finger. If the feedback ceases, the cause is a poorly fitting earmold. If it persists the cause is somewhere else in the system. If the earmold tubing is removed from the ear hook or sound outlet and the feedback ceases when the sound outlet aperture is occluded, then the leak is in the tubing or its connection to the hearing aid or to the earmold. With a body-type aid a frequent source of leak is the coupling between the receiver and the earmold. If feedback persists through these tests it is likely that the feedback is occurring internally, perhaps as a result of deterioration or damage to the acoustical isolation of the microphone or receiver.

(e) When the hearing aid is in place in the user's ear feedback should not be present, except at unusually high gain settings. The user should be able to wear the hearing aid at the preferred gain setting without presence of feedback while listening, chewing, yawning, or moving the head. If feedback does occur under these conditions, the most likely cause is the earmold, which may be too small or have vents that are too large. By gently applying pressure to the earmold while it is in the ear or by occluding the vent, the cause can be determined. If feedback ceases under these conditions, earmold modification or replacement is desirable. No hearing aid user should be required to use a gain setting based primarily on the threshold of feedback.

If the inspection and listening tests described above reveal malfunctions, the owner of the hearing aid should seek repair. Some of the causes of hearing aid malfunction may be remedied by the audiologist or the hearing aid dispenser with minimal delay and cost. Other problems require attention at an appropriately equipped repair facility. Whenever possible, a replacement hearing aid should be made available to the user while repairs are underway.

Environmental Acoustics

The successful use of a hearing aid often depends on the environment in which it is worn. The modern world is a noisy place. As technology increases the noise levels associated with daily life also rise. All forms of transportation, electrical appliances, motorized farm equipment, and many recreational pursuits have significant levels of noise associated with their use. The fact that we live in close association with large numbers of neighbors at home, work, play, and school makes it virtually impossible to avoid unwanted noise. These high levels of ambient noise have pronounced effects on communication for people who have hearing loss and, particularly, for those wearing hearing aids. Hearing-impaired individuals frequently complain of an inability to understand speech in moderate levels of background noise, such as that produced by traffic, electrical appliances, music, or competing speech. The complaint is common from individuals with mild-to-moderate hearing impairments and from hearing-aid wearers, no matter how severe the loss. Hearing aids and auditory-training units amplify sound, whether it is unwanted noise or speech, and the reduced redundancy resulting from poor signal-to-noise (S/N) ratios (see next section) combined with a deficient auditory system poses serious problems in speech perception. Important information-bearing speech elements, such as fricative consonants, are masked by noise, making auditory perception of them even more difficult than in quiet. As a result, environments that are acoustically suitable for normally hearing people may be unsuitable for acceptable communication by the hearing impaired.

Signal-to-Noise Ratio. Acoustic conditions are usually described in terms of the signal-to-noise ratio (S/N), a term that refers to the difference between the decibel level of a primary signal (for our purposes, speech) and the background noise in which it occurs. A positive S/N ratio (+10 dB, for example) indicates that the signal is 10 dB more intense than the noise. A negative S/N ratio (−5 dB) indicates that the noise is 5 dB more intense than the signal. The higher the positive number, the more favorable the listening environment. Since the level of normal conversational speech is approximately 60 to 70 dB SPL at a distance of 1 meter, the environmental noise level must remain below that intensity if the S/N ratio is to be positive. Maintaining a low environmental noise level is especially important for the hearing aid user because the input level of the primary signal at the hearing aid microphone is often less than 60 to 70 dB SPL. This occurs because the distance between the speaker's mouth and the microphone frequently is greater than 1 meter, with a consequent reduction in the intensity of the sound as it travels from speaker to listener. If distance between the speaker's mouth and the microphone of the hearing aid or auditory training unit varies as it does between normally hearing people involved in communication, it is essential that the environmental noise level be kept as low as possible to minimize its interference with the speech signal.

Although normally hearing individuals may be able to carry on satisfactory conversations at signal-to-noise ratios at or close to zero (Webster, 1969) the same is not true of the hearing impaired. A signal-to-noise ratio of at least +15 and preferably +20 dB or more is necessary for hearing-impaired listeners (Gengel, 1971; Gengel and Foust, 1975). If the signal-to-noise ratio is +10 dB or less, hearing-impaired listeners may prefer not to use amplification and to rely on visual cues instead (Gengel, 1971). Tillman, Carhart, and Olsen (1970) reported severe disruption of speech intelligibility for hearing-impaired individuals listening in noise through a hearing aid even at a signal-to-noise ratio of +18. Unfortunately, the S/N ratios in most public buildings do not approximate those necessary for easy communication by hearing-impaired listeners. Although all hearing-impaired individuals require more positive signal-to-noise ratios for acceptable communication than normally hearing individuals, the situation is most critical for children who are learning to use their hearing for the acquisition of language and speech, and for elderly people whose auditory performance breaks down quite easily under difficult listening conditions.

Environmental Noise Sources and Levels. Measures of noise levels from various sources and in various locations where communication occurs have been reported. Table 4.2 shows the levels reported by several investigators. These data indicate that hearing-impaired school children and adults often must communicate in environments that are unacceptable for efficient communication even by normally hearing individuals.

Recommendations have been made by Kryter (1970) regarding the maximum allowable noise levels for various locations as shown in Table. 4.3. Kryter's suggestions are based on noise levels that allow easy communication by normally hearing people without annoyance. They would enhance communication by hearing-impaired people even more.

Table 4.2 Measures of Noise Levels Reported for a Variety of Locations and Sources [decibel levels reported in terms of sound-level meter-weighting scales employed (A, B, or C)]*

Location or Source	*Noise Level*	*Investigator*
Empty classroom	55 dB B	Sanders, 1965
Occupied classroom	59–69 dB B	Sanders, 1965
Occupied classroom	63 dB C	Paul, 1967
Hotel meeting room	58 dB A	Beranek, 1956
Executive office	47 dB A	Beranek, 1956
Home		
Garbage disposal	74–81 dB A	Kryter, 1970
Washing machine	57–65 dB A	Kryter, 1970
Vacuum cleaner	74–79 dB A	Kryter, 1970
Lawnmower	66 dB A	Kryter, 1970
Traffic		
Diesel truck	77 dB A	Kryter, 1970
Freight train	93 dB A	Kryter, 1970
Subway	82–95 dB A	Kryter, 1970

*See definition of sound-level-meter in the glossary for explanation of A, B, C scales.

Table 4.3 Noise Levels Proposed by Kryter (1970) for Acceptable Communication by Normally Hearing People

Location	*Proposed Maximum Ambient Noise Level*
School rooms	35 dB A
Meeting rooms without amplification	45 dB A
Apartments and hotels	38 dB A
Homes	40 dB A
Offices	35–50 dB A
Concert halls	28 dB A

Reverberation. Another source of interference with speech perception is room reverberation. Reverberation occurs when sound waves are reflected from surfaces instead of being absorbed by them. It is worst in rooms that have many hard, flat surfaces such as tiled floors, windows, blackboards, and nonporous walls. When a person speaks in such a room, the sound waves travel in several directions until they strike a surface, are reflected, travel in another direction and strike another surface. At any given time in a reverberant room the sound waves present consist of direct waves from the source and many reflected waves. If room surfaces are highly reflective the intensity level of the propagated signal will change very slowly and thus may remain audible in the environment for a period of time following cessation of the signal at the sound source. In a nonreverberant environment, such as an anechoic chamber (without echo), sound energy will drop to zero as soon as the last wave produced has passed the point of observation. Any audible energy present after that time is due to reverberation caused by sound waves encountering a reflective surface.

While some amount of reverberation is desirable to produce pleasing sound quality and "liveliness" in a room, it is undesirable if it exceeds a certain amount. Reverberation is measured by determining the length of time, in seconds, for the sound power to decrease to one-millionth (60 dB) of its initial value after the source has stopped (Beranek, 1949). For example, if it takes one and a half seconds following cessation for a 100-dB SPL signal to decrease 60 dB from its original intensity level, the reverberation time is recorded as 1.5. The shorter the reverberation time, the better the listening environment and the less interference with speech signals.

Reverberation and Speech Perception. Reverberation reduces the intelligibility of speech by a masking phenomenon. If the reverberation time of a room is 1.5 seconds some portion of the energy associated with an acoustic event may remain audible for 1.5 seconds after termination. Some syllables of speech will be masked by preceding syllables that are being reflected around the room at suprathreshold intensity levels. Perception of consonants is most likely to suffer under these conditions because they are of lower intensity than vowels and contain higher frequency components. Reverberation of the low-frequency vowel components will mask high-frequency, low-intensity consonant sounds. The situation is made worse by the fact that the sound absorption characteristics of a typical room have a more pronounced effect on high frequencies than on low ones. The combination of absorption of high frequencies and reflection of low frequencies reduces the intelligibility of sounds in a reverberant room.

For normally hearing people, the optimal room reverberation time is between 0.75 and 1.0 seconds (Knudsen and Harris, 1950; Moncur and Dirks, 1967). Shorter reverberation times are necessary, however, if hearing-impaired listeners are to communicate effectively. Discrimination scores for hearing-impaired listeners may decrease from 97 percent at a reverberation time of 0.0 second to 80 percent at the "good" reverberation time of 0.9 second and 67 percent at 1.6 seconds in a quiet room (Moncur and Dirks, 1967). When noise *and* reverberation are present, scores for hearing-impaired listeners are dramatically lower (from 67 percent at 0.0 to 30 percent at 1.6 seconds). Unfortunately, a reverberation time of 1.6 is not uncommon in schoolrooms (Thomas, 1960; Tolk, 1961), while the optimal reverberation time for hearing-impaired listeners is below 0.5 second (John, 1960; Niemoller, 1968).

When the listener is using a hearing aid, long reverberation times are even more detrimental to speech perception. The interaction of noise, reverberation, and monaural hearing aid use may result in dramatic reductions in speech discrimination according to Finitzo-Hieber and Tillman (1978). Their findings for hearing-impaired children wearing monaural hearing aids are summarized in Table 4.4. These data show the decreases in discrimination scores that occurred as S/N ratio and reverberation time were made poorer. Optimal performance was achieved by a combination of reduced reverberation time and lowered level of background noise.

Table 4.4 Decreases in Percentage Discrimination by Noise Alone, Reverberation Alone, and by Combination of These Two Variables for Hearing-Impaired Children

	Reverberation Time in Seconds		
S/N Ratio in dB	*0.0*	*0.4*	*1.2*
+12	13.0	22.8	41.8
+ 6	23.5	30.8	56.0
0	44.0	55.2	71.8

From Finitzo-Hieber and Tillman, 1978.

Discrimination scores for these children averaged 87.5 percent in a quiet, sound absorptive room but fell to 15.7 percent when the S/N ratio was 0 and reverberation time exceeded 1.0 seconds. Finitzo-Hieber and Tillman suggested that a S/N ratio of +6 dB would be minimally favorable for normally hearing children in a room whose reverberation rate was 0.4 second, but a S/N ratio of at least +12 dB would be necessary for hearing-impaired children in the same room.

Control of Room Acoustics. There are several ways in which rooms may be made more favorable listening environments. The most effective approach would be to design and build them with proper acoustical treatment in the form of absorbent materials and optimal dimensions. Once a room is in use, however, there are less effective modifications that can be employed that will still improve the listening environment. To achieve this, the following steps should be taken.

1. Measures of the noise level and reverberation time should be obtained when possible.
2. Sources of noise should be identified. These often include traffic outside the room and activities within the room, such as noises generated by furniture movement, papers rattling, people talking, appliances, and pencil sharpeners.
3. Whenever possible, the noise sources should be minimized by rerouting traffic, changing location of the room to be used by hearing-impaired listeners, and eliminating noise sources as follows.
   (a) Equip furniture with rubber coasters.
   (b) Remove aquariums or other small appliances to another area.
   (c) Install carpeting on floors and/or walls. If the entire floor cannot be carpeted, use throw rugs or carpet squares at intervals.
   (d) Install acoustic tile in ceilings or on walls.
   (e) Hang drapery material along flat surfaces, such as large walls.
   (f) Modify heating and cooling systems to reduce vibration and motor noise.
   (g) Close doors and windows to minimize noise from outside the room. If necessary, improve the seal on these openings by installing weather strips or using carpet in doorways.
4. Consider the use of special auditory equipment to improve the S/N ratio at the listener's ear. Appropriate equipment is discussed in the following section.

AUDITORY TRAINING SYSTEMS

There are times when the use of special amplification equipment is preferable to the use of a personal hearing aid. These occur primarily under three conditions: when use of amplification is temporary, when special provisions must be made to include vibrotactile stimulation as well as auditory, and when it is important to improve the S/N ratio experienced by the listener. The type of auditory training equipment to be used should be chosen according to the purpose for its use.

Auditory trainers have the same general components as hearing aids. Most of them are larger than personal hearing aids and therefore more noticeable when worn. Auditory training units are often equipped with earphones as well as hearing aid receivers and can be used with a well-fitting earmold or with the headset. Use of earphones is convenient primarily for temporary use.

Before the technology of hearing aid components was advanced, the larger size of auditory trainers allowed the use of microphones and receivers with broader frequency responses and amplifiers that provided greater gain than could be obtained through personal hearing aids. This is no longer true, and the advantages of auditory trainers over personal aids today involve the improved S/N ratio that can be provided at the ear of the listener.

The purchase and maintenance of auditory training equipment should be managed by an audiologist. Performance specifications of auditory training units may not be in conformance with ANSI standards for hearing aids, and when installed, may vary in performance (Hardick, 1976; Matkin and Olsen, 1970).

Some auditory trainers can be equipped with a bone conduction receiver as well as earphones. These units are often used with profoundly hearing-impaired children whose reception of auditory information is limited. The vibrator is placed on the wrist, head, arm, or hand to facilitate the perception of low-frequency speech energy. The tactile information provided is useful to some children as an aid to developing and monitoring their own speech.

There are four major types of auditory training units in use today.

Hardwire Auditory Trainers

Also called group auditory trainers, hardwire units consist of one or more microphones wired to a large amplifier that delivers the amplified signal to several sets of earphones. These earphones are wired into the amplifier, and the signal provided by each earphone is adjusted by individual control boxes located on a desk or stand designed to accommodate them. The control box contains gain and tone controls usually for each earphone separately so that an optimal signal can be provided to each ear. The amplifier is also designed to accept input from a phonograph, tape recorder, or other signal sources.

Hardwire units were used most often in classrooms for hearing-impaired children prior to the mid-1960s. They provided higher fidelity amplification than was available through hearing aids and allowed use of media equipment with hearing-impaired students. Most systems did not provide microphones for each child, so child-to-child communication was not facilitated well. If the teacher used the microphone appropriately, the S/N ratio at the child's ear could be controlled satisfactorily.

The major disadvantages of hardwire units are (1) the limited mobility of teacher and student in the classroom, (2) the lack of flexibility for use outside of the classroom, (3) the frequent mechanical problems associated with broken cords and damaged receivers, and perhaps most important of all, (4) the failure to provide a satisfactory means for child-to-child communication or self-monitoring of speech. These disadvantages led to discontinuation of the use of hardwire units by most schools when other systems became available.

Desk Auditory Trainers

Single, self-contained hardwire units, called desk trainers, are used primarily to provide temporary amplification during special activities or for special purposes. These include speech therapy, tutoring sessions, or occasions when listening is enhanced by temporary use of amplification, such as when the listener is some distance from the speaker.

Desk trainers are portable, hand-carried units that must be placed near the listener. All components of the unit are contained in a case to which earphones are connected by wire. Because the microphone is located in the case, the unit acts like a large nonworn, personal hearing aid. The nature of the acoustic environment and the distance between the speaker and the listener determines the S/N ratio at the listener's ear. Although it is portable, the desk unit must be hand carried from place to place. This type of unit is really only satisfactory for temporary or intermittent use.

Induction-Loop Auditory Training Units

To overcome the lack of mobility associated with the hardwire units and the lack of control over the S/N ratio allowed by desk units, the induction-loop system was developed. A classroom or portion of one is enclosed by a wire loop attached to an amplifier that is fed by a teacher's microphone. A magnetic field is set up within the loop. The teacher's speech is amplified and fed through the wire loop into the magnetic field. The child wears a personal hearing aid equipped with a telecoil; when the aid is set on T, the signal from within the loop is picked up and fed to the receiver of the hearing aid. The signal is controlled by the volume control of the personal hearing aid.

The induction loop system increased the mobility of children within the confines of the classroom because no wires were required between the child's receiver and the amplifier. The teacher's mobility remained the same as with the hardwire arrangement.

Theoretically, the signal from the teacher's microphone is fed to all areas within the loop equally. The S/N ratio is controlled effectively when the hearing aid is set on T only. Use of both the telecoil and microphone settings of the hearing aid allow the children to receive input from both the teacher's microphone and from their own voices and those of their classmates. Under this condition, any noise in the environment is also amplified, but does not interfere greatly with reception of the teacher's signal under ordinary circumstances.

This type of system is relatively inexpensive to install and use. Children wear their own personal hearing aids, and all children within a classroom can be served by a single loop, teacher's microphone, and amplifier. There are several serious disadvantages to the loop system, however, described as follows.

1. The signal is not always equal within the loop. "Dead" spots occur within which the signal is significantly weaker than in other parts of the room.
2. The signal received by the telecoil varies in strength depending upon whether the coil is parallel or perpendicular to the floor. When a child bends over, the signal level received by the hearing aid fluctuates.
3. The signal often "leaks out" of the area enclosed by the loop into adjoining rooms or areas. This can be confusing and distracting to hearing aid users in adjacent areas unless it is carefully controlled. In addition the loop sometimes picks up noise from high-tension wires or radio waves nearby.
4. The frequency response of the auditory training system is limited by the response of the telecoil on the personal hearing aid. Manufacturers do not report this information as a general rule, and hearing aids are quite variable in this regard (Matkin and Olsen, 1970).

Frequency-Modulated (FM), Radio Frequency Auditory Training Units

The development of FM auditory trainers overcame many of the disadvantages experienced by users of earlier auditory training units. The systems perform as tiny radio transmitters (the teacher's microphone) and receivers (the children's hearing aid receiver unit). Using ultra-high-frequency bands that have been designated as educational transmitting frequencies, the teacher's microphone transmits a frequency-modulated signal into the air. The microphone is worn on the teacher's body at a prescribed distance from the mouth. The antenna is a small wire hanging from the microphone. The signal is received by the child's unit, which is tuned to the same frequency as the teacher's microphone. This receiver unit resembles a large hearing aid (see Figure 4.6). It is equipped with self-contained microphones, volume controls, and hearing aid-type receiver or earphones. No wires are necessary, because it operates on batteries and receives radio signals from the atmosphere.

To avoid interference (cross-talk) with other auditory trainers being used in the same area, the transmitting frequency of each set of units (teacher's microphone and

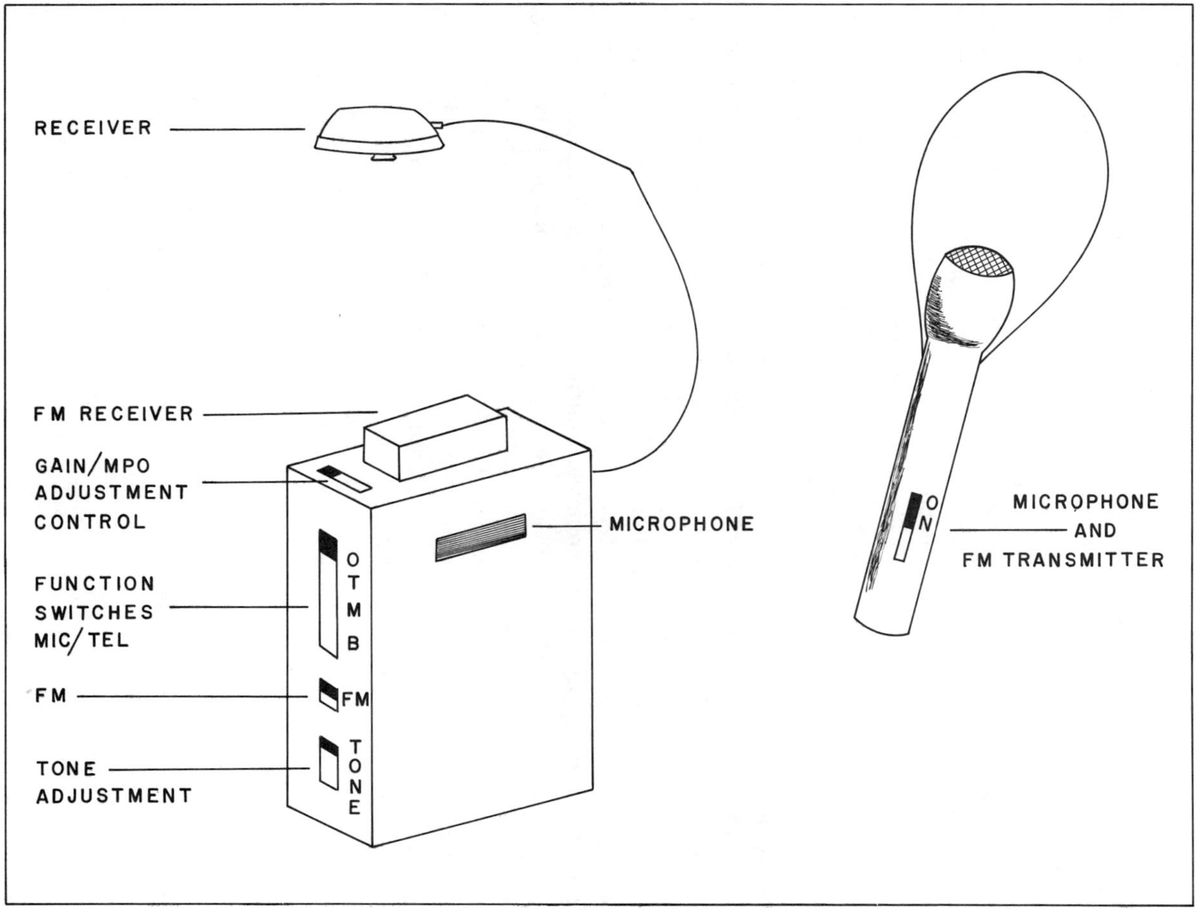

Figure 4.6. A typical FM receiver and wireless FM microphone-transmitter. The unit contains an environmental microphone as well as telecoil and FM reception. Other adjustments permit individual variations in gain, MPO, and frequency response (tone adjustment).

children's receivers) is controlled so that no two sets in a given school operate on the same frequency band. If desired, several teachers may be equipped with microphones; children change receivers as they move from class to class. Because the receiver unit contains microphones, the teacher's signal can be received alone or in combination with signals from the immediate environment when the external microphones are turned on.

The FM systems allow excellent mobility for teachers and students, both within and outside the classroom. It is not unusual for teachers to communicate from the classroom to the playground or other areas in the school, giving directions or getting the attention of children not immediately present. Fortunately for the teacher, the child cannot turn off the radio signal, only the external microphones. Unfortunately, teachers sometimes forget to turn off their microphones during recess, coffee breaks, or other noninstructional times. Children may hear interesting gossip or other comments from the teacher's lounge under these circumstances, a situation that may result in education of a nonconventional sort!

A major benefit can be derived from use of the FM systems with mainstreamed children or adults attending classes, lectures, or other events in large, noisy rooms. Although the distance between the speaker and the listener is great and the acoustic environment is poor, the signal from the microphone is delivered full strength at distances of several hundred feet. Noise in the immediate environment is minimized, especially if the environmental microphones are not activated. Because public school classrooms seldom have acoustic conditions favorable to hearing-impaired listeners, it is difficult for many children to benefit from instructional activities in the average classroom while wearing a personal hearing aid. The FM auditory trainer can provide a more favorable listening environment, and it can be carried from room to room with ease. Teachers need no special training in its use nor is it inconvenient to employ.

There are two disadvantages to the FM units. Their conspicuous size makes them unacceptable to some older children and adolescents, and support and counseling from an understanding adult is often essential if they are to be used. The greatest disadvantage, however, is their cost. FM units are much more expensive to provide to students than the other types of systems. It may be necessary to demonstrate their advantages to administrators before their purchase will be considered. Davis, Shepard, Stelmachowicz, and Gorga (1980) developed a videotape demonstration of the effects of noise on listening under various conditions of amplification that can be used for this purpose.

CONSUMER INFORMATION

There are several important facts about the manufacture and sale of hearing aids that consumers should know for their own protection. Many of these facts are not widely publicized and may not be generally available to the hearing-impaired public, at least not in a form they are likely to encounter. For example, government regulations governing the sale of hearing aids are a matter of public record, but most people do not attend to them as a matter of course.

Until the late 1960s almost all hearing aids were sold to the public by hearing aid dealers whose special training and experience with hearing assessment and habilitation ranged from zero to good. The services and business practices employed varied considerably from dealer to dealer. It was not unusual for a dealer to set up a temporary office in a motel for a week or two, sell hearing aids, then leave town, leaving no forwarding address. If the aids were unsatisfactory for any reason, the buyer had little recourse.

Hearing aid dealers are no longer the sole dispensers of hearing aids. Audiologists frequently dispense hearing aids from a variety of employment settings, including private practice, clinic, hospital, and university settings. Several "mail order" businesses will sell directly to consumers on recommendations from an audiologist. The advantages to these methods of hearing aid dispensing are related to the training required for audiologists as compared to that for hearing aid dealers.

Beginning in the early 1960s, governmental agencies and legislatures, spurred on by a strong consumer movement, moved to develop rules and regulations governing the manufacture and distribution of hearing aids. The Food and Drug Administration (FDA) developed rules that include the following provisions:

1. Performance characteristics of hearing aids must be specified clearly according to standard measurements and requirements.
2. Manufacturers and dispensers must inform consumers of the limitations of hearing aids with regard to the restoration of normal hearing.
3. Hearing aids may not be sold to users under the age of 18 unless their ears have been examined by a physician within six months prior to purchase. Hearing aids may be sold to adults without a physical examination only after they have been encouraged to have a medical examination and have decided against doing so. In the latter case, adults must sign a waiver provided by the dispenser.

In addition to the FDA regulations, the Federal Trade Commission (FTC) has also proposed guidelines for hearing aid sales and the Health Care Financing Administration (HCFA) has suggested rules by which the purchase of hearing aids by governmental agencies will be governed. At this writing, these sets of regulations have not been finalized. Among other provisions, the FTC rules require a 30-day "cooling off period," during which a hearing aid buyer can cancel the purchase agreement without serious penalty.

These regulations are designed specifically to prevent some of the abuses that occurred when the sale of hearing aids was not regulated in any way. These abuses included high-pressure sales tactics, misrepresentation of the benefits to be derived from use of amplification, refusal to refund money when the hearing aid was unsatisfactory, and sale of hearing aids without adequate assessment.

In addition to federal legislation, many states require that hearing aid dispensers be licensed. Licensure acts usually describe the sales practices required in a given state. Consumers who believe that they have been subjected to unfair business practices or misrepresentations should contact their state attorney general for information about legal requirements and remedies peculiar to that state.

REFERENCES

ANSI, *American National Standard for Specification of Hearing Aid Characteristics,* S3.22-1976. New York: American National Standards Institute, 1976.

Anonymous, Twenty-fourth annual facts and figures, *Hearing Aid J.,* 32, 5, 1978.

Bauer, B., Electroacoustic transducers. In S. Gerber (Ed.), *Introductory Hearing Science.* Philadelphia: W. B. Saunders Co., 1974.

Beranek, L., *Acoustic Measurements.* New York: John Wiley and Sons, 1949.

Beranek, L., Criteria for office quieting based on questionnaire ratings studies, *J. Acous. Soc. Am.,* 28, 833–852, 1956.

Brackmann, D. and House, F., Direct stimulation of the auditory nerve. In J. Northern (Ed.), *Hearing Disorders.* Boston: Little, Brown and Co., 1976.

Causey, G., Current developments in hearing aids. In M. Rubin (Ed.), *Hearing Aids: Current Developments and Concepts.* Baltimore: University Park Press, 1976.

Davis, J., Shepard, N., Stelmachowicz, P., and Gorga, M., Effects of classroom noise on the use of amplification (a videotape), Department of Speech Pathology and Audiology, University of Iowa, 1980.

Finitzo-Hieber, T. and Tillman, T., Room acoustics effects on monosyllabic word discrimination ability for normal and hearing-impaired children, *J. Speech Hearing Res.,* 21, 440–458, 1978.

Frank, T. and Gooden, R., The effect of hearing aid microphone types on speech discrimination scores in a background of multi-talker noise, *MAICO Audiol. Library Series,* 11, 5, 1973.

Gaeth, J. and Lounsbury, E., Hearing aids and children in elementary school, *J. Speech Hearing Dis.,* 31, 283–289, 1966.

Gengel, R., Acceptable speech-to-noise ratios for aided speech discrimination by the hearing impaired, *J. Aud. Res.,* 11, 219–222, 1971.

Gengel, R. and Foust, K., Some implications of listening level for speech reception by sensorineural hearing impaired children, *Language, Speech and Hearing Services in Schools,* 6, 14–20, 1975.

Griffing, T. and Dahlberg, K., Modular ITE aids—More than an alternative, *Hearing Instruments,* 29, 24–25, 1978.

Hardick, E., Rationale for inclusion of auditory training units under standards and rules applicable to hearing aids, *J. Acad. Rehab. Audiol.,* 10, 58–91, 1976.

Hawkins, D., Earmold acoustics and modification for mild and moderate hearing losses, *J. Acad. Rehab. Audiol.,* 12, 30–46, 1979.

House, W. and Urban, J., Long term results of electrode implantation and electronic stimulation of the cochlea in man, *Ann. Otol. Rhinol. Laryngol.,* 82, 504–517, 1973.

John, J., The efficiency of hearing aids as a function of architectural acoustics. In A. Ewing

(Ed.), *The Modern Educational Treatment of Deafness*. Manchester, England: Manchester University Press, 1960.

Knudsen, V. and Harris, C., *Acoustical Designing in Architecture*. New York: John Wiley and Sons, 1950.

Kryter, K., *The Effects of Noise on Man*. New York: Academic Press, 1970.

Langford, B., Coupling methods. In M. Pollack (Ed.), *Amplification for the Hearing Impaired*. New York: Grune and Stratton, 1975.

Lentz, W., Speech discrimination in the presence of background noise using a hearing aid with a directionally sensitive microphone, *MAICO Audiol. Library Series*, 10, 9, 1972.

Lybarger, S., Earmolds. In J. Katz (Ed.), *Handbook of Clinical Audiology*. Baltimore: Williams and Wilkins Co., 1972.

Matkin, N. and Olsen, W., Induction loop amplification systems: Classroom performance, *Asha*, 12, 239–244, 1970.

Michelson, R., Electrical stimulation of the human cochlea, *Arch. Otolaryngol.*, 93, 317–323, 1971a.

Michelson, R., The results of electrical stimulation of the cochlea in human sensory deafness, *Ann. Otol. Rhinol. Laryngol.*, 80, 914–919, 1971b.

Moncur, J. and Dirks, D., Binaural and monaural speech intelligibilitiy in reverberation, *J. Speech Hearing Res.*, 10, 186–195, 1967.

National Association of Earmold Manufacturers, NAEL standard terms for earmolds, *Hearing Dealer*, 13, (December) 1970.

Nelson, E., How the NAEL serves the hearing aid dispenser, *Hearing Aid J.*, 31, 12, 1978.

Nielsen, H., A comparison between hearing aids with directional microphone and hearing aids with conventional microphone, *Scandinavian Audiology*, 2, 1973–176, 1973.

Niemoeller, A., Acoustical design of classrooms for the deaf, *Amer. Ann. Deaf*, 113, 1040–1045, 1968.

Niemoeller, A., Silverman, S., and Davis, H., Hearing aids. In H. Davis and S. Silverman (Eds.), *Hearing and Deafness*, 3rd edition. Chicago: Holt, Rinehart and Winston, 1970.

Olsen, W., Physical characteristics of hearing aids. In W. Hodgson and P. Skinner (Eds.), *Hearing Aid Assessment and Use in Audiologic Habilitation*. Baltimore: Williams and Wilkins Co., 1977.

Paul, R., An investigation of the effectiveness of hearing aid amplification in regular and special classrooms under instructional conditions, Ph.D. Dissertation, Wayne State University, 1967.

Porter, T., Hearing aids in a residential school, *Amer. Ann. Deaf.*, 118, 31–33, 1973.

Sanders, D., Noise conditions in normal school classrooms, *Except. Chil.*, 31, 344–353, 1965.

Schell, Y., Electroacoustic evaluation of hearing aids worn by public school children, *Audiol. and Hearing Educ.*, 2, 7–15, 1976.

Simmons, F., Electrical stimulation of the auditory nerve in man, *Arch. Otolaryngol.*, 84, 2–54, 1966.

Simmons, F., Mongeon, C., Lewis, W., and Huntington, D., Electrical stimulation of acoustical nerve and inferior colliculus, *Arch. Otolaryngol.*, 79, 559–567, 1964

Smith, K., Earmolds and hearing aid accessories. In W. Hodgson and P. Skinner (Eds.), *Hearing Aid Assessment and Use in Audiologic Habilitation*. Baltimore: Williams and Wilkins Co., 1977.

Studebaker, G. and Zachman, T., Investigation of the acoustics of earmold vents, *J. Acous. Soc. Am.,* 47, 1107–1115, 1970.

Thomas, H., Architectural acoustics as a fundamental factor in the design of schools for the deaf. In A. Ewing (Ed.), *The Modern Educational Treatment of Deafness.* Manchester, England: Manchester University Press, 1960.

Tillman, T., Carhart, R., and Olsen, W., Hearing aid efficiency in a competing speech situation, *J. Speech Hearing Res.,* 13, 789–811, 1970.

Tolk, J., Acoustics, intelligibility of speech and electroacoustic systems in classrooms, *Proceedings of the Second International Course in Paedoaudiology.* The Netherlands: Groningen University, 1961.

Vernon, J., Mahoney, T., and Schleuning, A., Implantable hearing aids. In J. Northern (Ed.), *Hearing Disorders.* Boston: Little, Brown and Co., 1976.

Warren, M. and Kasten, R., Efficacy of hearing aid repairs by manufacturers and by alternative repair facilities, *J. Acad. Rehab. Audiol.,* 9, 38–47, 1976.

Webster, J., Effects of noise on speech intelligibility. In W. Ward and J. Fricke (Eds.), *Noise as a Public Health Hazard: Asha Reports No. 4.* Washington, D.C.: American Speech and Hearing Association, 1969.

Zink, G., Hearing aids children wear: A longitudinal study of performance, *Volta Rev.,* 74, 41–51, 1972.

PART Two

CHILDREN

CHAPTER 5

Early Intervention

The effects of hearing loss on the communication, language, educational, and social development of hearing-impaired children are well documented and are discussed in detail in the following chapters. Differences of opinion exist among professionals about many aspects of remediation for hearing-impaired children, but there is one area in which there is total agreement: *the earlier hearing loss is identified and remediation begins,* the better. Development of the ability to listen and the use of verbal symbols is dependent on early intervention, including the use of amplification. If effective auditory and language stimulation are to occur, children must be identified as having hearing loss before the language deficit is severe. Hearing loss is invisible, however; unless it is predicted as a result of certain prenatal or birth factors, it is usually not suspected until a child fails to learn to talk at a normal age. By this time (around 1 year or later), a serious delay in language development has already occurred. In the last 20 years, procedures used to identify and assess hearing impairment in children have improved. As a result it is now evident that hearing loss is a more common impairment than previous estimates indicated.

INCIDENCE OF HEARING IMPAIRMENT IN CHILDREN

Estimates of the number of hearing impaired children in the population range from 1 to 2 per thousand to 50 per thousand, depending on the definition of hearing impairment that is used. Most census figures are based on the number of children enrolled in special educational programs. Rawlings and Trybus (1978) reported that a total of 60,231 children are served in residential or day schools for the deaf or multiply handicapped, self-contained classes in the public schools, or regular classes with part-time educational services. Forty percent of them are enrolled in public school programs. These figures are misleading, however, because they include only those children receiving special services. They represent the most severely hearing-impaired children and agree with the widely used figure of 1 ''deaf'' child per 1000 births.

Children with mild to moderate hearing losses are usually excluded from these totals. National demographic data have not been collected for these children, but estimates based on population patterns have been reported by Berg and Fletcher (1970). Based on data extrapolated from census figures of 1967, they estimated that there were 1,146,555 hearing-impaired children of school age in the country. Of these, 636,975 were estimated to have mild hearing losses ranging from 26 to 40 dB, 353,875 to have moderate hearing losses (41 to 55 dB), 141,550 to have moderately severe losses (56 to 70 dB), and 14,155 to have severe hearing losses (71 to 90 dB). Berg and Fletcher estimated that 150,000 hearing-impaired children in the public schools were in need of extensive language, communication, academic, and counseling services. Another 950,000 needed less extensive but essential services, including hearing aid selection and orientation, vocabulary enrichment, and communication therapy.

School census figures in states in which audiologists conduct hearing conservation programs in the public schools indicate that the totals published by Berg and Fletcher underestimate the number of hearing impaired children in the schools. For example, data provided in 1977 by the Iowa Department of Public Instruction (whose schools employ more than 50 audiologists) show a total of 30,825 children with *known* hearing losses. The estimate for Iowa reported by Berg and Fletcher was 15,844 children.

In 1963, Eagles, Wishik, Doerfler, Melnick, and Levine reported an extensive study of the hearing levels of school children in the Pittsburgh area. Their data indicate an incidence of 50 children per 1000 whose hearing levels fall below the normal range in one or both ears. Although many of these children may have hearing losses that are not educationally significant, it is probable that at least half of them do. Unfortunately, the actual effects of different degrees and types of hearing loss on language and academic achievement are difficult to determine because of a lack of empirical data on large numbers of children.

The available data suggest that there are at least 20 times as many children with mild to moderate hearing losses as children with severe to profound losses. The numbers vary from one estimate to another because of the variability in the criteria used to define hearing loss. Several studies have shown that children with mild (15 to 30 dB) hearing losses exhibit reduced language skills and academic achievement when compared to children who have hearing better than 15 dB (Ling, 1969; Holm and Kunze, 1969; Quigley and Thomure, 1968; Needleman, 1977). It now seems reasonable to assume that children whose hearing levels are greater than 15 dB may be at risk educationally, although many children with mild hearing losses exhibit average or better than average achievement. If all of these children are included in incidence figures, there are probably more than two million of them in the public schools.

EARLY INTERVENTION PROGRAMS

Because the effects of hearing loss are so serious, the need for early remedial programming has been recognized for many years. The need to establish a means of communication with young children was top priority long before the advent of the electronic hearing aid, but appropriate personnel and services often were not available. Residential programs for deaf children existed in most states, but local programs were scarce.

Historical Development

Until the 1960s, most established educational systems limited preschool enrollment to children over the age of 3 years. Three factors contributed significantly to a change in this policy and the establishment of special programs for infants and toddlers: the development of improved hearing-testing techniques for babies from 0 to 3 years; the improvement in hearing aid electronics, which allowed extended low-frequency amplification, more durable hearing aids, and higher fidelity; and the rubella epidemic of 1964–1965, which resulted in the birth of approximately 20,000 severely hearing impaired children, many of whom were multiply handicapped.

Clinic-Based Programs. The earliest programs for young preschoolers were found in speech and hearing centers. The prototype for many of them was the John Tracy Clinic in Los Angeles. Established by Mrs. Spencer Tracy in 1943 as a reaction to her own frustrated attempts to obtain professional advice and services for her deaf son, the John Tracy Clinic serves children in the Los Angeles area on a daily basis, provides intensive short-term programs for parents and children from other localities, and disseminates a correspondence course for the parents of young deaf children (John Tracy Correspondence Course, 1968). The latter consists of a series of lessons for parents to conduct at home. Parents are encouraged to describe their experiences in letters to the clinic, which are answered individually by teachers of the deaf.

The John Tracy Clinic employs an oral method of teaching and emphasizes the use of lipreading and listening as a means of early communication. Parents are taught to devise games and use daily activities that allow many repetitions of words, phrases, and short sentences. The free correspondence course is a popular service throughout the world and has been printed in 16 languages. Recently, a new correspondence course for the parents of deaf-blind children has become available.

The major goal of the early intervention programs developed in speech and hearing centers and hospital settings was the development of lipreading and speech skills. Preacademic or readiness activities were not employed until programs were developed in educational settings (Moores, 1978). Programs in the early 1960s were of two major types: *Clinic therapy sessions* and *home training*.

Clinic Therapy Sessions. Usually conducted by speech-language pathologists, early therapy sessions in speech and hearing clinics emphasized the development of oral communication skills. Much time was spent on sensory training activities that consisted of visual and tactual matching games. Pairs of items were presented, such as two shoes, two pipes, two toy cars. Upon the presentation of an item, the child was required to choose its mate from an array of items. When this could be done visually, items were placed in a bag and the child chose the matching pair by feeling the shapes within the bag. Visual matching of colors, shapes, objects, and pictures was accomplished, with the latter becoming gradually more detailed and the required discriminations becoming more difficult. Figure 5.1 shows items requiring fine visual discrimination. The child's task was to identify the pictures that match or to choose the one that differed from the rest. These activities were designed to prepare the child to make the minute visual distinctions required for lipreading.

Lipreading activities required the child to identify objects or gross actions from the spoken word. Initial attempts to teach words through lipreading involved simple, highly visible words, such as *ball* or *airplane*. When one word could be consistently identified, another, visually dissimilar one was added and the distinctions between the two were made. The stimulus words were spoken in phrases and short sentences as often as possible to facilitate learning of the patterns of connected language (Harris, 1963).

As hearing aid technology improved, audition was emphasized as a tool for communication. In some programs, lipreading activities were abandoned and greater stress was placed on the use of auditory clues. A few programs stressed a unisensory approach, in which visual information was not provided (Pollack, 1970).

I had this kind of training

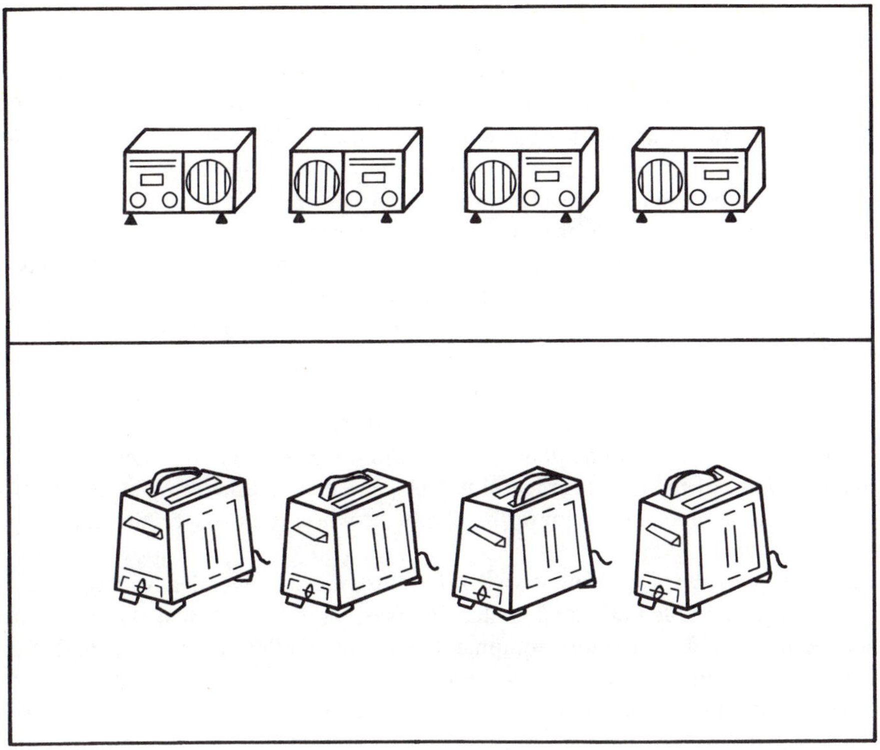

Figure 5.1. Examples of stimuli requiring fine visual discrimination.

The clinician spoke directly into the child's ear or held a card in front of the face to prevent the child from lipreading. Matching activities were replaced by auditory stimulation using a variety of sounds, but usually concentrating on the spoken word in sentence contexts.

The parents' role in clinic programs for very young children was to observe the activities, occasionally carry them out under the clinician's supervision, then use them at home daily.

Home Training Programs. As programs for hearing-impaired children proliferated, the usefulness of everyday activities associated with the child's home life for language stimulation became apparent.

To teach parents how to use daily events effectively, training sessions were shifted from clinic rooms to one of two settings. The child's home was used if it was near enough to the speech and hearing center to allow home visitation by a clinician. Families who lived in other geographic areas were trained in a home setting provided by the clinic. Stationary houses or mobile homes were used, whether adjacent to or near the clinics or, in the case of mobile homes, in various communities removed from the clinic. Parents and child were made comfortable in the home, and clinicians demonstrated the use of ordinary homemaking activities as language stimulation resources. The advantages to the use of a home setting are obvious. The natural environment allows for the identification of noises or activities that could interfere with use of amplification or maintaining the child's attention, as well as those that can be used to call attention to sound or are of high interest value. For example, the young child's fascination with bathroom fixtures and items such as soap, toilet paper rolls, and water have good potential for teaching the concepts of hot, cold, wet, dry, roll, splash, and pull, in addition to the names of the items involved. At the same time, the acoustic properties of bathrooms are not conducive to auditory perception and must be taken into account.

The parents' role in language stimulation is more easily demonstrated within a home setting than in a clinic. It is sometimes difficult for parents to generalize clinic activities to home use, but demonstrations within a familiar environment clarify the ongoing nature of the language learning task. Parents are asked to plan stimulation activities and demonstrate them to the clinician, who offers advice and encouragement.

These two types of clinic-based programs offered several advantages. They provided considerable individual contact between parent, child, and clinician. They used the most modern auditory equipment available. Children with varying degrees of hearing impairment received services, a fact that contributed to a concentrated effort to make maximum use of residual hearing. Services were available in communities that did not have formal educational programs for hearing-impaired children.

The scarcity of educational personnel such as teachers of the deaf, was a disadvantage of these early clinic-based programs. The training and skills of the speech-language pathologists and audiologists who staffed the programs resulted in an emphasis on the development of oral communication skills alone. Activities designed to foster cognitive, social, or educational development usually were not included. Nevertheless, these first clinic-based programs contributed enormously to the early treatment of hearing-impaired children. Their successful preparation of many children for subsequent educational procedures served as an impetus for the development of programs within educational settings. Furthermore, children who were successful in learning a verbal symbol system before they were old enough to attend school tended to achieve higher academically than children whose knowledge of language was developed later (Balow and Brill, 1975).

School-Based Programs. Studies of the educational achievement of hearing-impaired children published in the 1960s called attention to the need for systematic multifaceted intervention during the first 3 years of life. Coupled with improvements in testing techniques and hearing aid technology, these data provided an impetus for the development of early intervention programs that were within educational settings or staffed by educators of the deaf. According to Moores (1978), the evidence that the average deaf adult in the United States was unable to read at the fifth-grade level and lacked basic linguistic and communicative skills created an atmosphere of dissatisfaction with the status quo in education of the deaf.

Perhaps the most important factor in the rush to develop infant programs for the hearing impaired was the explosion of knowledge regarding the acquisition of language by normal children that occurred in the 1960s and early 1970s. Psychologists, linguists, and speech scientists reported empirical data showing that the learning of basic language skills begins at birth and proceeds rapidly, resulting in mastery of the major syntactic, semantic, and morphological rules of language before the age of 4 years. For the first time, the enormity of the language deficit associated with hearing impairment and its probable nature became evident. It seemed obvious that the key to improved linguistic functioning lay in the early (before age 3 years) development of a symbol system to which rules could be applied and that would allow reception and expression of information about the world and relationships within it.

There were few prototypes for very early language and cognitive intervention and no available data regarding the effectiveness of various procedures. All of the existing programs emphasized the development of oral skills (speech and lipreading) through stimulation by the spoken word alone; the educationally based programs continued this tradition. Facile use of a symbol system often was developed slowly by children with severe to profound hearing impairments. The desired level of knowledge of language rules and semantic relationships was not forthcoming for many children. Eventually, experimentation with the use of alternate forms of communication, including manual signs, was begun in infant and preschool programs.

As principles of early childhood education evolved from research with hearing children they were incorporated into preschool programs for hearing-impaired children. The use of Piagetian tasks for cognitive development began. Readiness activities associated with educational tasks were developed for young children. Procedures focused on the development of motor-perceptual as well as language skills. These experiences served to broaden the base of the early intervention programs and to prepare children better for later educational tasks.

Early Use of Amplification. By the time early intervention programs became a reality, the effects of the use of residual hearing on learning were becoming apparent. Until this time, many audiologists had been quite conservative in their approach to selecting amplification for infants and toddlers. As a result many children, identified at age 18 months or 2 years, did not receive hearing aids for more than a year after identification. Reports by Wedenberg (1967), Whetnall and Fry, (1964), Pollack (1970), and others had a significant impact on amplification selection procedures. It became obvious that the foundation of habilitation for hearing-impaired children is the early selection and use of appropriate amplification. No other action has greater potential for aiding development of communication and language skills. The effective use of residual hearing is so important that amplification must be selected as early as possible, based on as much information regarding the hearing loss as can be obtained, and monitored carefully and often by parents and professionals.

When possible, procedures used in the selection of hearing aids for adults should be used with children. If their language skills will allow, speech reception and discrimination scores may be the basis for comparing hearing aids. For nonverbal children, however, many of the procedures used with adults are not possible. Neither comparisons of speech scores, with and without amplification, nor subjective judgments of sound quality are easily obtained. Measures of tolerance for sound may not be possible. The audiologist must rely on audiological assessment data, electroacoustic measures of the hearing aids to be considered, experience with selection of hearing aids for adults with similar-appearing hearing losses, and careful observation of the child in question as the basis for hearing aid selection. The process must be an ongoing one and is best accomplished in conjunction with a parent-infant program or some other structured remediation process.

It is outside the scope of this discussion to describe in detail hearing aid selection for young children. Ross (1975), Matkin (1977), and Liden and Kankkunen (1973) provide excellent discussions of the procedures and problems involved. It is important to note, however, some relevant principles and issues.

Adjustment Problems. The selection of amplification should involve a cooperative effort on the part of the physician, audiologist, parents, clinicians or teachers, and child. Medical clearance must be obtained before the aid is purchased. Many audiologists recommend a trial period for every child, during which systematic observations can be made by adults in a variety of situations. Observations include making note of the sounds responded to while the aid is worn and any symptoms of fatigue or irritability associated with use of the hearing aid. Unless a supply of loaner aids is available, trial periods may not be possible without purchase. If the aid selected allows for flexibility in frequency response, power, and gain settings, most problems that arise can be alleviated by adjustments of these factors (Ross, 1975).

Parents and teachers should be taught to perform a listening check and visual inspection of the hearing aid daily, using the procedures described in Chapter 4. The importance of regular monitoring cannot be overemphasized because hearing aids are easily damaged and young children cannot report changes in their functioning. Earmolds will be outgrown frequently (every three to six months for toddlers) and must be replaced promptly when feedback becomes a regular problem. Care of the hearing aid should be emphasized along with instructions for obtaining repairs when necessary.

It is not unusual for body hearing aid receivers and earmolds to fall out of the ears of small children easily. In stubborn cases, it may be necessary to tape the receiver to the pinna or the cord to the mastoid process to prevent pull on the earmold. Sometimes it is necessary to remove the receiver from the earmold, attach it to an adapter, and wear it with a shell mold and tubing. The receiver can be taped behind the ear. This arrangement will change the frequency response delivered to the ear, however, and should be monitored carefully.

Some children are distracted by the presence of the hearing aid and pull on the cord or receiver whenever it is placed in the ear. Downs (1967b) described an adjustment procedure for children, involving use of the hearing aid for short (five minute) periods, several times a day and gradually increasing the time the hearing aid is in place. Within six to eight weeks, children should be wearing the aid all day, except for naps and rough play. Ross (1975) disagrees with such a schedule, saying that it calls too much attention to the hearing aid and drags out the adjustment process unnecessarily. He recommends putting the hearing aid on and leaving it on. Most young children adjust quickly and easily to the presence of the hearing aid, if their parents accept the aid and feel comfortable with it. If parents are hesitant about putting the earmold in place or expect the child to remove the aid, its presence can create a battle of wills. In that case, parents must be helped to recognize their behavior and to modify it. Under these circumstances, Downs' suggestion for keeping the hearing aid in place will be helpful.

When infants and toddlers resist wearing a hearing aid in the absence of obvious reasons, it is usually a sign of poor tolerance for amplified sound. Reducing the MPO or changing the frequency response of the aid may result in better acceptance. A few children cannot use amplification because of severe tolerance problems. The use of a bone vibrator as a receiver will sometimes provide useful vibrotactile information when auditory input is intolerable. Every effort should be made to find a hearing aid that can be tolerated, because even minimal auditory information may be useful in the reception of language and the monitoring of speech production.

Monaural Versus Binaural Fittings. Several areas of disagreement exist among audiologists regarding the type and number of hearing aids to be recommended for children. The questions of monaural versus binaural fitting and body versus ear level type are the most widely argued. There are two common approaches to the first question.

1. Select a single aid initially, monitor its use, and recommend a second hearing aid when adjustment to the first is complete. Proponents of this approach do not assume that all children are candidates for binaural hearing aids, especially if the hearing losses in the two ears are dissimilar, particularly with regard to speech perception. Some audiologists fit monaurally in order to monitor the effects of amplification on pure tone thresholds. There is some evidence that the use of powerful amplification results in temporary, possibly permanent, threshold shifts in some persons (Ross and Lerman, 1967). If a child is quite susceptible to damage to residual hearing, wearing an aid in each ear initially could result in damage to both ears before the effects are recognized. To avoid this, some audiologists prefer to fit monaurally until possible effects on residual hearing are determined.

2. Select binaural aids for all children in whom hearing can be measured in both ears. Proponents of this approach *do* assume that every child is a candidate for binaural amplification. It is difficult to obtain objective data on the advantages of binaural amplification, especially in nonverbal children. The experiences of adults are used to predict those of children, many of whom later report preferring binaural fittings. Matkin (1977) suggested that children who have useful hearing across several frequencies and no tolerance problems benefit most from binaural amplification. Children whose hearing is restricted to the low frequencies (500 Hz and below) show few advantages of binaural over monaural hearing aids.

Ear Level Versus Body Aids. The question of whether to select ear level or body hearing aids for children revolves around several factors, of which age is probably the most important. It is difficult to keep ear level aids in place on children under about 2½ years. Infants who spend much of their time lying down are particularly unsuited to using a head-worn aid. Toddlers lead a relatively rowdy life, falling and bumping into objects regularly. In addition, they assume more prone and upside-down positions than the average person. Head-worn aids are often dislodged and misplaced by young children as a result. Body aids, in addition to being sturdier and less easily damaged, may be fastened in place in a harness worn under the clothing. There is less chance that the aid will fall off, and its controls are less available for experimentation by the child.

Another factor to be considered is the degree of hearing loss. At one time, ear-level aids lacked sufficient gain to be used effectively by people with severe to profound hearing losses. Modern hearing aid technology has produced head worn aids that can deliver sufficient amplification for most losses, no matter how severe. Feedback problems occur more often than with body aids, however, because of the close proximity of the microphone to the receiver and the necessity for a tight seal at the ear. Because children's ears grow rapidly in early childhood, their use of powerful ear-level hearing aids results in more feedback problems than experienced by adults.

On the other hand, the use of ear-level hearing aids has several advantages. True binaural hearing can be provided by the use of an aid on each ear. Placement of the microphones at ear level allows for more natural reception of sound, including the possibility of using head shadow effects as localization cues. Development of the ability to use subtle auditory cues such as this to provide knowledge of the world appears to foster cognitive development and may be important to the total growth and development of a young child.

MPO Considerations. One of the most important considerations in selection of amplification for any hearing impaired person is the MPO of the aid to be worn.

Because young children cannot verbalize discomfort associated with loud sound, it is essential to avoid excessive power in aids selected for them. Many body hearing aids are designed to produce sound levels in excess of 140 dB SPL. Such levels are known to be intolerable to normally hearing persons and to result in damage to hearing; such powerful instruments should not be recommended. Hearing aids selected for children should not exceed MPO's of 120 to 125 dB (Ross, 1975; Madell, 1976).

Nursery and Preschool Programs

By the age of 3 or 4 most children are ready for participation in an organized nursery or preschool program. Several different types of programs exist, varying in the nature of the activities engaged in by children and the strategies employed by teachers. It is outside the scope of this book to describe these programs in detail. In general, they may be categorized as emphasizing preacademic and readiness work or social interaction and free play. In the former, structured activities involving visual-motor development, matching, and phonics are included. Special materials, such as readiness workbooks, are used and children are expected to work toward defined goals that lead to academic skills. Many 4- and 5-year-old children in preacademic programs learn to read and write numbers, the alphabet, and simple words.

Free-play programs provide a wide range of unstructured experiences. Toys, clay, puppets, puzzles, and other materials are available for free use by children. The teacher's role is less an activity leader and more a play facilitator. Group activities, such as story time, occur but constitute a small proportion of the day's procedures.

Language stimulation is the primary purpose of both types of program. In the readiness programs, specific language is taught in groups during number work, reading readiness and phonics work, story time, lipreading, listening, and writing activities. In the less structured programs, language stimulation is provided by teacher-child interaction during free play, story time, and group games and activities, such as nursery rhymes and finger or puppet play.

It is often beneficial for hearing-impaired children to attend preschool classes with their hearing peers. Although they may have difficulty communicating orally, they can participate in many play activities with them. Interaction with groups of hearing children during play provides a type of language and auditory stimulation that is not available in most other situations. The role models provided by hearing children are important. Their use of fluent speech as a communication tool with each other demonstrates its relevance to the hearing-impaired child's life far more effectively than an adult's speech can. If speech is not yet under the control of the hearing-impaired child, it is important to monitor placement carefully for signs of withdrawal, aggression, bewilderment, or rejection by the other children. If these occur and cannot be ameliorated within a reasonable time, the child probably should be removed from that preschool program, at least temporarily. It is unusual, however, for young children to fail to establish some form of communication during daily contact with other children, and the benefits are worth the effort involved.

Modern Parent-Infant Programs

Attempts to institute the earliest possible habilitative services to children resulted in the development of parent-infant programs by a variety of institutions and agencies. These programs stress the role of the parent as a teacher in a natural setting but are not necessarily provided only in home settings. Modern parent-infant programs often involve as much "therapy" for parents as for children, who may also be enrolled in nursery school or other educational programs.

Ideally, enrollment in a parent-infant program should occur immediately following the diagnosis of hearing impairment, but this does not happen for many families. Diagnosis is often delayed and spread over an extended period of time while parents are referred to various professionals and agencies. Typically, parents suspect hearing loss before the child is a year old. They consult the family doctor or pediatrician for confirmation. Because hearing impairment is invisible, not easily recognized on brief contact, and a low-incidence condition, many physicians discount the parents' fears until they become insistent.

The first referral is usually made to an otolaryngologist (a specialist in ear, nose, and throat disorders). Many communities do not have these specialists, so parents must be referred to physicians in other, often distant, communities. If the family has financial restraints, a service agency such as a Department of Social Services or Crippled Children's Services may become involved. Services must be approved, the paperwork increases, appointments are scheduled and coordinated, and time passes. If the otolaryngologist has the necessary equipment and personnel trained in pediatric audiology, hearing testing can be accomplished at the time of the first visit. If not, another referral is made to an audiologist for hearing assessment. If initial attempts to test a young child's hearing are successful, a hearing aid evaluation may be recommended; if not, further testing may be required before the results are shared with parents and their fears confirmed. Unless the otolaryngologist and the audiologist are familiar with the remedial services available in the family's home community, referral for follow-up educational services may not be made. In some cases, such referrals are not possible locally due to the limited services offered within a small community.

Parents report extreme frustration during this series of events, which are typical of those experienced by parents of hearing-impaired children. They are convinced that "something is wrong," but no one seems to take them seriously or to know what to do about the problem. Speech-language pathologists, audiologists, and teachers of the deaf often criticize physicians for not being alert to the possibility of hearing loss in young children or for failing to refer families to speech and hearing centers immediately. However, at least part of the unfortunate delay is the responsibility of speech and hearing personnel, whose services are not visible in the community because of insufficient public relations effort. Worse, some audiologists do not offer remedial services themselves and do not consider it their professional responsibility to locate them for the clients they see. It is not surprising, therefore, that enrollment in a parent-infant program does not always occur as early as possible.

Guidelines for Developing Parent-Infant Programs. Parent-infant programs may be sponsored in any setting in which adequate personnel and services are available. Planning should include consideration of the following factors.

Personnel. The most effective early intervention programs are provided by a team of professionals. Because hearing impairment affects almost every aspect of a child's development, it is important that the team include professionals who are trained to provide guidance to parents regarding social, cognitive, educational, and language development. Under ordinary circumstances parents do not have to be concerned with the specifics of early child development; normal children learn about their world and the symbol systems that represent it without special assistance. They are accepted as normally functioning members of the family and generally receive the support necessary to develop adequately. Once a diagnosis of any handicapping condition is made, however, family life is affected to some extent. Anxiety and other emotions occur, along with uncertainty as to how to handle the child effectively. The emotional state of the parents influences their interaction with the child, often without their being aware of it. Constructive, early guidance by professionals can lessen emotional trauma and uncertainty and assist parents in the serious task that they face.

Several different types of professionals should be included in the parent-infant program staff. Assessment of hearing status is important for planning and should be accomplished by an *audiologist*. This team member is also responsible for selecting appropriate amplification, training parents to monitor it, and offering guidelines for its use at home. The audiologist should direct the auditory management of the child, including early auditory stimulation activities. Periodic reassessment of hearing status and hearing aids is also the responsibility of the audiologist.

The *psychologist* is an important member of the parent training team, responsible for measuring intellectual status and observing the child's behavior, personality traits, and perceptual-motor functioning. The psychologist can explain aspects of child development that enable parents to understand and manage specific behavior effectively. In addition, the psychologist may serve as a counselor, a parent group facilitator, and a source of emotional support for parents.

The third team member is an *educator of the deaf*. This person is knowledgeable about the educational problems associated with hearing loss and the methods and procedures appropriate for use with hearing impaired children. Responsibilities of the teacher include explaining the specific techniques to be used and training the parents to engage in readiness activities at home.

Although many teachers of the deaf are trained to teach speech, the *speech-language pathologist* has more extensive training regarding the speech mechanism, its functioning, and the various aspects of speech that may require remediation. This professional is also the most knowledgeable member of the team concerning the structure, acquisition, and disorders of language. The responsibility for helping parents understand the language learning task faced by hearing-impaired children and teaching them useful procedures for language stimulation at home falls to the speech-language pathologist.

Finally, the parent-infant team should include a *hearing-impaired adult,* at least as a consultant. This team member represents the consumer of services and provides the parents with input that cannot be provided by hearing team members. Questions concerning expectations for the future are often answered by the mere presence of the hearing-impaired adult. Considerable care must be taken in choosing the individual for this role. The purpose is to provide a realistic role model, neither too idealistic nor too fatalistic. The choice of the particular adult may vary according to the characteristics of the children enrolled in the program. Parents of children with moderate losses should be provided a different role model than parents of children with profound losses. It is not fair to either group to introduce a representative of the other as typical. The impact made by these adults on parents is often unpredictable, but if they are representative of the population being served, the program's credibility is enhanced. Reactions by the parents should be elicited and discussed, preferably by the psychologist.

Organization. Parent-infant programs may be ongoing and long term or brief, intensive sessions, depending on their location and purpose. When sponsored by a local educational agency or speech and hearing clinic in an urban community, the program may be maintained on a permanent basis. The number of families to be served usually remains steady as children move in and out of the program because of age, location of residence, and other factors. Under these circumstances, a staff may be employed exclusively for the parent-infant program. Group and individual work with children and parents, home visits, regular parent meetings, and a coordinated educational program from infancy to high school are possible. Each family may be served regularly, either once or twice a week or daily. The pace of the program can be tailored to the needs and characteristics of the families.

There are many advantages to an ongoing program. Information can be assimilated more easily by parents over time; misunderstandings can be identified and cleared up; support is available to parents whenever needed; periodic reassessment can be an integral part of the program; and educational methods are coordinated with those used in the nursery school, kindergarten and upper educational levels.

Many parents of hearing-impaired children do not live in urban communities or in areas that can support a permanent program. Parents in rural areas and small cities generally receive limited support services from few, if any, local professionals. In many ways, these parents have a greater need for a parent-infant program than those who have a variety of services readily available. Delay of diagnosis is often longer and the resulting frustration and anxiety are higher. These parents must also worry about finding services for their children once the diagnosis is made. They often have no idea where or how to begin.

To serve parents such as these, periodic, intensive parent-infant programs have been developed in some communities. The duration of these programs ranges from three days to two weeks. Families either commute or arrange temporary living accommodations for the required period. Activities are planned for several hours each day for parents and children. The pace is often rapid and the advantages mentioned for the permanent program are not possible. Nevertheless, a well-planned, short-term program can provide parents with considerable information, support, and resources that will enable them to make decisions about obtaining future services in other communities or to lobby for those services locally.

The same expertise is necessary for both ongoing and short-term programs. Because local services may not be comprehensive, children attending short-term programs often undergo complete assessment of their psychological and communicative status while their parents receive training in their management. Such a concentrated program requires a great deal of effort by all team members.

Goals. Early intervention programs are based on the following goals:

1. To make parents more aware of the nature and effects of hearing loss on communication, language, social, and academic skills and achievement.
2. To acquaint parents with remedial and educational procedures currently in use with hearing-impaired children.
3. To make parents aware of their roles in the child's education and development.
4. To train parents to stimulate children at home with language and auditory activities.
5. To make recommendations regarding future education and training, based on assessment data.
6. To help parents locate and contact appropriate training programs available to the family.
7. To increase parents' knowledge and effectiveness as consumers of professional and commercial services.
8. To help parents express and accept their feelings about having a hearing-impaired child.

Components. To accomplish the goals listed above, early intervention programs should include at least the following five program components.

1. Information giving. Didactic information should be given during relatively brief sessions. It is difficult to avoid giving too much information at one time during intensive parent-infant programs, but every effort should be made to space information-giving sessions carefully. Sessions should be topic oriented, organized around a few basic points, and include time for questions and discussion. Depending on the length of the program and the time available for these sessions, the following topics may be included:

(a) How language develops normally, including the role of audition.
(b) Modes of communication used by the hearing impaired (speech, lipreading, listening, manual communication).
(c) Specific effects of hearing loss on language and communication.
(d) Specific effects of hearing loss on educational achievement.
(e) Educational methods and settings in current use with hearing-impaired students and their relation to onset and degree of hearing loss.
(f) Use of amplification, including cost and care of the hearing aid, effects of noise on auditory reception, and limitations of hearing aids.
(g) Materials available for parents (books, games, toys).
(h) The ear and hearing loss.

2. Demonstration of activities for children and parents. Parents may observe demonstrations from another room, or they may be present during the activity. If children are seen individually, it is often effective for the parent to be present, observe an activity, then exchange roles with the clinician or teacher, who guides the parent through a similar activity. If children are seen in groups, time should be provided for individual practice sessions with each parent-child combination. Many parents interact nonverbally with their hearing-impaired children and must be encouraged to speak or make interesting noises associated with play activities.

Sometimes parent-child interaction reveals parental behavior that contributes to negativism or frustration on the part of the child. Of course, the reverse is also true. These patterns of interaction are usually well-established, and their nature may not be understood by the parents. It is helpful, therefore, to videotape parent-child interactions and use them as part of the parent training. The psychologist and parents may view the videotapes together, identifying and counting types of behavior that enhance or detract from good parent-child interactions and cooperation. A discussion of alternate behaviors often provides parents with insight into their habitual behavior and practical methods of avoiding excessive conflict and frustration.

During demonstrations and guided practice sessions, the clinician should reiterate the importance of auditory and language stimulation in the normal development of communication skills. Procedures should include techniques associated with the educational method recommended. For example, if the proposed educational program emphasizes lipreading skills, activities should include those designed to increase visual reception of speech. If manual communication is a part of the educational procedures to be employed, parents should be shown how to combine speech and sign effectively.

Activities carried out in the home are especially effective in training parents. The child's own toys and possessions constitute the materials used. Individual interests centered around daily routine ensure that stimulation will be relevant and therefore more likely to be attended to and remembered. The variety of opportunities for language stimulation within the average home can best be demonstrated in that setting. If the parent-infant program cannot occur in the home, the clinic rooms used should replicate a home setting, if possible. Otherwise, the therapy room should be made comfortable and inviting, designed to put parents and child at ease.

3. Assessment of the children. Evaluation should include intellectual, problem solving, and social assessment; investigation of communicative patterns and language status; hearing testing; hearing aid selection; and evaluation of aided auditory behavior. The results of all tests and observations should be explained to the parents in easily understood terms. When possible, demonstrations of hearing loss, benefits and limitations of hearing aids, language forms that can or cannot be comprehended by the child, or other aspects of child's status should be provided. Examples should be related to everyday activities. For example, a child with a 55-dB hearing loss will probably not hear speech at normal conversational levels unaided but should hear loud speech, car horns, loud thunder, a book falling from a table, and other moderately loud sounds. A child who appears to be comprehending single words, but not two- and three-word combinations, is more likely to understand the names of things and a few action verbs than adjectives or short phrases. The latter example can be related to giving directions or teaching new vocabulary. The more practical the examples, the more meaningful they will be to parents.

4. Discussion of the parents' feelings and concerns. Most professionals are comfortable with information giving, explanations, and demonstrations; they often limit parent contacts to these important activities. Equally important to the child's early development and the parents' successful handling of it, however, is the emotional status of parents. Their confidence in the professionals involved and the procedures employed significantly influences their subsequent behavior. Parental doubts, anxieties, resentment, confusion, and frustration will interfere with their relations with the child, other family members, and professionals to the detriment of the early training program. Therefore, an essential component of the parent-infant program is parent counseling as it relates to the parents' feelings about themselves, the child, and the tasks they are expected to accomplish. Parents of handicapped children undergo painful emotions as they react to the diagnosis of their children. The emotional stages common to this process include denial, anger, guilt, and frustration. A discussion of these emotions as evidenced by the parents of hearing-impaired children can be found in Chapter 11, along with some guidelines for parent counseling and support. The principles discussed there are applicable to professional-parent contacts in early intervention programs.

In brief, intensive programs there is never sufficient time to cover all the important pertinent information. It is tempting, therefore, to spend all available time imparting facts and advice. This temptation should be resisted firmly, and time should always be allocated for discussions of parental concerns. Some parents force such discussions by bringing up bothersome points repeatedly until the professionals deal with them. Parents rarely express spontaneously the emotion underlying the events they describe, but the incidents and the way they are reported offer evidence of strong feelings.

An example of this behavior follows. The young father of a 3-year-old, moderately hearing-impaired boy reported that he had known previously only one person with a hearing loss, a man who could not talk, was uneducated, and considered peculiar by the people in the town where he lived. He wandered the streets, lived on welfare, and frightened children. ''Of course, he could have had something else wrong with him too,'' the father said. The story was repeated without obvious emotion to every staff member involved in the program. The fact that the anecdote was told repeatedly, however, was evidence of the importance of its content to the father. He did not say, ''I am afraid that my son will turn out that way,'' but his anxiety was real, and he needed to express it. Careful probing in an unhurried parent counseling session gave him the opportunity to talk about his concerns. It also gave the counselor an opportunity to set his mind at ease, since his son's use of amplification and prognosis were excellent.

Another example of the manner in which concerns are expressed obliquely by parents is easier to recognize and interpret. A couple from a rural area reported that they suspected that their daughter was hearing impaired by the time the child was 1 year old. A trip to the pediatrician resulted in a casual disregard for their concerns. The experience was repeated six months later. They requested a referral to a specialist, were told one would be made, went home and waited. Two months later they inquired about the referral, were chastised by a nurse for being overanxious, and discovered that no appointment had been made. Two tries later, they saw a specialist, who referred them to a distant medical center. They were referred to a parent-infant program when the child was 3 years old. These parents felt angry, betrayed, hostile, and desperate. It took no urging for them to express these emotions, but they needed to release them before they could concentrate on planning and future activities.

5. Provision of written materials for home use. Regardless of whether the program is short and intensive or ongoing, allowing regular contacts between professionals and children, written materials should be provided to parents. It is not possible for parents to remember everything that is discussed during their visits with professionals; the major points need to be covered more than once. Books, pamphlets, and lists of material or activities can be used by parents at home to clear up facts, reinforce important points, or guide them in carrying out suggestions for stimulation in the home. Although some materials are available commercially, through the Alexander Graham Bell Association for the Deaf or the National Association of the Deaf, they tend to be biased in one direction or another regarding the educational methodology that should be employed. They should be screened carefully so that a balanced presentation can be given. When appropriate, providing materials that represent both points of view (oral-aural versus total communication) will encourage intelligent decision making on the part of parents. Their reactions to these two philosophies should be discussed openly. Chapter 10 includes a description of the educational methods currently in use with hearing-impaired children.

It is often most effective to develop written materials based on the particular early intervention program provided. Each topic of discussion during parent sessions can be included in a booklet, which reiterates important points that have been made. For example, facts about hearing aids, their care and use, and how to monitor them at home can be accompanied by the name(s) of the aid(s) recommended; the addresses of the dispenser and a repair service; and a list of items needed for hearing aid care (such as a battery tester, hearing aid stethescope, bag of silica gel); and an address where these and other items may be purchased. The more individual the materials, the more meaningful and useful they are likely to be to parents. It is not necessary that a different parent information booklet be written for each set of parents. Basic information remains the same for all, but details relevant to individual children can be inserted at appropriate points. Most important, this type of booklet can describe actual resources rather than general ones that may not be available locally.

Two of the most important sections of the parent booklet are those containing a listing of resource materials and specific activities to be carried out by parents. Appendix A at the end of this chapter contains a sample list of resource material for parents. Appendix B gives suggestions for auditory training activities in the home. Suggestions for other language stimulation activities can be found in Appendix C. These lists should not be considered complete. The suggestions provided in each of them should be supplemented by an audiologist, speech-language pathologist, or a teacher of the deaf who is familiar with the child and family involved.

GUIDELINES FOR CHOOSING EDUCATIONAL AND HABILITATIVE APPROACHES

Early intervention with children having hearing loss is important for two major reasons. First, it contributes to early language stimulation and growth, which may minimize the detrimental effects of hearing loss on language development and educational achievement. Second, it provides an opportunity to identify the remedial procedures most appropriate for individual children *before* they have experienced failure, resulting in frustration and discouragement for both parents and children.

The Problem

There are no simple guidelines for making educational recommendations. The major decision to be made for infants is whether or not the child should be exposed to some form of manual communication (sign language and fingerspelling) in addition to spoken language. The controversy surrounding the use of sign with hearing impaired children is surprisingly strong and emotional. A discussion of the major arguments for and against the use of manual communication is reviewed in Chapter 10. Simply stated, they revolve around the presumed effects of the use of manual communication on the development of speech, lipreading, and social and academic skills. Educators who advocate the use of sign language assert that no detrimental effects result from its use and that it enhances lipreading and academic and social development. Opponents of sign language believe that it will prevent the development of listening and speech skills and make it impossible for children who use it to function well among hearing people. The empirical data available tend to support the arguments of those who favor the use of manual communication, but research is hampered by the number and complexity of the factors that influence the development of hearing-impaired children.

Many children have sufficient residual hearing to allow them to learn language through the auditory system. In view of the dominant role played by audition in the natural development of language, these children should be encouraged to use their hearing maximally and to minimize the use of vision as a language receptor. Those children whose residual hearing is insufficient for speech recognition must rely on visual input as a major means of language reception. Therefore, they should be exposed to manual communication as soon as their hearing status is confirmed. The problem, of course, is to identify which children fall into each of the two groups early enough in life to avoid their spending the optimal language learning years in a program ill suited to their needs.

In the past this diagnostic problem was approached by placing all young children in oral-aural programs that included no use of sign. If they failed to make progress, transfer to another type of program was made, usually after several years. The argument that "every child should be given a chance to be oral" seemed persuasive, at least before data became available that demonstrated the importance to eventual language competence of the first three years of life. Increasing numbers of educators are unwilling routinely to risk the failure of large numbers of children, especially in view of the data supporting the use of sign as a viable receptive and expressive language mode. Moores (1978) sums the problem up neatly. "For children with whom it is difficult to predict a potential for developing language auditorily, educators have two alternatives. If they believe the base of language lies in the auditory mode and that visual presentation inhibits this, they will recommend a straight auditory emphasis. The auditory failure later would be programmed into multisensory systems. If they believe the base of language lies deeper, they would consider modality to be relatively unimportant and, when in doubt, would provide simultaneous auditory-visual presentation.

If the base of language really is auditory, the first approach would serve the auditory children educationally and lose the others. The second approach would lose all children. If the base of language goes deeper, the first alternative would save the auditory children and lose the others. The second alternative would save all children. Given the present state of knowledge, educators making decisions regarding methodology must do so in the face of great uncertainty. In thinking through the problem, they must be aware that if their orientation is wrong, their decisions will have lasting detrimental effects on children.''

Because the base of language is poorly understood and hotly debated, many educators do not feel comfortable making educational decisions without using more practical criteria. The development of pragmatic guidelines for choosing appropriate educational programs for children while they are very young is an urgent concern.

Criteria for Selecting Educational Procedures.

The controversy surrounding the use of manual communication has resulted in a dearth of objective criteria that can be used in choosing the most appropriate educational approach for a given child. Authors tend to come down on one side of the issue or the other. There are two exceptions to this general rule.

Liden and Kankkunen (1973) suggested that the difference between aided and unaided pure tone thresholds provides data that may aid in decisions concerning educational methodology. They described three types of test scores obtained for children. The first involved a large difference in thresholds across frequencies obtained in the unaided and aided conditions. Figure 5.2 shows an audiogram of this type. The second type reveals a large difference between aided and unaided thresholds at frequencies through 1000 Hz, as shown in Figure 5.3. The third type shows responses to sound only at frequencies below 500 Hz and reveals no difference between aided and unaided thresholds as shown in Figure 5.4. Liden and Kankkunen suggested that children whose test results are of the first type have considerable residual hearing and are excellent candidates for the oral-aural approach. Children in the second category also have usable residual hearing and are candidates for the oral-aural approach, but their language development will be slower and the eventual educational outcome is questionable. Children whose test results are of the third type probably receive only vibrotactile stimulation from sound; they are not candidates for the oral-aural method and should be exposed to manual communication from the outset of their education.

Northern and Downs (1974) suggested a deafness management quotient

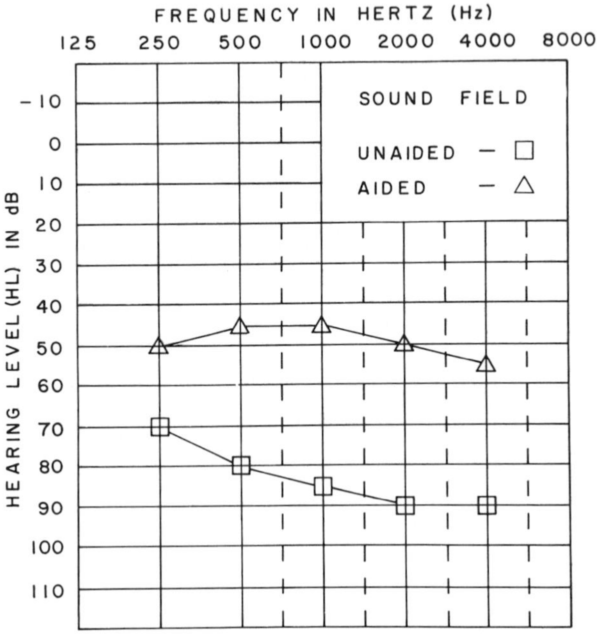

Figure 5.2. Audiogram depicting a large difference between unaided and aided thresholds for pure tones across frequencies from 250 to 4000 Hz.

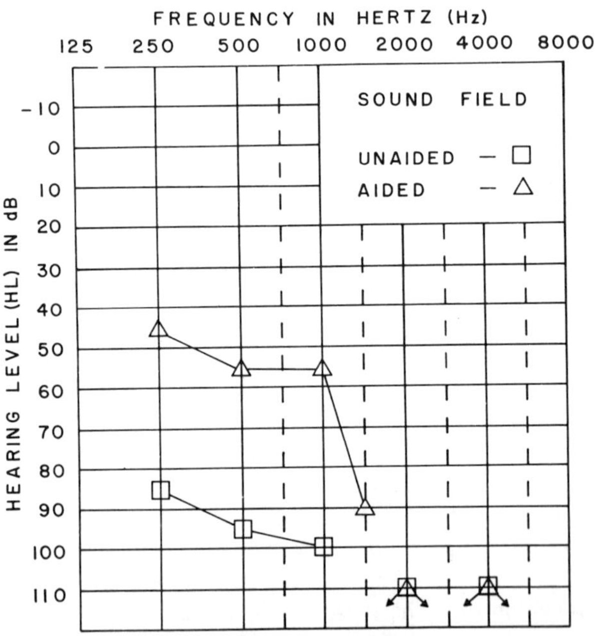

Figure 5.3. Audiogram depicting a large difference between unaided and aided thresholds for pure tones in the low and midfrequencies (250 to 1500 Hz).

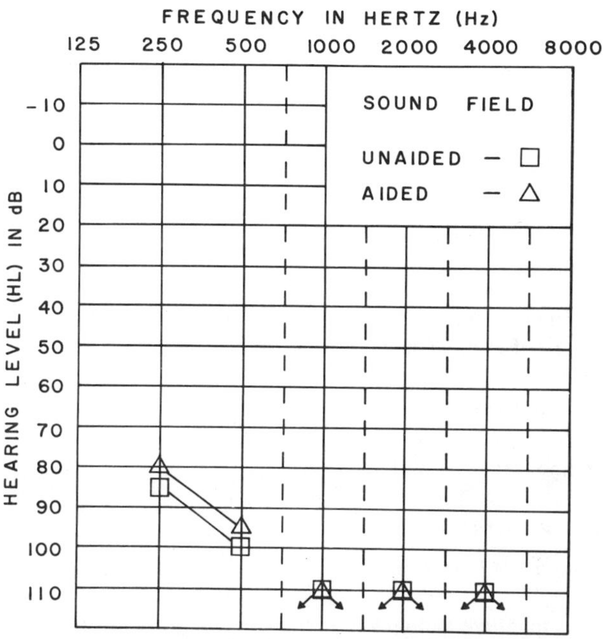

Figure 5.4. Audiogram depicting no difference between unaided and aided thresholds for pure tones.

(DMQ) as a point of departure for the development of placement guidelines. The DMQ consists of a 100-point scale based on five factors: residual hearing (30 points), central intactness (30 points), intellectual factors (20 points), family constellation (10 points), and socioeconomic status (10 points). Table 5.1 shows the DMQ rating criteria for each of the five factors. The scale was validated by applying it post hoc to young adults whose records and current functioning levels were available. The results indicated that a DMQ of 81 or greater was necessary for successful completion of an oral-aural education. Success was measured in terms of effective oral communication and preparation for a vocation or further education on completion of high school.

The DMQ represents a good first effort to quantify decision making. Unfortunately, some of its factors require subjective judgments outside the realm of many professionals. For example, judging a family's level of support to the child is difficult without considerable contact with the family over time. Socioeconomic status is often difficult to assess, and its effects are not well documented. Certain of the intellectual factors (such as perceptual dysfunction) may not lend themselves to diagnosis early in life. These disadvantages would be minor except for the skewed nature of the scores necessary for oral success. When a reduction of only 20 points on a 100-point scale indicates a poor prognosis for achievement in one type of

Table 5.1 Suggested Scale for Direction of Deafness Management Quotient (DMQ)—Total: 100 Points

Residual Hearing: 30 Points Possible

0 = no true hearing
10 = 250–500 < 100 dB
20 = 250–500–1000 < 100 dB
30 = 2000 < 100 dB

Central Intactness: 30 Points Possible

0 = diagnosis of brain damage
10 = known history of events conducive to birth defects
20 = perceptual dysfunction
30 = intact central processing

Intellectual Factors: 20 Points Possible

0 = MR < 85 IQ
10 = average > 85 − 100 IQ
20 = above average: > 100 IQ

Family Constellation: 10 Points Possible

0 = no support
10 = completely supportive and understanding

Socioeconomic: 10 Points Possible

0 = substandard
10 = completely adequate

Auditory program leading to oral: 81–100 points

Total communicative program: 0–80 points

Reprinted with permission from J. Northern and M. Downs, *Hearing in Children,* The Williams and Wilkins Company (1974).

program, there is little margin for error. Indeed, this is the point: there is little margin for error with severely to profoundly hearing-impaired children. Only those with adequate residual hearing, intact central processes, good intellect, and strong family support will be able to succeed in programs that do not supplement auditory input with nonambiguous visual symbols, such as sign.

The DMQ is not designed for use with children whose hearing losses are moderate or severe, rather than profound, but it does help focus attention on the factors that are important to any hearing-impaired child's success. The following observations and guidelines are offered as a supplement to the DMQ.

Residual Hearing. Generally the child with the most residual hearing is the best candidate for an oral-aural approach. Professionals disagree, however, as to how much residual hearing is necessary for language to be learned efficiently through the auditory system. The disagreement is based not only on philosophical differences and different interpretations of the terms "residual hearing" and "language learning," but on the heterogeneity of hearing-impaired children. Audiograms alone cannot be used to predict the successful use of hearing. Hearing for speech, including the ability to discriminate speech sounds, is more important than pure tone thresholds and is sometimes poorly related to them. Unfortunately, it is difficult to test speech perception skills in children before they have been exposed to auditory stimuli for a period of time.

Two promising approaches to the development of speech discrimination testing procedures for young children are underway. Erber and Alencewicz (1976) described a word-discrimination test for use with young children that uses monosyllabic, spondaic, and trochaic words. The test is designed to identify children who respond to auditory presentations by "hearing" and those who respond by "feeling." Children who rely on tactile sensation to interpret sound vibration receive different kinds of information from the spoken word than those who receive and process words auditorily. If the dominant process can be established for each child, educational programming can be based on objective data. The word discrimination task cannot be administered to children, however, until they are familiar with the words in the test. At the present time, the task is useful only with children who are 3 to 4 years old and who have been enrolled in educational programs for some time. The test is not helpful, therefore, in making initial educational placement decisions.

Eilers, Wilson, and Moore (1977) studied speech perception in infants and toddlers using a conditioned response to a change in phoneme perception. When presented with spoken phonemes at a repetition rate of one per second, normally hearing infants can be trained to respond quickly to a shift from one phoneme to another. Data from hearing-impaired children have not yet been reported, but they would provide important information regarding the relation of speech perception to hearing loss characteristics. The ability to detect differences between phonemes or syllables would be evidence of useful residual hearing for speech discrimination. Its absence would suggest caution in relying on audition as the primary input system for educational purposes.

In spite of the variability among children, there is evidence that the ability to identify words auditorily is related to the degree of hearing loss as measured by pure tones. Erber (1974) presented spondee words to hearing-impaired children whose pure tone averages ranged from 52 to 127 dB (ANSI, 1969). He reported that children tended to score high (70 percent or better) or low (below 30 percent). The 500–1000-2000 Hz pure tone average was a good predictor of the ability to recognize spondee words auditorily. Children whose hearing thresholds were less than 85 dB scored high; children whose thresholds were 100 dB or more scored low. Children whose hearing losses fell between 85 and 100 dB exhibited a wide range of scores and predictability was poor.

These data suggest that pure tone thresholds can be used as gross estimates of the usefulness of a child's residual hearing for speech recognition through audition. Because pure tone data are obtainable from very young children, tentative decisions regarding appropriate educational methods can be made early. Generally speaking, children whose hearing thresholds are better than 85 dB should receive maximal auditory stimulation and be monitored carefully for evidence that an auditory-verbal feedback loop is being established. The acoustic information contained in the speech signal should be useful to these children, especially if they have hearing across a broad range of frequencies. As a result, they will be able to make use of voicing, manner, nasal, and place information as described in Chapter 2. If they are successful in learning to differentiate among phonemes the use of sign will probably not be necessary for adequate development of language and academic skills.

Children whose hearing losses are greater than 100 dB, especially those who have residual hearing for only a restricted range of frequencies (a ''corner'' audiogram, for example) should be stimulated with speech and sign simultaneously. These children will not be able to use place information for speech perception and will even be severely limited in the amount of low-frequency information that can be used for speech perception. They will require visual information in some form as a supplement to audition; sign provides the least ambiguous form of visual information available, but other visual clues will also be helpful, such as fingerspelling, cues, or gestures.

Because of the importance of early language stimulation and the absence of evidence that sign is detrimental, children whose hearing losses fall into the ''gray area'' of 85 to 100 dB should be exposed to both speech and sign. Hearing losses of this magnitude will affect the perception of manner and place information as discussed in Chapter 2. Because the same degree of hearing loss does not affect people the same way, some of these children will be able to establish effective auditory-verbal feedback loops while others will not. It makes more sense to provide both auditory and visual information to such children than to take a chance on questionable auditory abilities.

Careful monitoring of all children is important; modifications in the procedures employed should be made when they seem warranted.

Intelligence. Data are not available that relate intelligence directly to achievement in different types of educational programs. Experience indicates, however, that intelligence is more of a factor in achievement in auditory programs than in total communication programs. This observation is supported by logic. Because auditory programs provide less redundancy and fewer nonambiguous message cues, children must be able to synthesize information, predict missing data from those available, and make decisions based on less sensory information than that provided by total communication programs. Well-developed cognitive processes will assist in the task; without them, progress may be slow and achievement reduced.

Many of the schools for the deaf that advocate an auditory approach to education are private institutions. As a result, the children accepted as students are screened regarding hearing status, intelligence and family constellation. It is no accident that the mean IQ of children in classes within private schools is frequently above average, in spite of the fact that hearing-impaired children often score poorly on intelligence tests and that deafness is associated with a number of other handicapping conditions that affect intellectual functioning.

The influence of intelligence on language development and educational achievement is confounded with other factors, but it is an appropriate criterion to apply when choosing an educational program for a child or a child for an educational program. Other things being equal, children whose intellectual functioning is below average should be enrolled in programs that provide a maximum of language stimulation through all sensory systems and a minimum of ambiguity. Like all children, they will rely on the most meaningful information available. The increased redundancy provided by multisensory input simply allows them more "looks" at the information, making processing easier and more complete.

Other Handicapping Conditions. Multiply handicapped children present a difficult educational task. Regardless of the nature of the handicap in addition to hearing loss, it will usually affect the child's experiences in some limiting way. The limitations imposed will help determine the choice of educational program to be employed. Orthopedically handicapped children may not have free use of their hands; oral communication or use of a language board may be most expedient and the only feasible means of language expression. Conditions affecting the mobility of the articulators (dysarthria) may preclude speech production but leave speech reception relatively unaffected. Sign or some other visual output may be necessary for expression but not for reception. Visual defects may preclude the use of fine visual distinctions (as in lipreading); total blindness will preclude visual input of any kind. Auditory or tactile information must be maximized for children thus affected.

Family Considerations. The most commonly used measure of family status is an estimate of socioeconomic standing. Although important in a general sense, the economic status of a family is not a good indicator of the level of emotional support that will be available to the child. Several other factors are more important. These include marriage stability; relationships among parents, parents and children, siblings, parents and extended family, and parents and the community; attitude of the family toward educational institutions; ability of the parents to work through their emotional reactions to the child's hearing loss; employment status of the mother; and levels of expectation parents hold for their children. For single parent families, questions surrounding employment conditions and adjustment to the single state are important.

Although there are exceptions, parents who have serious life problems unrelated to the hearing-impaired child generally will spend less time stimulating the child and will be less involved in the educational process. The burden of training rests primarily on professionals under these circumstances. Follow-up work at home may be sporadic and tentative, so the educational procedures employed probably should not depend heavily on parental participation. Placing the responsibility for success on parental effort is likely to result in guilt or hostility on the part of parents and frustration on the part of the professionals. Early recognition of family problems that may reduce the effectiveness of home-based activities may prevent inappropriate placement and reduced success for the child.

Any educational program is more effective if parents and other family members remain actively involved. Failure to do so results in reduced input to the child and fewer learning experiences. It is difficult to estimate which type of program is most severely affected by lack of parental involvement. Children in total communication programs progress most rapidly when their parents learn sign and use it consistently in conjunction with speech (Schlesinger and Meadow, 1972). Children in auditory programs benefit most from frequent, meaningful auditory stimulation at home, in the park, at the store, and so on (Pollack, 1970). Involvement of families may be a more important factor in decisions of residential versus local placement than in the matter of educational philosophy. Nevertheless, an awareness of the probable contribution to be made by given family members should be helpful to professionals in setting goals for specific children. At the least, it should prevent the establishment of unrealistic objectives and the development of unnecessary hostility between parent and professional that will be detrimental to any program.

Type of Program Available Locally. A pragmatic consideration in making recommendations for future educational programming concerns the nature of the facilities available in the family's home community. A continuum of services involving a choice of educational approaches is desirable for any community but exists in only a few. Small communities usually lack the resources to provide a variety of services, and many large communities choose to limit the existing programs to one educational philosophy. Under these circumstances, professionals must be sensitive to both the needs of the child and the reality of the situation.

For borderline children whose chances of success in either oral-aural or total communication programs are reasonable, referrals to existing local programs of either type can be made comfortably, as long as there are provisions for close follow-up and reevaluation. For children for whom an oral-aural approach seems to be clearly the method of choice, the advantages of such a program should be outlined and suggestions for determining how well audition is being stimulated in the local program should be given to parents. The parents of profoundly hearing-impaired children, who appear to need manual communication as an adjunct to spoken language, should be counseled regarding these needs and suggestions given for determining whether or not progress is occurring in programs that do not provide for them. In any event, frequent reevaluation is necessary to determine the effectiveness of the procedures being used.

It is important that professionals avoid prejudicing parents against existing local programs. The counseling task is delicate; sufficient information about the child's status and needs must be provided to allow intelligent decision making without excessive bias. Some children cannot be served appropriately within the local community because of insufficient resources. Professionals have an obligation to help parents understand this reality, but their input must be *based on objective data and experiences with the program in question*. It is difficult enough for parents to contend with a diagnosis of hearing loss and the associated decisions that must be made, without their being prejudiced against the local program at the outset of the child's training.

Teaching parents to be evaluators of their children's progress will contribute more to successful education than lectures for or against any educational philosophy. When parents have little choice in where they are located, and available programming is not appropriate for their child's needs, they must be given support and encouragement as they gradually come to realize that local education is not possible for the child. Some time may be lost in such cases, but the eventual resolution will be more acceptable to parents and therefore more beneficial to the child. In some communities changes in educational philosophy and programming have occurred as a result of unsuccessful attempts to serve some children. Initial willingness on the part of parents to cooperate rather than criticize is an effective way to foster change.

When relocation seems advisable and parents are able to manage it, they should be encouraged to visit other programs that appear appropriate and to compare them to the local one. The final decision must be made by parents with assistance from professionals. Dogmatic decisions by professionals are presumptuous and often detrimental to the child and the family.

REFERENCES

Balow, I. and Brill, R., An evaluation of reading and academic levels of sixteen graduating classes of the California School for the Deaf, *Volta Rev.*, 77, 255–266, 1975.

Berg, F. and Fletcher, S., *The Hard of Hearing Child, Clinical and Educational Management*. New York: Grune and Stratton, 1970.

Downs, M., The establishment of hearing aid use: A program for parents, *MAICO Audiol. Library Series*, 4, 1967(b).

Eagles, E., Wishik, S., Doerfler, L., Melnick, W., and Levine, H., Hearing sensitivity and related factors in children, *Laryngoscope*, Special Monograph, 1963.

Eilers, R., Wilson, W., and Moore, J., Developmental changes in speech discrimination in infants, *J. Speech Hearing Res.*, 20, 766–780, 1977.

Erber, N., Pure-tone thresholds and word-recognition abilities of hearing-impaired children, *J. Speech Hearing Res.*, 17, 194–202, 1974.

Erber, N. and Alencewicz, C., Audiologic evaluation of deaf children, *J. Speech Hearing Dis.*, 41, 256–267, 1976.

Harris, G., *Language for the Preschool Deaf Child*. New York: Grune and Stratton, 1963.

Holm, V. and Kunze, L., Effect of chronic otitis media on language and speech development, *Pediatrics*, 43, 833-839, 1969.

Liden, G. and Kankkunen, A., Hearing aid procedures in young deaf and hard of hearing children, *Scandinavian Audiology Suppl.*, 47-54, 1973.

Ling, D., Rehabilitation of cases with deafness secondary to otitis media. In A. Glorig (Ed.), *Otitis Media*. Springfield, IL: Charles C Thomas, 1969.

Madell, J., Hearing aid evaluation procedures with children. In M. Rubin (Ed.), *Hearing Aids: Current Developments and Concepts*. Baltimore: University Park Press, 1976.

Matkin, N., Hearing aids for children. In W. Hodgson and P. Skinner (Eds.), *Hearing Aid Assessment and Use in Audiologic Habilitation*. Baltimore: Williams and Wilkins Co., 1977.

Moores, D., *Educating the Deaf: Psychology, Principles, and Practices*. Boston: Houghton Mifflin, 1978.

Needleman, H., Effects of hearing loss from early recurrent otitis media on speech and language development. In B. Jaffe (Ed.), *Hearing Loss in Children*. Baltimore: University Park Press, 1977.

Northern, J. and Downs, M., *Hearing in Children*. Baltimore: Williams and Wilkins Co., 1974.

Pollack, D., *Educational Audiology for the Limited Hearing Infant*. Springfield, IL: Charles C Thomas, 1970.

Quigley, S. and Thomure, R., *Some Effects of a Hearing Impairment on School Performance*. Urbana: Institute of Research on Exceptional Children, University of Illinois, 1968.

Rawlings, B. and Trybus, R., Personnel, facilities, and services available in schools and classes for hearing impaired children in the United States, *Amer. Ann. Deaf*, 123, 99-114, 1978.

Ross, M., Hearing aid selection for preverbal hearing impaired children. In M. Pollack (Ed.), *Amplification for the Hearing Impaired*. New York: Grune and Stratton, 1975.

Ross, M. and Lerman, J., Hearing aid usage and its effect upon residual hearing: A review of the literature and an investigation, *Arch. Otolaryngol.*, 86, 57-62, 1967.

Schlesinger, H. and Meadow, K., *Sound and Sign: Childhood Deafness and Mental Health*. Berkeley: University of California Press, 1972.

John Tracy Correspondence Course for Parents of Preschool Deaf Children. Los Angeles: John Tracy Clinic, 1968.

Wedenberg, E., Experience from thirty years, auditory training, *Volta Rev.*, 69, 588-594, 1967.

Whetnall, E. and Fry, D., *The Deaf Child*. Springfield, IL: Charles C Thomas, 1964.

APPENDIX A
Resource Materials for Parents

ORGANIZATIONS

Alexander Graham Bell Association for the Deaf
1537 25th Street, N.W.
Washington, D.C. 20007

American Speech-Language-Hearing Association
10801 Rockville Pike
Rockville, MD 20852

International Association of Parents of the Deaf
814 Thayer Street
Silver Spring, MD 20900

John Tracy Clinic
806 West Adams Boulevard
Los Angeles, CA 90007

National Association of the Deaf
814 Thayer Street
Silver Spring, MD 20900

BOOKS

Jean Simple,
Hearing Impaired Preschool Child–
A Book for Parents
Charles C. Thomas, Springfield, IL, 1970, pp. 36–84.

Gives two series of lesson plans for the preschool child to work on speech and language. The lessons are simple and thoroughly explained. They are designed for a child one year and older. Appendix A gives a list of reading materials and other sources of ideas. Appendix B lists children's books by age level which would be helpful in training session. Appendix C gives an outline for a program in auditory training for the preschool child.

What's Its Name?
Alexander Graham Bell Association
1537 25th Street, N. W.
Washington, D. C. 20007

A workbook designed for parents and teachers of hearing-impaired children that stresses auditory training. It contains materials ranging from pictures of one-syllable words to nursery rhymes.

Sister James Lorene Hogan
The ABC's of Auditory Training
St. Joseph's Institute for the Deaf
1483 82nd Boulevard
St. Louis, MO

A classroom manual for ages 5 to 9; discusses the ability of deaf children to respond to sound.

Edgar G. Lowell and Marguerite Stoner
Play It By Ear
Educational Materials Dept.
John Tracy Clinic
806 West Adams Boulevard
Los Angeles, CA 90007

Auditory training games for young deaf and hard-of-hearing children ($3.50).

Parent Education Film Series
Educational Materials Dept.
John Tracy Clinic
806 West Adams Boulevard
Los Angeles, CA 90007

Parent attitudes and communication for deaf children. Free to parent groups.

Baby's 1st Total Communication Book, 1974.
Center for Deafness
600 Waukegan Road
Glenview, IL 60025
Book I, Food & Clothing $3.50
Book II, Toys & Animals $3.50
Auditory Tapes—$5 per set
Teacher's Guide—$7.50
Student Handbook
1. Beginners (I & II) $2.75
2. Intermediate (I & II) $2.75

Uses signs and fingerspelling and contains 40 lessons of vocabulary with practice sentences—supplementary teacher guide, student handbook and cassette tapes available.

Consonant Picture Cards
Ideal School Supply Co.
Oak Lawn, IL 60453

Good for articulation and language work, they have clear pictures for each consonant sound and are color coded so that they can be sorted according to initial or final consonant. These picture cards can be used to help a child associate the sounds of consonants with their written symbols.

Joan M. Sayre,
Helping the Child to Listen and Talk—Suggestions for Parents and Teachers
The Interstate Printers & Publishers, Inc.
Danville, IL 61832

A booklet of suggestions and illustrations presented to help give teachers and parents a better understanding of the child with a speech and/or hearing problem. Provides suggestions for ways to stimulate the child to listen and speak at home and at school.

The Family Circus (for developing thinking skills). Developed by
Sister Mary Walter, O.S.F., Ed. M.
St. John's School for the Deaf
3680 S. Kinnickinnic Avenue
Milwaukee, WI 33207

Uses cartoons and captions to introduce various questions gradually. Part I includes sentence construction; Part 2 develops thinking skills through the use of "why" questions. Thinking skills are developed on three levels:

1. Studying the picture for literal facts.

2. Interpreting the cartoon; relationships, inferences, outcome.
3. Critical thinking; judgments, imagining, sensing emotions.

Recipes for Fun
Cole, Haas, Heller, & Weinberger, 1970
Par Project
576 Hill Terrace
Winnetka, IL 60093

Easy activities to do at home, using odds and ends for games of "make believe, making things, party fun, exploring, learning games, music and rhythm."

Communication with the Deaf,
Powrie Doctor, Ed.
American Annals of the Deaf
5034 Wisconsin Avenue, N. W.
Washington, D. C. 20016

A discussion of various modes of communication and teaching procedures used with deaf children.

TOY CATALOGUES
(WRITE TO THE FOLLOWING)

Community Playthings
Rifton NY 12471

Judy Company
310 N. Second Street
Minneapolis, MN 55401

Playskool Manufacturing
3720 North Kedzie
Chicago, IL 50518

Creative Playthings
P. O. Box 1100
Princeton, NJ 08540

Childcraft
155 East 23rd Street
New York, NY 10010

Creative Playthings, Western Division
5757 West Century Boulevard
Los Angeles, CA 90045

Fisher Price Toys, Inc.
606 Girard Avenue, East
East Aurora, NY 14052

Childhood Guidance Products, Inc.
200 Fifth Avenue
New York, NY 10010

APPENDIX B
Suggestions for Auditory Stimulation Activities

AWARENESS OF SOUND

1. Call attention to sounds around the house, including the vacuum cleaner, running water, the telephone, the washing machine, and other applicances. Identify each sound and react to it by pointing to your ears, smiling, "listening," and so on. Place the child near the sound and encourage similar reactions.

2. Associate sounds with animals. This can be done first with picture books (you imitate animal sounds) and later with real animals the child encounters.

3. Use music and noisemakers to illustrate the presence and absence of sound. Encourage the child to clap, sway, or march when the music is "on," to stop when it is "off."

LOCALIZATION OF SOUND

1. Have someone call the child's name from one side of the head. Turn the child's head to help him or her to locate the sound.

2. Activate musical toys and have the child locate them in the room. Music boxes, radios, alarm clocks, and wind-up toys can be used for this activity.

3. Play hide and seek with family members. Using a blindfold, have the child locate someone who is calling his or her name repeatedly.

IDENTIFICATION AND DISCRIMINATION OF SOUND

1. Using noisemakers or toys that make different sounds, play a game in which the adult activates a single toy and the child activates and listens to the same toy. When two toys have been sounded repeatedly, arrange them behind the child's back, activate one and have him or her turn around and choose it from the group of toys. This can be done also with animal sounds, musical instruments, sounds of common objects in the home (alarm clock, pot and spoon, kitchen timer, for example) and speech (using the names of toys or objects). When the child can identify the source of the sound consistently, gradually add other items to the game.

2. Using the activity described above, gradually increase the distance between the noise sources and the child to encourage listening at a distance.

IMITATION OF SOUND

1. Play games with the child that involve the repetition of a sound, word, or phrase. Encourage imitation of the sound by taking turns in the game. For example, place a toy on the high-chair tray or table in front of the child. Push it off onto the floor, saying "Uh-oh" with exaggerated inflection. Replace the toy and repeat the sequence. This basic format can be applied to many activities, such as stationery hide and seek (saying "Peek-a-boo" or "Where's (Name) ? There she is," as you cover and uncover your eyes).

2. Encourage active play with toys that can be associated with a given sound. Dollhouse activities can start with the doorbell, "Ding-Dong," and "Who's there?" Airplane, car, and animal sounds can be made by adult and child as they manipulate these and other toy objects. Specific sounds can be stimulated well in play activities. For example, the train goes "ch-ch-ch," the popcorn goes "p-p-p," and an engine goes "mmmmm."

APPENDIX C
Suggestions for Language Stimulation Activities

1. Use story books with clear pictures and simple text. Identify the characters and their actions in simple terms. ''This is Mary. This is Bob. Mary is crying. Why is she crying? She is hurt.'' Identify animals by name and the sound they produce. Encourage the child to imitate the animal's actions and sounds and to associate them with each animal name.

2. Talk about activities as you do them in the home, at the store, and in the car. Name the objects and actions involved. ''I'm setting the table. This is a fork. Put the plate here,'' and so on.

3. Teach nursery rhymes or finger plays with distinct rhythms and act them out as you say them.

4. When dressing the child, name the clothes, body parts, and actions involved. ''Here is your sock. Put the sock on your foot. The sock is on your foot.''

5. Identify body parts. ''Where is your nose? Here it is.''

CHAPTER 6

Language and Speech Characteristics

TSA (Technical Sythetic Assessment Test)
Peobody Language Assessment Test
Distar Language Series
Apple Tree Language Series

I. Principles of Language Learning

- **A.** Role of Audition in Learning Communicative Behavior
- **B.** Language Acquisition as a Remedial Approach

II. Language Development and Use

- **A.** Knowledge of Vocabulary and Word Class Usage
- **B.** Knowledge of Grammar

III. Speech Characteristics

- **A.** Effects of Mild to Moderate Hearing Impairment on Speech
- **B.** Effects of Severe to Profound Hearing Impairment on Speech
- **C.** Intelligibility

Language represents the means by which humans communicate all but the simplest messages to each other. It is such a natural part of human behavior and is learned so early in life by the vast majority of humans that it is often taken completely for granted.

PRINCIPLES OF LANGUAGE LEARNING

Linguists have theorized that the capacity for learning language is an innate human trait (Lenneberg, 1967), one that exists in all persons regardless of their actual ability to use language in overt ways. Studies of language develoment in young children (Brown and Bellugi, 1964; Braine, 1963; Ervin, 1964) have revealed the following principles of language acquisition:

1. Although the expression of language through spontaneous speech begins at approximately one year of age, much knowledge about language, including some of its prosodic features, is learned prior to the utterance of the first "words." To some extent, comprehension of linguistic components occurs prior to expression of the same elements.
2. Children's first utterances consist of a limited number of word classes, which are combined in unique ways to form short sentences.
3. Young children do not appear to be imitating adult grammar. Instead they seem to be testing hypotheses about relations between grammatical constituents such as subjects, predicates, objects, and others. As their utterances are reinforced by adult speakers, they gradually discard hypotheses that do not match the adult grammar of the language being learned.
4. The indispensable ingredient in language performance is adequate exposure to a corpus of language against which to test hypotheses. Parental speech is the usual source of exposure and, for hearing children, no special precautions must be taken to provide adequate exposure.
5. Language learning proceeds rapidly during the first few years of life. There is evidence that the capacity to acquire language may peak between the ages of 2 to 4 years (Lenneberg, 1967). Children who are learning normally appear to have learned all of the basic rules of language structure prior to age 4½ or 5 (Berko, 1958; Menyuk, 1969). Beyond that age, language learning consists of refinements of the basic rules. Furthermore, there is reason to believe that the capacity to learn a first language efficiently diminishes appreciably by adolescence (Lenneberg, 1967; Menyuk, 1969).
6. The necessary exposure to parental language normally occurs through the auditory system. Infants are bathed in a variety of sounds from birth, spoken language being one of them. Babies do not have to "listen" for exposure to occur; much general knowledge is absorbed without obvious effort on the child's part.

The foregoing principles represent a very limited synopsis of normal language learning; it is beyond the scope of this book to discuss in depth the acquisition of language by children. The reader is encouraged to pursue such knowledge, however, because an understanding of language learning in normally hearing children forms a basis for understanding the language deficits experienced by hearing-impaired children.

Role of Audition in Learning Communicative Behavior

In light of the principles listed above, it is obvious that hearing-impaired children run the risk of failing to learn language at the normal time or rate, because the learning of language is primarily an auditory event. Its common code is composed of sounds that vary in minute and important ways and of combinations of sounds into units of varying size (syllables, words, and phrases). These units are grouped into patterns associated with differing ways of expressing meaning (various sentence structures). Overlaid on the sound and sound combinations that form the basis of a spoken language are the prosodic features that provide subtle clues to shades of meaning, the emotional state of the speaker, and the importance of the message to be delivered. In some cases prosodic features of stress and timing are used to clear up ambiguities between utterances that are identical with regard to the sounds they contain. For example, the sentence "They gave her baby food," will be interpreted differently when stress is placed on the words "baby" as opposed to "food" or when "food" is preceded by a slight pause. Spoken language is a sequential event; sounds are produced rapidly and their correct sequencing is essential to meaning. The difference between "cats" and "cast" is one of minor sequencing, but the difference in meaning is profound. The human auditory system receives and analyzes sequences of sounds quickly and accurately. Consequently, spoken language and audition are inextricably bound together; the facile learning of the former is dependent on the latter.

Not only do infants *hear* spoken language from birth, there is growing evidence that they can discriminate auditorily among speech sounds immediately following birth (Eimas, 1975). Within a few months an infant is already a sophisticated listener who receives and uses auditory information as an essential part of growth and development. As an example, consider the normal infant who wakens from sleep and begins to fret as a reaction to hunger. As the mother prepares the feedings, she makes certain sounds, some of them caused by objects such as bottles and pans, and others produced by the mother herself. Soothing statements ("Hush, hush, Mommy's coming") occur, and the sound of her footsteps as they move toward the baby's crib are available for interpretation by the infant. Within a short time after birth, infants react to the sounds of approaching footsteps and increasing loudness of the voice by decreasing crying behavior. Within a few months, they learn to turn to face the door; when older they stand and reach out before the mother is visible to them. Thus the infant learns to anticipate events on the basis of auditory information and previous experience. A sense of timing is developed and an orderliness of events is established, primarily as a result of audition.

As the child grows older and language develops, relatively subtle knowledge is obtained along with the growth of vocabulary and grammar that we normally associate with language learning. Features such as sarcasm, which often involves reversal of meaning signaled by tone of voice and stress patterns, are almost entirely auditory in nature. (For example, "I like that," spoken with emphasis on the final word, which has a rising and then falling inflection, carries anything but approval as a message.) Comprehension of puns is dependent upon subtle shifts in sound combinations or an understanding of multiple meanings of words. Each of these high-level linguistic activities is dependent on hearing as a foundation for its development.

More important to the development of well-adjusted children is the early learning of the mores and customs associated with the society in which they live. Knowledge of acceptable behavior, especially verbal behavior, is learned by *overhearing* important interchanges between adults as much as by individual experience. Children learn not to repeat gossip to the person discussed, not to ask adults their age, not to use profanity or obscenity under certain circumstances, how to make up excuses to avoid unpleasant tasks ("Mabel, I'd love to go to the lecture with you but I have a terrible headache tonight"), how to say one thing and mean another ("I don't really want to play golf, dear, but I have to please the boss") and so on.

While we may react negatively to the idea of "teaching" children such behavior, it is necessary for smooth acceptance into society. Try to imagine a young person who is totally honest and says what is thought all the time. ("My, Mrs. Jones, you look older every time I see you. Are you sick?" or "I don't want to go to the lecture with you, Mabel; you bore me"). While there are some people who can and do make such statements regularly, the general population operates by a set of unwritten, unspoken guidelines for "polite" behavior, most of which were learned by children through close observation of adult interactions.

The degree to which the types of linguistic knowledge described above are available to hearing-impaired children depends to a large extent on the status of their individual auditory systems. The more severe the hearing loss and the earlier the onset of hearing impairment, the more reduction there is in exposure to the corpus of language surrounding them. If the hearing loss is not identified early, the optimal time for learning language may be past before habilitative procedures, including amplification, are provided. In cases of moderate-to-profound hearing loss identified after the age of 12 to 18 months, the language deficit is probably already severe. When we consider that a hearing baby "listens" to parental speech for about a year before producing the first words, moves rapidly through the production of simple sentences before the age of 2, and incorporates such linguistic rules as the formation of plurals, possessives, verb tenses, use of proper pronouns, compound and complex sentence structures, and question formations, into spontaneous speech patterns by the age of 5, the range of potential language problems of hearing-impaired children becomes clear.

In fact, the most obvious difference between young children who hear normally and those who do not is their development of speech and language skills. Speech is only one form of language, but it is the most obvious one. It is not unusual for family members to become suspicious of hearing loss in children initially because of their failure to speak at the expected age. While absent or disordered speech is the most noticeable of the possible language deficits, it is not the most important in terms of assessment and habilitation of language disorders in hearing-impaired children. Because children generally comprehend a given linguistic component before they are able to express it spontaneously, the hearing-impaired child's grasp of linguistic elements and rules must be measured independently of the ability to express them through speech. Many deaf children exhibit functional knowledge and use of concepts and grammatical relations through gestures, for example, even though they give no evidence of being able to comprehend or produce spoken language. On the other hand, understanding the speech of others and producing intelligible speech themselves are important skills for hearing-impaired children to master. When well developed, these skills allow for greater ease of communication with peers, family members, teachers, and other persons with whom they come in contact.

Communication with others in some form is essential to every aspect of human life. Because communication is based on the use of codes or symbol systems (i.e., language), language knowledge and use form the basis of most human endeavor. Development to self-concept and an understanding of the relationship between the self and the environment are dependent on communicative interaction within the environment. Educational achievement is totally language based. Vocational achievement depends on the educational level attained and the development of the ability to work with and for others. It is virtually impossible to overemphasize the importance of language skills to the development of individuals and thus to the development of hearing-impaired individuals.

Language Acquisition as a Remedial Approach

The development of language skills should constitute the major purpose and the focus of habilitation of hearing-impaired children. This task would be much easier if all hearing-impaired children exhibited similar well-defined language deficits and responded equally well to a standard set of habilitative procedures. Unfortunately, the hearing-impaired children who require remedial services are an incredibly heterogenous group. Their hearing losses range from mild (15 dB HL) to profound (no measurable hearing) and may be conductive or sensorineural. Their hearing losses may have been discovered in infancy or after they have failed one or more grades in school. They may or may not wear amplification. If they do, it may have been selected by one of a variety of persons on the basis of extensive or little assessment of hearing. The amplification worn may or may not be adequate or functional. The degree of hearing loss may remain constant or fluctuate periodically. The pure-tone threshold configuration varies from child to child. A given child's family may be knowledgeable and supportive or disinterested and confused. Hearing-impaired children may have additional handicapping conditions or they may have "simple" hearing loss. They may have received extensive habilitation in the past or they may have received none at all. In short, hearing-impaired children present the clinician with as wide a variety of characteristics as can be imagined. Planning a program for them is a challenge and must be based on an individualized approach.

Information concerning language development in hearing-impaired children is much more available for those classified as deaf than for those with mild or moderate hearing losses. Identification of the latter group usually occurs later and they vary markedly with regard to degree of hearing loss, age of onset, amount and type of audiologic intervention, and environmental setting. As a result they cannot be grouped easily, and collection and interpretation of data are quite difficult. Profoundly hearing-impaired children (especially infants and toddlers) are more easily identified and grouped, making possible the collection of more information in a systematic manner. Even so, well-controlled studies that describe specific language characteristics of these children have become available only recently.

Since the designations "deaf" and "hard of hearing" are made arbitrarily by professionals, it is wise to determine how these terms are defined by individual authors before attempting to interpret the data reported. In reviewing the literature in this area, it is futile to establish rigid definitions of either of the terms and attempt to force existing data into them. In the following discussion, attempts will be made to define the populations involved, but there will be considerable overlap within many of the studies.

LANGUAGE DEVELOPMENT AND USE

Attempts to describe the language characteristics of hearing-impaired children have resulted in a minor controversy over the nature of the language problems exhibited. Some professionals refer to the language skills of hearing-impaired children as being *delayed,* while others classify them as being *deviant.* A third approach labels the language deficits as being *different,* in the sense that a dialect is different from standard English. The controversy appears to be esoteric, since the label applied to the language problems of this population is not reflected in the treatment approaches recommended for use with them. Persons who prefer the term *delay* point to the similarities in the sequences of development of language forms and concepts between deaf and normally hearing children. Proponents of the term *deviant* cite studies that reveal usage of certain language forms by the deaf in a manner unlike that of normally hearing children of any age. Both positions are supported by data, but for neither do the data appear conclusive.

Regardless of the terminology used, hearing-impaired children who have no other impairment can be said to have the purest form of language disorder. Its cause is well understood and no assumptions regarding dysfunction of portions of the central nervous system need to be made. Studies of normal language development in children indicate that language is normally learned early in life as a result of extensive auditory experience. It is not necessary to *teach* specific language forms or content to children, only to expose them to them daily. It follows naturally that reduced exposure to language because of hearing loss during the early years of life will result in less efficient learning of language. The important questions to be asked are as follows. (1) What are the specific language deficits that result from reduced auditory input? (2) How is the degree of hearing loss related to the specific deficits incurred?

The answers to the first question could be organized in several ways. For example, effects of hearing loss on receptive versus expressive language offers one way of approaching the question; knowledge of language forms versus content is another. Each of these assumes an artificial division of language skills that cannot be supported by experience or evidence. It is possible to talk about the semantics or the syntax of a language as though these were separate entities as long as we remember that, in actual use, vocabulary and structure are interrelated. The meaning of a given word is influenced by its relation to other words within an utterance or to the situation in which it is used. To make matters more complex, the prosodic features of an utterance, such as stress, are capable of determining its meaning. It is obvious, then, that attempts to categorize language elements into mutually exclusive classes will not be very satisfactory. Nevertheless, categories such as reception, expression, syntax, and semantics offer useful general guidelines for discussion purposes, if we remember the limitations inherent in the use of such terms.

The answer to the second question is important, but largely unknown. Most of the research into the effects of hearing impairment on language development has involved the use of severely or profoundly hearing-impaired subjects. Studies of children whose hearing losses are mild or moderate are relatively rare, probably because they are less easily identified and located for research purposes. In the discussions of studies that follow, the subjects are identified in the way the original authors described them, using the terms "deaf" and "hard of hearing" as they were originally used.

Knowledge of Vocabulary and Word-Class Usage

Knowledge of the lexical components of language by hearing-impaired children has been investigated in several ways. Administration of vocabulary or concept tests, analysis of elicited language samples, and use of experimental tasks involving word association or cloze procedures have all been employed. The descriptions of word usage that result from all of these procedures are remarkably consistent. Hearing-impaired children appear to differ from normally hearing children in the rate and degree to which they learn the meaning of words.

Studies Using Vocabulary Tests. Young and McConnell (1957) administered the *Ammons Full Range Picture Vocabulary Test* to matched pairs of hearing-impaired and normally hearing children, 8 and 14 years of age. Although the hearing losses ranged from mild to moderately severe, not one of the hearing-impaired children scored as high on the test as the matched control. In one case, two children whose IQ test scores were only three points apart exhibited a difference of 42 points on the vocabulary test.

Davis (1974) investigated the performance of 6- to 8-year-old hearing-impaired children on the Boehm Test of Basic Concepts (*BTBC*). The *BTBC* is a task in which the child identifies pictures representing 50 concepts considered necessary to satisfactory academic achievement in kindergarten through second grade. The concepts represent vocabulary used in directions and curriculum for these three grades, including such items as *next to, separate, matches, top, after, few, as many as,* and similar words and phrases. Results indicated that children whose hearing losses do not exceed 50 dB (ANSI, 1969) scored significantly higher than children whose hearing losses fell between 51 and 70 dB, but significantly lower than normally hearing children. Only one-third of the children with the milder hearing losses and none of the children whose losses exceeded 50 dB scores above the 50th percentile; 91 percent of the latter group scored below the 10th percentile. Although the number of concepts correctly identified increased with age, the mean percentile rankings for the hearing-impaired children fell sharply, indicating that the gap between them and their hearing peers increases as time goes by. The children showed a growth of only three concepts per year from age 6 to 8, and they did not exhibit orderly patterns of development in their knowledge of the 50 concepts. While normally hearing children showed consistent patterns of concept knowledge as the difficulty of the items increased, the hearing-impaired children showed almost random knowledge of the word involved. An order of difficulty for them could not be established.

Usage of a given word in a single context measures only one dimension of vocabulary knowledge. Because a word may have several different meanings and serve different language functions, another dimension of vocabulary knowledge is necessary for good linguistic performance. Investigation of the understanding and use of analogies, multiple meanings of words, and synonyms reveals that deaf children lag behind normally hearing children in vocabulary knowledge and usage by from 3 to 8 years by age 14 (Templin, 1966). While normally hearing children exhibited a regular, consistent increase in knowledge of the multiple meaning of words as they became older, deaf children showed no systematic improvement in their performance with increasing age. Vocabulary development in the deaf appears to differ significantly from that in normally hearing children; they know fewer word meanings and do not "know" them as well as much younger children.

Using Language Samples. Rather than administering vocabulary tests, some investigators have measured vocabulary knowledge and growth by examination of language samples collected from deaf children. Results of these investigations are similar to those obtained with the use of vocabulary tests. Schultze (1965) reported a study involving 32 deaf children from 12 to 17 years of age; their written language samples totaled 20,383 words. The most commonly used word was "the" (1433 times); only 34 words were used more than 100 times. These words were predominately pronouns, prepositions, and verbs. Because the vocabulary of the subjects in Schultze's study had been studied in a similar manner three years previously, she was able to estimate vocabulary growth levels for the group. Her results indicate that although the total number of different words used by deaf children had more than doubled in a three-year period, they exhibited vocabulary usage similar to that of first-grade students just learning to read.

An analysis of the language samples of 19 preschool deaf children (Griswold and Commings, 1974) revealed that their expressive vocabulary is made up primarily of nouns, pronouns, verbs, modifiers, prepositions, and question words. Nouns accounted for 55 percent of the total vocabulary used by the youngest children; modals, demonstrative pronouns, and articles were not used. The question words used most frequently were "when" and "what." The preschool deaf children in this study exhibited smaller vocabularies than normally hearing children, but used a surprisingly large array of word classes. The greatest disparity between words used by the deaf and normally hearing preschoolers lay in the use of function words such as demonstrative pronouns, auxiliary or modal verbs, connectives, and verb tenses. Because these are the word classes that are most deficient in older deaf children as well, it appears that hearing impairment affects vocabulary development in a selective manner, the nature of which is obvious in early childhood.

Several studies of deaf children have used the type-token ratio (TTR) as a measure of vocabulary knowledge. TTR refers to the ratio between the number of different word classes (types) and the total number of words (tokens) in a language sample. Simmons (1962) and MacGinitie (1964) have reported reduced usage of prepositions, pronouns, adjectives, and adverbs in language samples taken from deaf children. Nouns and verbs constituted the word classes used most frequently.

Brannon (1968) analyzed spoken language samples of 30 normally hearing, 15 hard-of-hearing (27-66 dB ASA), and 15 deaf children (hearing losses greater than 75 dB ASA), by sorting the words they produced into 14 classes. Results of the study revealed that hearing-impaired children showed a reduction in the number of total words, types of words, and number of different words spoken. Normally hearing children used a total of 11,400 words, while children with mild-to-moderate hearing losses produced 5149 and deaf children produced only 4385 words.

Word-class usage by the two hearing-impaired groups was significantly different. The less severely hearing-impaired children used all word classes adequately with the exception of adverbs, pronouns, and auxiliaries. Deaf children used significantly fewer words in all classes than normals, except for conjunctions. The hearing-impaired children tended to overuse nouns and articles. Brannon concluded that hearing impairment interferes with the learnig learning of function words more than that of content words.

Use of Cloze Procedures. Another means of determining class usage by hearing-impaired children involves the use of a *cloze* procedure, in which words are omitted from written passages and subjects are asked to restore the missing words. MacGinitie (1964) presented a cloze task to 30 deaf and 30 normally hearing children, matched according to reading achievement. The deleted words included nouns, verbs, adjectives, adverbs, and function word types (such as conjunctions, prepositions, and auxiliaries). Deaf children were significantly poorer at restoring words in the sentences than normally hearing children, but the pattern of difficulty exhibited was similar for both groups.

Other investigators have reported several word classes to be used less frequently by deaf than by normally hearing children. Odum, Blanton, and Nunnally (1967) investigated the abilities of deaf adolescents (median hearing loss of 98 dB ASA) to use nouns, verbs, adjectives, conjunctions, and prepositions in sentence completion and cloze tasks. They found the performance of deaf subjects to be significantly poorer than that of normally hearing pupils in the fifth to sixth and twelfth grades. When every third, fourth, or fifth word was deleted from stories from fourth-grade readers, deaf students performed much more poorly than normally hearing ones. Although the performance of the deaf children improved as the interval between word deletions was increased, the performance of the normally hearing children did not. While the added contextual clues aided the deaf in predicting the form class of the deleted word, it did not help them predict the actual word that was deleted. Semantic words (nouns, verbs, and adjectives) were easier for the deaf to supply than syntactic words (indefinite articles, quantifiers, conjunctions, and prepositions) and required less context for accurate prediction.

Odum et al. (1967) concluded that the deaf employ language processing startegies that differ from normal hearers, particularly with regard to the use of syntactic words. Although there are fewer syntactic than semantic words in the language, and syntactic words are used more frequently, the deaf show a serious lack of knowledge of the semantic and idiomatic properties of function words. The impact of this fact on reading achievement and linguistic performance is substantial.

Use of Word-Association. Another means of studying semantic knowledge is through word-association tasks. When children are presented a word and asked to respond to it with the first word that comes to mind, the responses may be classified as syntagmatic (words from a different word class as the stimulus, for example, dog-bark) or paradigmatic (words from the same class, for example, dog-cat). The type of response given by a child changes with age, with syntagmatic responses occurring most often before age 5 to 7 and paradigmatic responses occurring most frequently beyond that age (Entwistle, 1966). Attempts to classify word associations made by hearing-impaired children have yielded contradictory results. Kline (1945) found similar patterns of syntagmatic-paradigmatic shifts in deaf and normally hearing children, while Jacobson (1968) found a decline in paradigmatic responses in deaf children as they grew older. Tweney and Hoemann (1973) hypothesized that the different results seen in these experiments could be traced to the fact that early studies required deaf children to respond to English words in written form. The effects of reading and writing the stimulus-response words on children whose first language may not be English could account for differences between deaf and normally hearing children and among the deaf subject groups themselves. Tweney and Hoemann repeated the classic word-association task by fingerspelling, speaking, and signing 18 ASL equivalents of nouns, verbs, and adjectives to 7- to 13-year-old deaf children (PTA = 80 dB or greater), who responded by speech, fingerspelling or sign. The deaf children exhibited increasing numbers of paradigmatic responses with age, but the shift from syntagmatic to paradigmatic occurred at a later age and to a lesser degree than for normally hearing children. The deaf children performed similarly when responding in English (speech or fingerspelling) and in ASL (sign). The authors interpreted this as evidence that linguistic and conceptual development through manual language can parallel processes that have been demonstrated in normally hearing children.

Fremer and MacGinitie (1969) presented a word-association task to deaf children, aged 11 to 18 and normally hearing chiidren, aged 9 to 14. The children were required to respond to a stimulus word with as many words as possible that were related to the stimulus word along some dimension. Results indicated that normally hearing children evidenced continued growth in the number of associations they made, while deaf children reached a plateau after the age of 14.

Summary of Studies of Word Usage. The studies of vocabulary development reviewed above indicate several important facts:

1. Hearing-impaired children exhibit reduced vocabulary knowledge when compared to normally hearing children at the same age regardless of the nature of the task presented.
2. The nature of the use of vocabulary by hearing-impaired children differs from that of normally hearing children. Although they may have knowledge of various form classes, they do not use them as appropriately as normally hearing children. This is particularly true of common function words of the language.
3. Hearing-impaired children do not understand the multiple meaning of words. They tend to attach one meaning to a given word and fail to process it accurately in a different context. The subtle relationships between words and their meanings are largely unknown to deaf children.
4. The degree of vocabulary deficit appears to be related to the degree of hearing loss. Use of certain form classes varies according to the severity of the hearing loss.

5. General vocabulary knowledge increases with age, but the gap between normally hearing and hearing-impaired children in word usage widens as the children grow older.
6. Knowledge of words and their meanings is "spotty" and less universal among hearing-impaired children than among the normally hearing. The latter children appear to experience systematic vocabulary growth that is related to universal experiences. The vocabulary of deaf children may be unduly influenced by teaching curriculum and strategies, rather than by natural language experience.

Knowledge of Grammar

Effective communication between persons involves more than understanding the meanings of single words. The relations among lexical items as they are combined into messages of varying lengths and structures largely determine message meaning. Very young children form combinations of words in an effort to communicate such relationships. These early sentences appear to begin with combinations of words from one or two categories, sometimes referred to as *pivot* and *open* classes. Pivot words refer to a small number of words similar to function words in adult grammar. Words in this class usually have well-defined positions in a grammatical sequence; they constitute a limited number of words such as *that, my, more, big, see*. Open words resemble content words of adult language and constitute a much larger class to which items are added quickly. Examples of open class words are *boy, milk, daddy, push*. Early utterances may combine pivot and open words, as in *see boy* or open and open words, as in *daddy push*.

Linguists do not agree on the psychological reality of the pivot-open classification of child grammar, but it offers a descriptive way of analyzing early two-word utterances. When young children move beyond the two-word utterance stage, their sentences are often described as being "telegraphic," because function words are omitted from the sentences produced in very much the same way they are omitted in telegrams. It has been hypothesized that the omission of words from utterances such as "Daddy go car" is a result of reduced memory span, but most linguists now agree that the omission of function words represents the child's grammatical stage rather than a chopped off version of adult structure. This observation is important when considering the use of syntax by hearing-impaired children. Their language is often described as being "telegraphic," but the nature of the "missing elements" is somewhat different. Although pivot class words (of function words) are learned and used very early by normally hearing children, they are often absent from the utterances of hearing-impaired children for many years.

Investigations of syntactic knowledge and use by hearing-impaired children have used a variety of experimental tasks and procedures. The majority of the work that has been reported involves the use of English by deaf children trained by oral-aural procedures. Only recently have children who have been trained with the use of sign language been the subject of studies of syntactic knowledge. Although the impact is not clearly understood, it can be assumed that the linguistic knowledge exhibited by deaf children and reported in the literature is significantly affected by the stimulus and response modes used by experimenters. Because of the nature of hearing impairment and its effect on the accurate reception of spoken utterances, much of the stimulus material is presented in written form; because of the effects of hearing impairment on speech production, the child's responses are also obtained in written form to enhance their intelligibility. The use of written materials affects the type of children included in studies, especially with regard to age and linguistic (English) status. Written samples of spontaneous language can seldom be obtained before the age of 8 from children with reasonably good knowledge of English. If stimuli are to be read, subjects generally must possess reading skills of at least second- or third-grade level. Children with severely delayed language may not be able to read or write well enough to produce reliable language samples or participate in experimental paradigms based on English knowledge until they are much older than their normally hearing peers.

These facts necessarily limit both the choice of subjects for studies of language skills and the methodology employed with them. The result is a body of literature on hearing-impaired children that describes the written language skills of older children who are well beyond the ages associated with peak language learning. It is therefore difficult to generalize findings to young children even though common sense indicates that the same characteristics exist in them to a greater degree. Because most available training procedures and materials are designed for use with young children, there may be some discrepancy between the direct needs of those being trained and those on whom the materials were based.

In addition, generalization of research findings for deaf subjects to children with less severe hearing losses is dangerous. It may lead to erroneous assumptions concerning their language deficits and their habilitative needs. The few existing studies of sentence usage by moderately hearing-impaired children provide very important information, especially when compared to data for deaf children.

Morphology. Morphology represents the system of rules by which the smallest meaningful units of language (morphemes) are combined to form words and to express variations in meaning. The production of grammatical sentences depends in part on the correct usage of morphological rules. Morphemes fall into two classes, free and bound. Free morphemes are lexical items, such as ball or run; bound morphemes are those language units that cannot stand alone, such as -s and **-ing**, but which change the meaning of words to which they are attached (e.g., balls, running). Bound morphemes are usually unstressed units of language; most of them have poor visibility and audibility. It can be hypothesized that their relative obscurity may make their learning by hearing-impaired children quite difficult. The observation that these children often omit the endings of words in their speech is probably related to their reduced ability to perceive and produce certain bound morphemes.

Few investigations of the morphological usage of hearing-impaired children have been reported. Cooper (1967) modified Berko's test (1958) and presented it to 140 deaf children (hearing losses greater than 70 dB ASA) and 76 normally hearing children ranging in age from 7 to 19 years. The paper-and-pencil task required the children to respond appropriately to inflectional and derivational morphological rules. Inflectional rules included regular and irregular verb tenses, plurals, comparatives and superlatives. Derivational rules included adjectival and adverbial endings and noun and verb derivatives. Stimuli were read by the subjects who pointed to the correct response on the receptive portion and wrote their answers for the production portion of the task. Results of Cooper's study reveal several interesting facts. Deaf females scored higher than deaf males in all age groups. The performance of deaf subjects was markedly poorer than that of normally hearing subjects, with 19-year-old deaf females scoring more poorly than 9- to 10-year-old normally hearing females and 17- to 18-year-old deaf males scoring more poorly than 7- to 8-year-old normally hearing males. Out of a possible score of 48, the average score for deaf males was 18.3, for normally hearing males, 32.9; for deaf females, 25.3, for normally hearing females, 37.2. Although scores for normally hearing males increased from ages 7 to 8 to 13 to 14, scores for deaf males did not improve after ages 9 to 10. Deaf females' scores continued to improve through ages 15 to 16, while normally hearing females' scores improved with chronological age throughout the age range tested. Correlational analyses revealed significant relationships between performance on the morphology test and reading and vocabulary scores for both groups of subjects. Error-response patterns for both groups were similar, with inflectional morphemes being easier than derivational ones and reception of morphemes being better than their production.

Gilman and Raffin (1975) investigated the use of eight inflectional morphemes by deaf children whose educational procedures included the use of Seeing Essential English (SEE) (Anthony, 1971) in the classroom. One purpose of the study was to determine whether or not deaf children exposed to a system of manual signs that represented English morphemes would be able to use certain morphemes appropriately. A second purpose was to identify those variables that might be related to morpheme usage. A written test involving a four-item multiple choice paradigm was administered to 20 severely hearing-impaired children (aged 8 to 12) whose hearing losses exceeded 80 dB HL. The morphemes plural **s,** possessive **'s,** present tense singular **s**, past tense **ed**, present progressive **ing,** adverbial **ly,** comparative **er,** and superlative **est,** were tested. Group performance for the children was above chance level on all morphemes except **est.** Age, hearing level, and years of experience with SEE were not significantly related to performance on the task; teacher consistency in use of the morphemes, reading level, and sex were significantly related to test performance.

The reliance on reading necessitated by the use of written tasks makes it difficult to separate this factor from others that may affect task performance. To determine whether knowledge of the morphemes tested by Gilman and Raffin was dependent on the ability to read them accurately, Raffin, Davis, and Gilman (1978) presented the same inflectional morphemes in a spoken and signed presentation to 67 deaf children being trained with SEE. The children viewed a video tape and judged the correctness of sentences that were signed and spoken simultaneously. The mean score was 34.4 (possible score of 48), a performance that was significantly better than chance at the .01 level. Only 4 of the 67 subjects failed to score above chance on the task. The authors compared the deaf childrens' performance on the eight morphemes to data from developmental studies of normally hearing children and concluded that deaf children exposed to SEE develop use of inflectional morphemes in the same general sequence as young normally hearing children. The number of years of exposure to the signed-English system was found to be the factor most closely related to knowledge of the morphemes. Neither age nor sex was related to performance on the task.

Syntax. Many different procedures have been used to investigate the use of syntax by hearing-impaired people. Written and oral language samples have been analyzed, and standardized and experimental tests have been administered.

Knowledge of Syntax in Written Form. One of the earliest attempts to investigate the differences between the structure of the language generated by deaf children and that produced by normally hearing children was reported by Heider and Heider (1940). They collected 1118 compositions written by deaf and normally hearing children in response to a short motion picture. Heider and Heider did not report hearing levels for their deaf subjects, all of whom were enrolled in residential schools for the deaf. Analysis of the compositions included measures of sentence length, sentence type, frequency of occurrence of certain word classes, and use of subordinate clauses. The authors concluded that, when compared to normally hearing children:

1. The deaf used shorter sentences of simple construction.
2. The deaf used relatively fewer verbs in clauses, but more in simple sentences.
3. The deaf used fewer forms requiring precision of meaning, such as connectives and prepositions, but they used relatively more prepositional phrases of other types.
4. The deaf used relatively rigid, unrelated units of language, that were seldom connected in any meaningful way.
5. The language of the deaf was similar to that of younger normally hearing children.
6. The deaf exhibited difficulty producing sentences that indicate possibility rather than actuality.

The approach used by Heider and Heider in their analysis of the compositions collected differs considerably from approaches used today, and their findings cannot be compared directly to more recent data. Nevertheless, this landmark study revealed characteristics of the written language of deaf children that have been corroborated many times since.

The most comprehensive attempts to investigate syntactic abilities in deaf children have been reported by Quigley and his associates at the University of Illinois (Quigley, Smith, and Wilbur, 1974; Quigley, Wilbur, and Montanelli, 1974; Wilbur, Quigley, and Montanelli, 1975). These investigators developed an experimental written test, which later became the Test of Syntactic Ability (*TSA*). The *TSA* was designed to examine in depth the rules underlying the comprehension and production of sentences by deaf children. Quigley and his associates reasoned that the so-called "deviant" language produced by deaf children is related to their use of generative rules of grammar that differ from those used by normally hearing children.

The experimental form of the *TSA* involved two basic tasks: *sentence completion tasks* and *sentence correction tasks*. Sentence completion was accomplished either by inserting a missing word freely or choosing a word from a multiple-choice array. Sentence correction tasks required the child to read a sentence and decide whether it was correct or incorrect. For some sentences, the child was required to rewrite the sentence to make it correct and in others the task was to choose a sentence or sentences that had the same meaning as the language sample given. The original test consisted of 10 tests, each designed to examine a particular English language structure such as negation, auxiliary words, pronominalization, and others.

The *TSA* was administered to approximately 450 deaf students (age 10 to 18 years) and 60 normally hearing students (age 8 to 10 years). A complete description of the *TSA* and a summary of research findings can be found in a final report by Quigley, Wilbur, Power, Montanelli, and Steinkamp (1976). The order of difficulty for the syntactic structures tested was similar for deaf and normally hearing children. Negation, conjunction, and question formation were the least difficult, and pronominalization, verb usage, complementation, and relativization were the most difficult for both groups of children. The order of difficulty for deaf and normally hearing varied slightly within the two groupings listed above. Deaf children exhibited a strong tendency to impose a S-V-O surface order on sentences, resulting in faulty comprehension of complex sentences.

One structure that appears to be particularly difficult for deaf children is the passive voice. Only about 50 percent of deaf adolescents understand passive sentences and only two-thirds of those can produce them (Schmitt, 1968; Power and Quigley, 1973). When confronted with passive sentences, most deaf children interpret them as S-V-O, active, declarative sentences, thereby receiving exactly the opposite meaning intended in utterances such as, "Mary was hit by Bill." The same type of misinterpretations occur also with sentences containing relative clauses.

Knowledge of Syntax in Spoken Form. In an effort to circumvent the reduced spontaneity that may result from requiring written responses from children, several researchers have investigated the spoken language skills of hearing-impaired children. Goda (1959) studied reading, writing, speaking, and lipreading skills of 56 deaf adolescents by analyzing both written and spoken language samples. Goda reported that written language, spoken sentences, and average reading level were significantly related to intelligence as measured by nonverbal tests. Deaf females scored consistently higher than deaf males on all measures. Goda concluded that all language skills are closely interrelated and the deaf child who performs well in one skill will probably perform well in others.

Using a sentence-recall task, Sarachan-Deily and Love (1974) investigated the use of syntactic rules by deaf adults whose language skills were taught to them in schools for the deaf after age 5. Recall of active, passive, negative, and passive negative sentences by deaf children revealed very different error types from those of the normally hearing controls, who deleted modifiers, substituted synonyms, or changed transformational structure of the sentences when recall errors were made. Half the errors made by deaf subjects involved the deletion of major sentence constituents, resulting in gross violations in English sentence structure. The authors concluded that deaf individuals whose language is learned after the age of five exhibit an unstable or a limited competence in English syntax.

Pressnell (1973) compared the acquisition and use of syntax by two groups of hearing-impaired children to that reported for normally hearing children. Children whose losses ranged from 50 to 92 dB (ANSI 1969) and children whose hearing losses were greater than 93 dB constituted the experimental group. The *Northwestern Syntax Screening Test* (*NSST*) was administered to each child, from whom Pressnell also collected a spontaneous spoken-language sample, which was scored according to Lee and Canter's *Developmental Sentence Scoring Analysis* (1971).

Pressnell's results indicated that hearing-impaired children's reception and expression of spoken sentences increased with age, but not as rapidly nor as consistently as that of normally hearing children. The greatest gains in expression of syntax occurred between the ages of 5 and 9 years. Analysis of the spontaneous language samples revealed that hearing-impaired children exhibit greatest difficulty in the accurate use of main verbs. Their performance suggests that hearing-impaired children may develop the use of verb forms in a different sequence from that of normally hearing children, possibly as a result of teaching procedures used with them.

The restricted use of verb forms was also studied by Wilcox and Tobin (1974). They presented tape recorded stimuli to children with moderate-to-severe hearing losses (47 to 88 dB, ANSI, 1969), and to normally hearing children, who were asked to perform three tasks: (1) repeat the sentence after hearing it and seeing a picture that depicted it, (2) recalling the sentence later by viewing the picture associated with it, and (3) repeating a separate set of sentences with no pictorial representation. The hearing-impaired children scored significantly poorer than normally hearing children on all three tasks; they exhibited greatest difficulty with the recall task. The verb forms of present perfect (have + en) and negative passive ("the cake was not baked by Mary") proved most difficult for the hearing impaired. With the exception of these two forms, the hearing-impaired children appeared to have developed the use of the verb forms tested in a sequence similar to normally hearing children.

Brannon and Murry (1966) investigaged the spoken syntax of children by eliciting spoken language samples (descriptions of pictures) from three groups of children: 30 normally hearing children, 15 children whose average pure-tone losses ranged from 27 to 66 dB ISO, and 15 children whose average pure-tone losses were greater than 75 dB. The language samples of the three groups differed with regard to the length and complexity of the sentences produced. As expected, the normal group exhibited language that was better than that of the less severely hearing-impaired group, which in turn was better than that of the group labeled as deaf. Substitution of incorrect words for the correct form was the most common syntactical error for both groups of hearing-impaired subjects; the tendency to omit function words increased with increased severity of hearing loss. Verb constructions accounted for the greatest number of errors for both groups of hearing-impaired children.

Tervoort (1967) obtained language samples from 48 deaf children in the United States and Europe, using a unique procedure. He divided deaf residential students into pairs and filmed their communication with each other during private, unmonitored conversation over a six-year period. Subjects ranged in age from 7 to 12 years when the study began. The resulting films were translated by the subjects themselves, other students, the experimenter, teachers, parents, and deaf adults. Sentences were analyzed with regard to length, means of expression (speech, fingerspelling, sign) and syntactic quality. The latter was defined as exoteric (grammatical) or esoteric (nongrammatical).

Tervoort's results indicated much greater use of nouns than any other word class. He interpreted this as evidence of the subjects' attempts to "symbolize their visual world through manual description," an easier task with nouns than other word classes. In general, information expressed through speech decreased as age increased, while that expressed through sign and fingerspelling increased steadily with age. The greatest gains in vocabulary occurred before the age of 14.

The length and quality of sentences increased as the children grew older. Thirty-five percent of all sentences were exoteric. These included sentences that were acceptably grammatical, but not completely so. The errors that occurred in acceptable sentences fell into four categories: (1) omissions of words ("I live Royal Center"), (2) inversions (reversals) of words ("Mother my sew dress"), (3) additions of superfluous words ("Wonder why Oswald shot to him"), and (4) substitution of words ("Who are she?"). The esoteric sentences could not be analyzed according to known linguistic rules. They were characterized by a free order of vocabulary items and an absence of morphological markers. Examples of esoteric sentences are: (1) "Tired I tired I I I track now" and (2) "My sister my sister false decorate girl make false decorate false decorate" (p. 1294). A shift toward grammaticality occurred with age and was most evident in the American schools; it coincided with a shift away from speech only as a mode of expression. Tervoort concluded that the deaf children studied were far more successful in developing language skills than speech skills. His data also indicated that increases in speech skill did not correlate with improved language skills.

These investigations of spoken language skills in hearing-impaired children reveal patterns of syntactic difficulty similar to those associated with written language samples. It is obvious that complex sentence structures are poorly understood and seldom produced by hearing-impaired children. What is not obvious is the nature of the processing difficulties that account for the poor performance observed. In an effort to determine the perceptual strategies employed by hearing-impaired children, Davis and Blasdell (1975) presented 12 pairs of sentences in which relative clauses were embedded medially to 24 hearing-impaired and 15 normally hearing children from 6 to 9 years of age. All sentences followed the same pattern, $N_1V_1N_2V_2N_3$, and pairs were identical except for the reversal of N_1 and N_2 and a word change of V_2. (An example of a sentence pair is: "The cat that hit the
N_1 V_1

ball ran down the steps." "The ball that hit the cat bounced down the steps.")
N_2 V_2 N_3 N_1 V_1 N_2 V_2 N_3

Four pictures were presented with each sentence presentation and the child's task was to choose the one picture that best represented the sentence. Figure 6.1 shows the pictures associated with the sentence pair given above. Results revealed a significant difference between the control and experimental groups' ability to process the sentences correctly, but both groups used similar strategies when they were in error. The most common error strategy was the interpretation of $N_1V_1N_2$ as the subject-verb-object of the sentence ("The man chased the sheep"). Hearing-impaired children exhibited a wider range of error responses than normals, the pattern of which caused the authors to suggest that visual and acoustic ambiguities strongly affect the hearing-impaired child's sentence processing strategies. These strategies, while similar to those of normally hearing children, seem less stable and more easily influenced by acoustic or semantic confusions.

Summary of Studies of Syntax. Certain generalizations can be drawn from the studies reviewed above.

1. Hearing impairment significantly affects the acquisition of grammatical rules for use in comprehension and expression of spoken and written language.

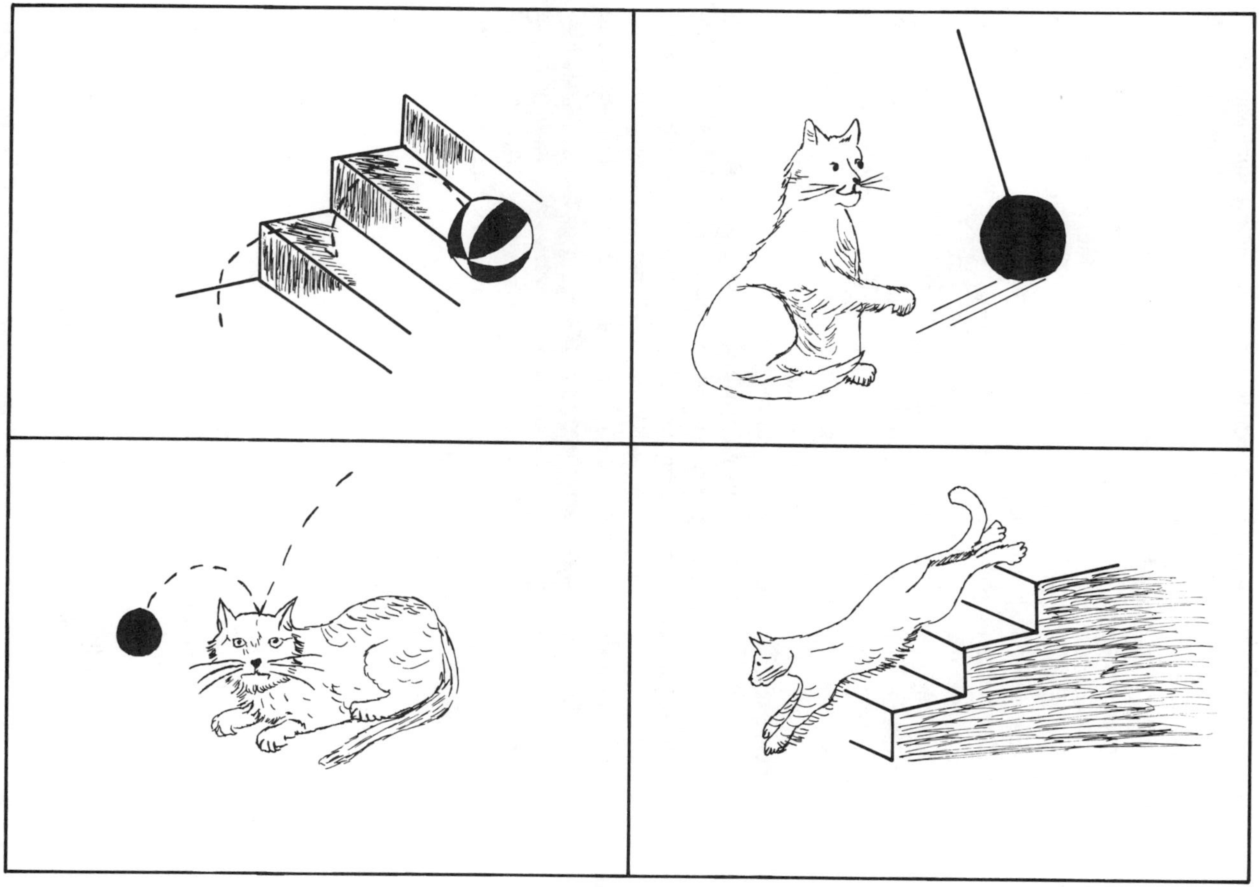

Figure 6.1. Picture array representing the sentence pair, "The cat that hit the ball ran down the stairs; the ball that hit the cat bounced down the stairs."

2. The severity of the deficit in knowledge of language structure appears to be related to the degree of hearing loss. Children with moderate-to-severe hearing losses appear to develop and use sentence forms more rapidly and more efficiently than children labeled as deaf by the investigators.
3. Sentences produced by hearing-impaired children contain a high proportion of content words, especially nouns, and few function words.
4. Hearing-impaired children tend to impose a S-V-O surface structure on complex sentences, resulting in their misinterpretation. Although young normally hearing children employ such a strategy also, they tend to abandon it earlier than do children with hearing impairment.
5. Hearing-impaired children appear to develop a poor understanding of deep structure grammatical rules as a means of comprehending complex sentences. As a result they misinterpret sentences presented to them and produce agrammatical sentences themselves. In the case of profoundly hearing-impaired children, they may never be able to use some types of complex sentence forms appropriately.
6. Although their syntactic skills improve with age, progress is painfully slow for some linguistic features. Greatest gains in knowledge occur before adolescence, when development of a variety of language skills appears to asymptote. The level at which the plateau in language learning occurs is probably related to severity of the hearing loss and the degree to which a language code is learned in the first three to five years of life. Hearing-impaired children who are identified late in preschool years or who receive inadequate services in infancy and early childhood may be doomed to a knowledge of language that is insufficient for adequate educational or vocational achievement.

SPEECH CHARACTERISTICS

The speech produced by hearing-impaired children is directly related to the severity of the hearing loss and the degree to which an auditory-verbal feedback loop can be established. Speech is learned normally through the auditory system. During the first few months of life, infants produce many exotic sounds, some of which are not components of the active language they will learn. The phonemics of that specific language occur so often, however, and are reinforced through audition so early, that within a few months of birth an infant babbles only those sounds that are a part of the language heard daily. This early, consistent exposure to the phonology of the native language is important to the eventual development of articulation skills and the intelligibility of speech.

At the same time that phonemes are being decoded and stored in memory, other aspects of speech are also being learned. These include voice inflections, rhythm of connected speech, stress patterns associated with different types of utterances, and other nonphonemic components of natural speech. The degree to which the acoustic information described above is available to an infant directly influences the nature of the speech that will later be produced. The use of even limited residual hearing may make the difference between intelligible and unintelligible speech.

Effects of Mild to Moderate Hearing Impairment on Speech

Children who do not hear normally usually experience difficulty in speaking clearly. Those who sustain mild to moderate hearing losses exhibit misarticulations similar to those of normally hearing children who have developmental disorders of articulation. They appear to develop and use speech sounds in the same order of difficulty as that experienced by normally hearing children (Oller and Kelly, 1974). Unless the hearing loss is severe, articulation of vowels develops normally and voice quality is not significantly different from normally hearing children (West and Weber, 1973). This fact is important; the effects of moderate hearing impairment on speech are quite different from those of severe or profound hearing loss as described in the next section.

The sounds most commonly misarticulated by children with moderate hearing impairments are fricative consonants (such as **s, z, sh,** and **th**), affricates (such as **ch** and **j**), and the initial liquid **r.** Their speech deviates from normal in three major respects:

1. Omission of final consonants.
2. Infrequent production of voiced fricatives.
3. Rare use of voiced, back, lingual consonants, such as **g, j,** and **ng** (West and Weber, 1973).

Effects of Severe to Profound Hearing Impairment on Speech

There are three major aspects of speech that are affected by severe hearing loss: phonation, articulation, and rhythm. Errors of each of these affect intelligibility adversely and contribute to the perception of what is often called "deaf speech" or "deaf voice."

Errors of Phonation. The most serious error of phonation that occurs in deaf speakers is the failure to coordinate breathing and speaking. Deaf children tend not to associated the breath stream with the production of speech unless they are taught specifically how to control it to provide a power source for speech. Deaf speakers may produce only one or two syllables per breath or attempt to speak while inhaling. Syllables and words are often grouped incorrectly because a breath is taken in the middle of words or phrases. Control of the breath stream for speech much be accomplished before other aspects of speech can be improved.

Forner and Hixon (1977) investigated the respiratory behavior of 10 profoundly hearing-impaired individuals. Their subjects exhibited normal respiratory functions during rest but several deviancies during speech acts. Normal phrasing was rare; instead, attempts at continuous speech resulted in "short stretches of speech . . . broken by inappropriate pauses" (p. 395). Less than one-third the normal number of syllables per breath were produced by these deaf speakers, and pauses for breath were not coordinated with the linguistic structure or meaning of the message being spoken. This lack of coordination results in frequent inappropriate pauses in speech, during which major quantities of air are expended, leaving an insufficient amount of air in the lungs to support the remainder of the speech act. The overall result of these respiratory differences is an inefficient use of the power source for speech. Deaf speakers tend to "run out of air"; they do not plan ahead for speech acts by breathing deeply and conserving the flow of breath in a manner appropriate to the message being spoken. Therefore, sentences are interrupted frequently by pauses that interfere with the linguistic characteristics of speech and make perception of the message difficult (Forner and Hixon, 1977; Monsen, 1979).

The voice produced by deaf speakers has been described as dull, monotonous, hoarse, nasal, harsh, breathy, strident, and strained. The perceptions resulting in such terminology probably have their origins in the pitch, loudness, and duration characteristics of the speech produced by deaf speakers. Some investigators have reported abnormally high pitch in deaf speakers, restricted use of pitch changes, and frequent pitch breaks during utterances (Angelocci, Kopp, and Holbrook, 1964; Boone, 1966; Black, 1971; Martony, 1968). Monsen (1979) reported that young hearing-impaired children have vocal fundamental frequencies within the normal range. Listener judgment of their voice quality appeared to be related primarily to the intonation contours used during speech. Most of the children whose voices were judged as having poor quality used two abnormal intonation contours, a *flat* contour and a *changing* one. The flat contour consisted of little pitch variation; the changing contour was characterized by rising and falling fluctuations in pitch within a single syllable (Monsen, 1979). Deaf speakers often have little control over the fundamental frequencies of their voices, exhibit few changes in pitch, and cannot control the pitch variations that do occur (Martony, 1968). Not only do these problems affect perceptions of voice quality, they also interfere with the stress patterns of speech that are produced by changes in pitch and loudness.

The loudness of the voice is poorly controlled by some deaf speakers, resulting in variable intensities that are unrelated to the content or emotional intent of the utterance. This can be distracting even when it does not affect intelligibility adversely (Angelocci et al., 1964; Calvert and Silverman, 1975).

Speech produced by deaf individuals is often characterized by hypernasality. Coordinating the movements of the soft palate, pharyngeal walls, and other oral structures for the production of oral versus nasal sounds is difficult for many deaf speakers. Unusual pharyngeal resonance patterns occur during speech as a result of a combination of retracted tongue position, hypernasality, and increased tension.

The quality is difficult to describe but easy to identify when heard. This combination of slightly aberrant movements of the oral mechanism probably accounts for what is described as "typical deaf speech."

Errors of Articulation. Children with severe to profound hearing losses misarticulate both vowels and consonants, making their articulation patterns unique.

Vowel Errors. Deaf children misarticulate vowels almost as frequently as consonants (Markides, 1970). They produce vowels that cannot easily be distinguished from each other because their formant structures are poorly defined. Spectrographic analysis of the speech of deaf talkers reveals that the first two formants occur within an unusually restricted range of frequencies (Angelocci et al., 1964). Deaf children apparently attempt to produce different vowels by making only minimal changes in the position and movements of the articulators, a limitation that may affect vowel formant transitions; Monsen (1978) reported small second-formant transitions for diphthongs produced by deaf speakers. The tongue often assumes a neutral position in the middle of the mouth, moving only slightly as different vowels are produced. This results in what has been called "neutralization of vowels" by deaf speakers (Hudgins and Numbers, 1942).

In addition to the lack of differentiation among vowels, deaf children may also prolong them to durations that are three to five times as long as those produced by normally hearing speakers, although there is considerable variability within and between deaf speakers (Monsen, 1974; 1979).

Consonant Errors. Deaf children produce fewer consonants and develop them later than normally hearing children; consonant production among preschool deaf children is similar to that of normally hearing children at 12 months of age. Studies of consonant production reveal a consistency of errors among deaf speakers (Hudgins and Numbers, 1942; Morley, 1949; Carr, 1953; Markides, 1970; Heidinger, 1972; Smith, 1972; Hutchinson, Kornhauser, Beasley, and Beasley, 1978) as follows:

1. Front, voiced consonants are produced more often than other less visible sounds, which are frequently misarticulated or omitted.
2. More errors occur on final than initial consonants; final consonants are often omitted.
3. Deaf speakers often confuse voiced-voiceless cognates.
4. Consonant production is often accompanied by hypernasality and/or audible nasal emission of air.
5. Consonants are frequently omitted from blends.
6. Neutral vowels are often inserted between abutting consonants including those of blends (guluve for glove); a neutral vowel is often added to the end of words ending in plosives (doguh for dog).
7. Coordination of phonation with consonant production is often faulty, resulting in inappropriate voicing of voiceless consonants and vice versa.

The speech of deaf children often contains consonants that cannot be identified easily. Even when they are formed correctly by the articulators, consonants are often distorted by inappropriate voicing, stress, and duration.

Errors of Rhythm. Abnormal patterns of speech rhythm may constitute the most deviant aspect of deaf children's speech. The smooth flow of speech, coordinated with respiration and phonation and characterized by appropriate intonation and stress, is dependent on fine coordination of the musculature of all the physiological systems involved in its production. This coordination is learned naturally through auditory feedback by children whose hearing is normal. When speech production is taught in the absence of useful hearing, such coordination is difficult to achieve.

Natural rhythm of speech involves normal rate, stress patterns, and intonation. It is influenced by breath control, which contributes to a smooth, uninterrupted flow of speech that is not slowed down by frequent pauses for breath (Forner and Hixon, 1977). The rate of speech produced by deaf children is lower than normal, ranging from 28 to 145 words per minute compared to a rate of 134 to 210 words per minute for hearing children (Voelker, 1938; John and Howarth, 1965). At least part of the prolonged rate observed can be attributed to faulty breathing patterns, which contribute to incorrect groupings of words. An abnormally slow rate of speech influences the rhythm of speech in several ways. Not only is speech slower, but the prolonged duration of syllables blurs distinctions between those that are stressed and unstressed. The abnormal duration of unstressed vowels tends to obliterate recognizable stress patterns (Calvert, 1962; Levitt, 1971). It is not unusual for a deaf speaker to place greatest stress on function words in a given sentence (such as "the" or "to") rather than on content words that convey greater meaning. The perceptual set of the average listener does not allow processing of the inappropriately stressed words as they are intended. Unless speech is highly intelligible the listener will try to interpret the stressed segments as content words, with serious effects on intelligibility.

Stress and intonation are also influenced by changes in the pitch of utterance. Attempts by deaf speakers to vary pitch often result in pitch breaks, especially in the middle of prolonged vowels, which interfere with the perception of normal stress patterns (Monsen, 1979). Some deaf speakers employ a "favorite intonation contour" (Stewart, 1969) for all utterances, regardless of meaning or structure. A universal intonation contour, composed of a single pattern of pitch, duration, and stress characteristics, would contribute to a listener's perception of deaf speech as monotonous, whereas a constantly changing intonation contour as described by Monsen (1979) interferes with judgments of voice quality as well as interfering with intelligibility.

Levitt (1971) described two types of rhythm errors: lack of rhythm and incorrect rhythm. The former occurs when all syllables are stressed equally, a likely occurrence when vowels are prolonged and breath groups of only one or two words are produced routinely. The latter occurs when stress differences are employed, but incorrectly. Unsuccessful attempts to control pitch and voicing and interruptions caused by running out of breath each contribute to improper stress patterns.

Intelligibility

Considering the fundamental nature of the problems deaf speakers have in producing speech, it is no surprise that their effort often results in speech that cannot be understood by the listener. Studies of the intelligibility of hearing-impaired subjects have yielded remarkably similar results. Although intelligibility varies widely among individual subjects in most studies, the average is consistently reported to be around 20 percent. An exception is the report by Monsen (1978) that indicated a mean intelligibility of 76 percent for 67 hearing-impaired children enrolled in the Central Institute for the Deaf. Both day and residential students are included in the reported research. Judgments of intelligibility have been made by teachers of the deaf, speech-language pathologists, and naive listeners. Spoken materials from which intelligibility ratings are measured have ranged from single phonemes to sentences. Although the variables of listener, material, degree of hearing loss, and educational setting influence intelligibility slightly, the findings are the same: only about one of every five utterances of deaf children and adolescents can be understood by hearing listeners. By contrast, more than 50 percent of the spontaneous utterances of the 4-year-old hearing-impaired child studied by West and Weber (1973) were intelligible. Table 6.1 shows the results of several studies of speech intelligibility.

The poor intelligibility of deaf children's speech has been of great concern to educators and clinicians for many years. Although the role of residual hearing in the development of good speech skills is widely recognized, specifics about how *much* hearing is required for what level of skill is largely unknown. It is dangerous to try to predict the eventual nature of the speech of an individual child; certainly it cannot be predicted on the basis of a pure-tone audiogram. Some children who have severe, but not profound, hearing losses exhibit poorer skills than children with poorer hearing. Conversely, some children with hearing losses of 90 to 100 dB develop excellent speech skills.

One factor related to pure-tone thresholds appears to be fairly reliable. Children who have measurable hearing at all frequencies, or at least at frequencies from 250 to 2000 Hz, are more likely to develop intelligible speech than children who have no measureable hearing above 500 or 1000 Hz. Children with these "corner" audiograms appear to experience great difficulty establishing the auditory-verbal feedback loop that is necessary for monitoring speech production.

There is much we don't know about the speech of hearing-impaired children. The effects of aberrant movements of the articulators on perceptual judgments, the relationship between specific hearing thresholds and intelligibility, and the relation-

Table 6.1 Summary of Speech Intelligibility of Deaf Speakers Reported by Various Investigators

Investigator	*Description of Subjects*	*Mean Intelligibility*
Brannon (1964)	20 day school students, 12–15 years old; hearing losses 75 dB or greater	20–25%
Nober (1967)	46 residential students, aged 3–15; 60 dB or greater	Results given in age norms 60–80 dB = 4 yr 80 dB or greater = 3 yr on test of articulation
Markides (1970)	58 day and residential students, 7–9 years; no hearing levels given	31% (teachers) 19% (naive listeners)
Heidinger (1972)	20 residential students, 10–14 years; 85 dB or greater	20%
Smith (1972)	40 day and residential; 8–10 and 13–15 years; 80 dB or greater at 1000 Hz	18.7%
Weiss, Goodwin, and Moores (1975)	60 preschool chldren from several day and residential programs; 75 dB or greater	37%
Monsen (1978)	67 students at Central Institute for the Deaf, age 11 and older	76%

ship between phonological, articulatory, and rhythm deficits and overall intelligibility are only poorly understood.

REFERENCES

Angelocci, A., Kopp, G., and Holbrook, A., The vowel formants of deaf and normal-hearing eleven-to-fourteen-year-old boys, *J. Speech Hearing Dis.*, 29, 156–170, 1964.

Anthony, D. and Associates, *Seeing Essential English Manual*. Anaheim, CA: Educational Services Division, Anaheim Union High School District, 1971.

Berko, J., The child's learning of English morphology, *Word,* 14, 150–177, 1958.

Black, J., Speech pathology for the deaf. In L. Connor (Ed.), *Speech for the Deaf Child: Knowledge and Use*. Washington, D.C.: A. G. Bell Association, 1971.

Boone, D., Modification of the voices of deaf children, *Volta Rev.,* 68, 686–692, 1966.

Braine, M., The ontogeny of English phrase structure: The first phase, *Language,* 39, 1–13, 1963.

Brannon, J., The speech production and spoken language of the deaf, *Lang. Speech,* 9, 127–136, 1966.

Brannon, J., Linguistic word classes in the spoken language of normal, hard of hearing, and deaf children, *J. Speech Hearing Res.,* 11, 279–287, 1968.

Brannon, J. and Murry, T., The spoken syntax of normal hard of hearing and deaf children, *J. Speech Hearing Res.,* 9, 604–610, 1966.

Brown, R. and Bellugi, U., Three processes in the child's acquisition of syntax, *Harvard Educ. Rev.,* 34, 133–151, 1964.

Calvert, D., Speech sound duration and the surd-sonant error, *Volta Rev.,* 64, 401–402, 1962.

Calvert, D. and Silverman, R., *Speech and Deafness*. Washington, D.C.: A. G. Bell Association, 1975.

Carr, J., An investigation of the spontaneous speech sounds of five-year-old-deaf-born children, *J. Speech Hearing Dis.,* 18, 22–29, 1953.

Cooper, R., The ability of deaf and hearing children to apply morphological rules, *J. Speech Hearing Res.,* 10, 77–86, 1967.

Davis, J., Performance of young hearing impaired children on a test of basic concepts, *J. Speech Hearing Res.,* 17, 342–351, 1974.

Davis, J. and Blasdell, R., Perceptual strategies employed by normal hearing and hearing-impaired children in the comprehension of sentences containing relative clauses, *J. Speech Hearing Res.*, 18, 281–295, 1975.

Eimas, P., Speech perception in early infancy. In L. Cohen and P. Salapatek (Eds.), *Infant Perception: From Sensation to Cognition* (Vol. 2). New York: Academic Press, 1975.

Entwisle, D., *Word Associations of Young Children*. Baltimore: Johns Hopkins Press, 1966.

Ervin, S., Imitation and structural change in children's language. In E. Lenneberg (Ed.), *New Directions in the Study of Language*. Boston: M.I.T. Press, 1964.

Forner, L. and Hixon, T., Respiratory kinematics in profoundly hearing-impaired speakers, *J. Speech Hearing Res.,* 20, 373–408, 1977.

Fremer, J. and MacGinitie, W., Content of controlled continuous word association. In J. Rosenstein and W. MacGinitie (Eds.), *Verbal Behavior of the Deaf Child: Studies of Word Meaning and Association.* New York: Teachers College Press, 1969.

Gilman, L. and Raffin, M., Acquisition of common morphemes by hearing-impaired children exposed to the Seeing Essential English sign system. Paper presented at the Annual Convention of the American Speech and Hearing Association, Washington, D.C., 1975.

Goda, S., Language skills of profoundly deaf adolescent children, *J. Speech Hearing Res.,* 2, 369–376, 1959.

Griswold, L. and Commings, J., The expressive vocabulary of preschool deaf children, *Amer. Ann. Deaf,* 119, 16–28, 1974.

Heider, H. and Heider, B., A comparison of sentence structure of deaf and hearing children, *Psychol. Monographs,* 52, 42–103, 1940.

Heidinger, V., An explanatory study of procedures for improving temporal features in the speech of deaf children, Ph.D. Dissertation, Columbia University, 1972.

Hudgins, C. and Numbers, F., An investigation of the intelligbility of the speech of the deaf, *Gen. Psychol. Monographs,* 25, 289–392, 1942.

Hutchinson, J., Kornhauser, R., Beasley, D., and Beasley, D., Aerodynamic functioning in consonant production in hearing-impaired children, *Audiol. Hear. Educ.,* 4, 23–31, 1978.

Jacobson, D., Word associations and usage of parts of speech by deaf children, Master's Thesis, University of Minnesota, 1968.

John, J. and Howarth, J., The effect of time distortions on the intelligibility of deaf children's speech, *Language and Speech,* 8, 127–134, 1965.

Kline, T., A study of the free association test with deaf children, *Amer. Ann. Deaf,* 90, 237–257, 1945.

Lee, L. and Canter, S., Developmental sentence scoring: A clinical procedure for estimating syntax development in children's spontaneous speech, *J. Speech Hearing Dis.,* 36, 315–340, 1971.

Lenneberg, E., Prerequisites for language acquisition, *Proceedings of International Conference on Oral Education of the Deaf,* Washington, D.C.: A. G. Bell Association, 1967.

Levitt, H., Speech production for the deaf child. In L. Connor (Ed.), *Speech for the Deaf Child: Knowledge and Use.* Washington, D.C.: A. G. Bell Association, 1971.

MacGinitie, W., Ability of deaf children to use different word classes, *J. Speech Hearing Res.,* 7, 141–150, 1964.

Markides, A., The speech of deaf and partially-hearing children with special reference to factors affecting intelligibility, *British J. Dis.,* 5, 126–140, 1970.

Martony, J., On the correction of voice pitch level for severely hard of hearing subjects, *Amer. Ann. Deaf,* 113, 195–202, 1968.

Menyuk, P., *Sentences Children Use.* Boston: M.I.T. Press, 1969.

Monsen, R., Durational aspects of vowel production in the speech of deaf children, *J. Speech Hearing Res.,* 17, 386–398, 1974.

Monsen, R., Toward measuring how well hearing-impaired children speak, *J. Speech Hearing Res.,* 21, 197–219, 1978.

Monsen, R., Acoustic qualities of phonation in young hearing-impaired children, *J. Speech Hearing Res.,* 22, 270–288, 1979.

Morley, D., An analysis by means of sound spectrograph of intelligibility variations of consonant sounds spoken by deaf persons. Unpublished doctoral dissertation, University of Michigan, 1949.

Nober, E., Articulation of the deaf, *Exceptional Children*, 33, 611–621, 1967.

Odum, P., Blanton, R. and Nunnally, J., Some "cloze" technique studies of language capability in the deaf, *J. Speech Hearing Res.*, 10, 816–826, 1967.

Oller, D. and Kelly, C., Phonological substitution processes of a hard-of-hearing child, *J. Speech Hearing Dis.*, 39, 65–74, 1974.

Power, D. and Quigley, S., Deaf children's acquisition of the passive voice, *J. Speech Hearing Res.,* 16, 6–11, 1973.

Pressnell, L., Hearing impaired children's comprehension and production of syntax in oral language, *J. Speech Hearing Res.,* 16, 12–21, 1973.

Quigley, S., Smith, N., and Wilbur, R., Comprehension of relativized sentences by deaf students, *J. Speech Hearing Res.,* 17, 325–341, 1974.

Quigley, S., Wilbur, R., and Montanelli, D., Question formation in the language of deaf students, *J. Speech Hearing Res.,* 17, 699–713, 1974.

Quigley, S., Wilbur, R., Power, D., Montanelli, D., and Steinkamp, H., *Syntactic Structures in the Language of Deaf Children.* Champaign-Urbana: University of Illinois Press, 1976.

Raffin, M., Davis, J., and Gilman, L., Comprehension of inflectional morphemes by deaf children exposed to a visual English sign system, *J. Speech Hearing Res.,* 21, 387–400, 1978.

Sarachan-Deily, A. and Love, R., Underlying grammatical rule structure in the deaf, *J. Speech Hearing Res.,* 17, 689–698, 1974.

Schmitt, P., Deaf children's comprehension and production of sentence transformations and verb tenses, Ph.D. Dissertation, University of Illinois, 1968.

Schulze, G., An evaluation of vocabulary development by thirty-two deaf children over a three year period, *Amer. Ann. Deaf,* 110, 424–435, 1965.

Simmons, A., A comparison of the type-token ratio of spoken and written language of deaf and hearing children, *Volta Rev.,* 64, 417–421, 1962.

Smith, C., Residual hearing and speech production of the deaf, Ph.D. Dissertation, City University of New York, 1972.

Stewart, R., The speech of children with high frequency losses of hearing, *Sound,* 3, 40–43, 1969.

Templin, M., Vocabulary problems of the deaf child, *Internat. Audiol.,* 5, 349–354, 1966.

Tervoort, B., *Analysis of Communicative Structure Patterns of Deaf Children.* Final Report, Project No. RD-467-64-65, Vocational Rehabilitation Administration, U.S. Department of Health, Education and Welfare. Groniger: University Press, 1967.

Tweney, R. and Hoemann, H., The development of semantic associations in profoundly deaf children, *J. Speech Hearing Res.,* 16, 309–318, 1973.

Voelker, C., An experimental study of the comparative rate of utterance of deaf and normal hearing speakers, *Amer. Ann. Deaf,* 83, 274–284, 1938.

Weiss, K., Goodwin, M., and Moores, D., *Evaluation of Programs for Hearing Impaired Children: 1969–1974.* University of Minnesota Research, Development and Demonstration Center in Education of Handicapped Children, Research Report No. 91, 1975.

West, J. and Weber, J., A phonological analysis of the spontaneous language of a four-year-old hard-of-hearing child, *J. Speech Hearing Dis.,* 38, 25–35, 1973.

Wilbur, R., Quigley, S., and Montanelli, D., Conjoined structures in the language of deaf students, *J. Speech Hearing Res.,* 18, 319–335, 1975.

Wilcox, J. and Tobin, H., Linguistic performance of hard-of-hearing and normal-hearing children, *J. Speech Hearing Res.,* 17, 286–293, 1974.

Young, C. and McConnell, F., Retardation of vocabulary development in hard of hearing children, *Except. Chil.,* 23, 368–370, 1957.

CHAPTER 7

Assessment of Language and Speech

Assessment of language and speech skills requires that the clinician obtain enough information about a child's use of language to allow a reasonably accurate description of the skills under the child's control. It is unlikely that a single test or a single observation will yield the information necessary for making judgments about any child. Therefore, the clinician must devise a means of collecting several types of information in an efficient way. Many clinicians consider the analysis of a language sample to be the most satisfactory means of obtaining a representative picture of language knowledge and speech production while others prefer informal interactions or the use of standardized tests. Under ideal circumstances, all three of these approaches should be used and the results combined for a complete picture of language and speech knowledge and usage. An ongoing evaluation, conducted during the first days of therapy, would allow for a variety of procedures to be employed. In diagnostic settings or under circumstances in which the clinician has limited access to the child, assessment procedures must be chosen that will allow collection of the maximum amount of information within a reasonable and limited time span.

ASSESSMENT OF LANGUAGE

With the exception of the Test of Syntactic Abilities (*TSA*) developed by Quigley and his associates (Quigley, Steinkamp, Power, and Jones, 1978), the language assessment tools available to the average clinician were not designed with the hearing-impaired child in mind, an important consideration when selecting them and interpreting their results. Test items generally have not been selected on the basis of their visibility on the lips, the likelihood that they may or may not be acoustically ambiguous, or the probability that they can be *heard* by anyone with reduced hearing. The nature of the linguistic items to be tested almost precludes consideration of the preceding factors. Because the purpose of most language tests is to compare the performance of a given child to established norms for groups of children, test items must represent aspects of the language considered to be (1) most important to its successful development and (2) most stable and predictable in the normal population. These include such basic components of language as noun-verb agreement and plural or possessive forms, represented by the presence versus the absence of an ''s'' on a noun or verb; tense changes, represented by differentiation of short, similar words (he/she); and syntax, represented by strings of words whose surface order must be received accurately for appropriate comprehension. These and other units of language cannot always be tested in ways that maximize the hearing-impaired child's chances of performing well.

Nevertheless, these language components are invariants, in that they cannot be substituted for in the correct usage of language. Past-tense markers consist of either unstressed *ed* or structural word changes; there are no readily acceptable alternatives for expressing that linguistic form, except through the use of a modal verb, whose structure also changes with tense. The same is true for most of the bound morphemes of English, the correct usage of which is necessary for appropriate linguistic performance. If we wish to compare the hearing-impaired child's development, comprehension, and use of important language structures, we must assess his or her functioning on the same structure we consider important for the normal child. Therefore, failure to test items because they are poorly visible or barely audible negates the purpose of language assessment and results in an inadequate evaluation of the child's language skills.

Factors Influencing Test Performance

Use of Visual Information. Children with hearing loss are visually oriented. Through a system of trial and error they have learned to use visual information to varying degrees of effectiveness; they depend on it as an adjunct to imperfectly received auditory information. For children whose hearing losses are not severe, reliance on visual cues will be less and the nature of the cues that are useful may be different from those used by children with severe and profound hearing losses. During language assessment, however, it is wise to assume that a hearing-impaired child will attend to and use whatever visual cues are available as an aid to test performance. With this in mind, there are visual cues that it is advisable to provide and others that should be avoided. The former are those that will provide an appropriate situation in which the child can perform optimally. The latter are those that may influence the child's responses either favorably or adversely with regard to test performance, because of their interpretation.

The testing environment should be arranged to allow for the easy use of appropriate visual cues. Lighting should be planned so that the examiner is clearly visible to the child throughout the testing session. Light sources should never be located behind the speaker, because this causes the face to become a silhouette against the light and diminishes the clarity of facial expression and lip movements. The examiner should be seated within the visual field of the child, who should not have to turn the head or body sharply when looking from the test materials to the examiner's face. If test items or instructions are to be spoken, the examiner should be certain the child is attending before presenting information. Hearing-impaired children frequently prefer to look over the test items (e.g., pictures or objects) before they are ready to attend to their spoken counterparts. Allowing the child time to become oriented each time the test array changes will enhance attending behavior and thus increase the chances for maximal performance.

As in all spoken communication with the hearing impaired, the examiner should speak clearly, without exaggeration of mouth movements. Because language testing will be done on a one-to-one basis, it is usually not necessary to speak loudly. Loud speech results in changes in facial movements that may hinder lipreading and in acoustic modifications that may introduce distortion.

The examiner should avoid giving several types of visual cues. Hearing-impaired children may attend to subtle pieces of information that are inadvertently provided by the examiner. For example, when administering a point-to-the-picture task, it is common for beginning clinicians to pronounce the test item, then look at the correct item on the test materials until the child makes a choice. An alert hearing-impaired child can simply follow the examiner's eyes and choose responses accordingly. Some children will interpret irrelevant information, such as the location of the clinican's hand as it rests on a test booklet, as a clue to the correct answer. The best way to avoid giving visual cues of this nature is to practice administering tests in a standard, neutral manner. In the case of point-to-the-picture tasks, the examiner should pronounce the item, look at the child, then follow the child's movements while pointing to the item of choice. When pages are turned, the clinician's hand should then be removed from the test booklet and the item administered as suggested above.

Use of Auditory Information. All but the most profoundly hearing-impaired children will use auditory information to some extent during language assessment. Under no circumstances should language tests be administered to hearing-impaired children who wear hearing aids unless they are wearing amplification suitable to their needs. Whatever steps necessary should be taken to insure that the amplification device in use is operating satisfactorily and its controls set appropriately for the testing situation. All language assessment should be performed in a favorable acoustic environment. Noise sources should be identified ahead of time and eliminated. These include noises that are apt to be overlooked by normally hearing persons, such as the hum of an electric clock or aquarium motor in an otherwise quiet classroom, the noise made by jangling jewelry worn by the examiner, noisy fluorescent lights, heating or cooling unit blowers, or traffic outside the testing area. These sounds do not have to be loud to interfere with test performance, especially if they are located near the microphone of the amplification device in use.

Auditory information that is unnecessary for test administration should be avoided. Running commentary by the examiner may confuse a child who must concentrate on auditory and visual information in order to decipher messages. Hearing-impaired children are often poor at judging the relevancy of available auditory input; irrelevant comments may not be recognized as such and then discarded as nonessential to the task at hand. It is advisable to limit spoken comments *during testing* to those most relevant to the task at hand. This doesn't mean that verbal encouragement or proper feedback should not be offered, only that it should be clearly identifiable as such and held to an acceptable minimum.

Asking Children to Repeat Responses. Because hearing-impaired children are accustomed to misunderstanding spoken messages more often than the average child, examiners must be cautious about requesting them to repeat answers, either verbal or nonverbal. While such requests are often the legitimate result of failure to understand the child, to see a hurried pointing response, or to be able to distinguish an ambiguous response, they may be interpreted by the child as evidence that the original response was incorrect. In their daily lives, hearing-impaired children often respond to messages inappropriately as a result of inaccurate message reception. When this happens, they may be asked to repeat or the person with whom they are communicating may indicate in some other way that their responses were faulty. Thus, an examiner's statement of, "Which one? Show me again," may be interpreted as evidence of an incorrect response. Hearing-impaired children frequently change their answers when asked to repeat, unless they are very certain of their reception and comprehension of the item presented. On a point-to-the-picture test involving an array of three choices, this kind of alternative response will increase the probability of the occurrence of a correct response by chance.

The best way to avoid the need for repetition of responses is to establish the rules for test administration before testing begins. Children should be told that they may see and hear each item the appropriate number of times (this may vary from test to test) before choosing a single response. The first response will be accepted and recorded by the examiner. Children should be encouraged to ask for repetitions of a test item if they feel they need it. (While most language tests are designed for single presentations of test items, it makes no sense to adhere rigidly to such a procedure when the child being tested has a peripheral hearing impairment. The purpose of language assessment with such children is not to test their ability to hear or to lipread, but to investigate the degree to which they comprehend and/or express language under optimal circumstances.) If it is absolutely necessary to ask for a repetition of the child's response, the examiner should return to the questionable items at the completion of the test.

Mode of Communication. Hearing-impaired children use a variety of communication modes. These vary with degree and nature of the hearing loss and educational philosophy involved and include lipreading, audition, speech, fingerspelling, signing, reading, and writing. The ability to *communicate* in any of these modes may be evaluated separately by tests designed to measure each. It is important to remember, however, that the assessment of *language* skills should focus on the sum of linguistic knowledge possessed by children, regardless of the mode(s) by which they receive and express it. Therefore, language test items should be delivered to hearing-impaired children via the mode(s) utilized by them in their daily lives. To assess language knowledge in children who are accustomed to communicating via speech and hearing, clinicians must provide an environment in which the child can see and hear speech optimally. It is equally as important for children whose normal communication mode includes manual communication (fingerspelling and sign) to be tested in an environment that is optimal to their comprehension. This means that examiners of these children must be prepared to present instructions and test items simultaneously in both spoken and manual form. To do otherwise penalizes children in a way and to an extent that is not defensible. Test results reflect the examinees' ability to lipread or to hear but not their language knowledge, and erroneous conclusions may be drawn that lead to inappropriate recommendations and remediation practices. In the past most speech-language pathologists and audiologists have not been prepared to communicate using manual communication. As a result, they have either avoided becoming involved in assessment of the severely hearing-impaired population, or they have evaluated children using only speech or writing as stimulus forms. Neither of these approaches is sufficient. Indeed, neither have been legal since the passage of P. L. 94-142 in 1975. Among its other provisions this federal law (The Education for All Handicapped Children Act of 1975) requires that all evaluation materials used with children be free of racial or cultural bias. When children have impaired sensory, physical, or communicative skills, they must be evaluated using assessment instruments that take these deficits into account. Evaluators have the responsibility to be aware of the characteristics that dictate the use of special testing procedures and to provide the latter for each child according to individual needs (P. L. 94-142, 1975).

Hearing-impaired children often exhibit serious language deficiencies and are in need of well-designed remediation programs such as those that speech-language pathologists and audiologists are trained to provide. Unless an accurate measure of linguistic knowledge can be obtained, however, the evaluation and the recommended remediation program may fall short of the child's needs.

There are two approaches that may be taken toward the assessment of children who utilize use communication. The first is for the examiner to become proficient enough in the use of sign and fingerspelling to administer tests and other procedures bimodally (using speech and manual communication simultaneously). This method of communicating is known as simultaneous or total communication. There are many advantages to this approach, not the least of which is increased rapport with the children being tested. Anxiety levels are significantly reduced when such children become aware that communication on *their* terms is possible. The pressure of the test situation is enough to alienate the average child without the added frustration of having only a portion of the usual information available as a tool of communication.

The second approach is to provide an interpreter to assist in evaluation procedures. While this is certainly preferable to evaluating the child through the use of speech only, it has some disadvantages. Control over the stimulus presentation is reduced, and interpreters must be trained to deliver stimuli exactly as they are spoken by the examiner. This may involve somewhat different use of sign than that to which most interpreters are accustomed. "Translation" of the stimuli into sign rather than "interpretation" is called for, and the difference between the two is an important factor. Of course, if the examiner does the signing, the same precautions must be taken, but there is less likelihood of inconsistency when a single person is involved.

Use of an interpreter also serves to divide the child's attention between two people. If the examiner wishes to engage the child in other activities (such as an examination of the oral mechanism or imitation of speech sounds) it may be difficult to obtain attention and cooperation. Once the interpreter becomes a source of information, most children will then rely on that person as the sole provider of instructions, stimuli, explanations, and, in a way, *permission* to perform. This can be avoided if the examiner is able to use simultaneous communication. In addition, there is some evidence that comprehension of a message is better when it is presented bimodally by a single speaker than when interpretations is provided (Caccamise and Blasdell, 1977).

Until recently the sign system used by most deaf persons, both adults and children, was American Sign Language (ASL). This form of manual communication did not allow for easy translation from English into sign and vice-versa. (Recall the various sign systems and their uses discussed in Chapter 3.) This fact complicated language testing and led to the wide use of written stimuli for testing hearing-impaired children. Using the written form allowed for a visible, nonambiguous presentation of the bound morphemes necessary to English grammar (such as **ed, ing,** and **s**), English word order, function words, and other aspects of English not easily represented by ASL. Of course, use of written stimuli assumed that the examinees could read well enough to comprehend the message, thus limiting the population to be tested to older children who had attended school for several years (and were, therefore, well past the age for which normative data on the tests were available).

Because of the varied nature of the communicative modes used by hearing-impaired children and the situational demands placed on them, a thorough assessment of their language skills should include presentation of stimuli through spoken, written, or manual modes or any combination of these that is appropriate for a given child. The test procedures chosen for a child should be dictated by the child's needs and experiences, not by the tests or procedures preferred by clinicians based on experiences with normally hearing children. Efforts to tailor the evaluation to the child under test will require flexibility on the part of clinicians. These efforts will also result in the collection of meaningful baseline data that can be used effectively in the planning of language remediation.

The Language Evaluation

Assessment of language skills in children requires accurate observation of linguistic behaviors. Observation may be based on limited exposure to a given child during a visit to a diagnostic center for assessment or long-term exposure in a classroom or therapy situation. The observer and the envirnment may be familiar to the child or they may be strange. The observation period may be brief or extended over several days or weeks. Formal assessment tools, such as published tests, may be used by one examiner, while another may prefer to rely on informal interaction with the child. None of these alternative options is sufficient by itself, and a combination of them is preferable if language status is to be depicted accurately. Generally speaking, more experienced examiners require less time to become familiar with a child, less time in analysis procedures, and use of fewer "test" instruments to objectify data. Inexperienced examiners tend to over-rely on tests and test scores to describe language behavior, and experienced examiners may not provide enough verifying data to support their observation-based conclusions. Language assessment procedures that lie somewhere between these extremes should be the goal of the clinician.

Steps in the Language Evaluation. Language assessment data may be used for a variety of purposes, most of which involve the planning and execution of remediation programs. Therefore, it is important to obtain more than a score or set of scores if adequate planning is to result. The nature of a child's responses to a given task is often as important as whether or not the response was correct and may be more important in planning a teaching strategy that is well-suited to the child. Therefore, the language evaluation should consist of several steps.

1. *General observation.* This is a process of systematically viewing and recording behavior under a variety of circumstances. The obtained observations can then be used as an important adjunct to test scores, especially as a clue to their validity. Interactions between the child and teachers, parents, peers, and siblings may reveal patterns of communicative skills and interactive behavior that will influence learing in structured situations. What is the child's strategy for communicating? Does it work? If not, does the child become frustrated and if so, what form does the frustration take? How do the parents or peers then react? How successful is the child in getting a point across? What seems to be the primary mode for reception of language or environmental information? How comfortable does the child seem to be in classroom, play, family, or evaluative situations? What types of activities hold interest and which ones appear to be of no interest? Is the child a group participant or a loner? Is the child accepted by other children? What is the relationship between the child's ability to communicate effectively and the level of acceptance and/or warmth exhibited by peers or family members? Does the child appear motivated to communicate with familiar and nonfamiliar persons?

The informal observations described above should be augmented by careful observation of behavior during test administration as well. Does the child appear to be sure of responses or hesitant and tentative? Are the instructions understood before testing begins? Do responses appear random? Does the child's attention wander frequently or is the child alert and observant throughout the testing? Does the child seem reluctant to participate in the tasks presented or anxious? What is the child's reaction to praise, encouragement, or the suggestion that a response was incorrect? If easily discouraged, can the child be influenced to continue the activity or does the control of behavior become a difficult problem?

Not only will observation of the behavior listed above provide a basis for interpreting the validity of obtained test scores, it will also suggest appropriate teaching strategies to be employed by the clinician. Potential behavior problems may be identified and behavior management procedures that seem suitable can be instituted at the start of the remediation program rather than after a period of struggle between child and clinician. Maximal use of the input modes preferred by the child at the beginning of therapy will provide the most supportive atmosphere possible and may make the difference between cooperation and refusal to cooperate. Opportunities for early success can be made available based on knowledge of the child's interests and skills obtained through observations; the importance of building a chance for immediate success into remediation programs should not be ignored and can be enhanced greatly by careful observations prior to therapy.

2. *Clinician-child interactions.* To determine specific characteristics of language use during ordinary interactions, the clinician should engage the child in cooperative tasks that indicate how information already possessed is used. Materials or information are presented that informal observation has revealed to be known to the child. The child should be asked to describe, to list attributes, to contrast, or to predict. Make a note of the ways in which knowledge is organized and the ability to answer questions such as "What will happen if . . ." or "Why do you think that happened?" Responses can be analyzed later with regard to their grammaticality if the session is recorded. The clinician should attend primarily to the practical usage of language under a semiformal condition, especially with regard to the semantics of the utterances and the levels at which the known words or information can be expressed. For example, is the child able to group nouns into categories according to class (animals, foods, furniture), some function (walks upright, swims, lives in forests), or orthographic similarities (words containing two *e's,* words having only one different letter between them such as "house" and "horse," and so on)? Can the child use imagination to move beyond the present set of circumstances ("what if", "suppose you were?")? How effectively can the child explain reasons for classifying in a certain way or predicting a certain outcome? If the clinician is relaxed and the materials are interesting, much information can be obtained about the habitual ways in which the child's language is organized and used. In addition, the child's approach toward self-expression can be observed. Is the child confident or uncertain? Is the child eager to explain answers or hesitant to venture a guess? Does the child dissemble in an attempt to avoid giving answers or making decisions? Is the child interested in some topics, disinterested in others? How intelligible are utterances? When an utterance is not intelligible, what strategies does the child use to increase communication? What appears to be the major mode of reception? How consistently does the child appear to use auditory or visual information separately and combined? How does the child respond to verbal reinforcement, to corrections?

At the end of the structured observation period, the clinican should possess important information about the child's characteristic approach toward the use of language as a basis for making decisions and as a basis for communication. Knowledge of how well language "works" for a given child will be a valuable aid in planning a therapy approach tailored to the child's interests and needs.

3. *Testing*. In choosing the tasks to be administered, the clinician must determine the kinds of information most essential to an understanding of the child's linguistic status. The more sophisticated the user of language, the greater the amount of objective information that can be obtained. Most clinicians, however, are limited in the amount of time they can spend in language assessment of a single child, and most children are limited in the patience they will exhibit in the face of extensive evaluation. It is important, therefore, to determine which aspects of language are the most important indicators for a given child and to obtain information about those aspects in as efficient a way as possible. This means that the language evaluation—the battery of tests, amount of observation, types of adjunct information, and interpretation of results—will consist of different tasks, emphases, and procedures depending on the child to be evaluated and the decisions to be made as a result of the assessment. For example, decisions regarding educational placement should be based on data that include knowledge of language known to be necessary for academic achievement at various grade levels. The decision to enroll a child in therapy should be based on a comparison of the child's language skills to those of other children of the same age and stage of development. Four-year-old children should be evaluated using a different set of tasks and procedures than 10-year-old children.

4. *Analysis of evaluation results.* After testing and observation are completed, the clinician should compare performance on the various tasks presented and arrange test results along some logical dimension. Error patterns on tasks should be identified; consistent errors should be catalogued, perhaps in developmental order. Language forms or concepts to which the child responded inconsistently across test procedures or in spontaneous use should be retested in a diagnostic teaching paradigm. If the child can demonstrate knowledge of a linguistic form such as the concept of negation, under some circumstances but not all, the discrepancies should be noted carefully and used as guidelines in planning remediation.

To use test results as a basis for treatment, tests will have to be analyzed beyond the typical scoring procedures suggested by test manuals. Standard scores, percentile rankings, and age equivalents are unidimensional pieces of information. Raw scores are numbers, meaningless without context or normative data to which they can be compared. The language delay experienced by hearing-impaired children results in the use of many language tests or procedures with them that were designed for younger children. Norms established on children from 3 to 7 years of age are of little value with a 9-year-old child; we already know that the child is not functioning at age level and the percentile score resulting from comparison to norms will not provide much useful information except as an indication of the seriousness of the delay. In the following section, suggestions will be given for use of test scores and norms for individual tests.

The most important information to be obtained from assessment procedures is a *description* of the language behavior of the child under a variety of conditions. That being the case, the outcome of all the procedures employed should be recorded in descriptive terms that can be used to communicate knowledge of the child's linguistic status to parents, teachers, and other professionals. What does the child know and under what circumstances is it known? Can objects or actions be identified that cannot be expressed? Under what circumstances does communication break down? What are areas of strength and weakness in language? How does the child respond to evaluation techniques? How would the examiner evaluate the validity or reliability of the results obtained? What are the implications of the problem areas identified? The outcome of assessment should be interpreted in light of those questions. This will entail a narrative description of the child's performance that may include the scores or percentile rankings derived from raw scores but should never be limited to them.

5. *Use of evaluation results to plan remediation.* It should be obvious that the purpose of diagnostic procedures is to determine the need for treatment and to furnish a basis for treatment. Unfortunately, many language tests are administered to children, scored, and the results recorded in a cumulative folder, never to be consulted again. This occurs most often in situations in which there are too few professional personnel to serve the needs of the children identified. Although the lack of personnel may continue to be a problem for years to come, it is unlikely that test scores will continue to be filed away so completely. P. L. 94–142 requires that an individual educational plan (IEP) be designed for every handicapped child who receives special services within a school system. Because language status is central to a child's academic functioning, it has become an integral part of the evaluation resulting in the formulation of an IEP. Goals for teaching and remediation must be established for each component of the IEP, and all speicalists and educators who serve the child in question cooperate in the development and execution of the IEP with the informed consent and participation of the parents. Audiologists and speech-language pathologists have the knowledge and expertise to provide valuable input to the development of IEPs and should develop the habit of presenting language performance information in a useful form as it relates to the educational needs and status of the child. Reporting that a child scores 26 on the *Boehm Test of Basic Concepts* will not be very helpful in planning for that child. Listing the concepts answered correctly and incorrectly, and arranging the latter into concepts of quantity, space, time, or other categories could contribute significantly to the development of remedial goals.

Children require remediation based on objectives and goals that are established *before* treatment begins and revised as therapy progresses. In essence, all observations of language behavior can and should be related to the child's communicative needs and environment for the purpose of planning remediation, to be carried out either by clinicians, teachers, or parents.

Language Tests. The following discussion provides a framework for selection of assessment tasks and procedures that may be relevant to a given hearing-impaired child. For purposes of discussion, tasks have been given categorized as receptive or expressive, and they have been further classified as primarily testing syntax (structure) or semantics (meaning). It is important to remember that most language tests and, indeed, most verbal utterances represent a combination of structure and meaning. The meaning of a sentence depends to some extent on its structure, and the purpose of structual modifications is to express meaning in different ways. For example, the message that John clobbered Bill can be expressed as "John hit Bill" *or* "Bill was hit by John." It cannot be expressed as "Bill hit John," so word order expresses intent in a clearly specified way. Although meaning and structure are closely intertwined, it is useful to attempt to separate them somewhat for testing purposes as long as the clinician is cognizant of the *gestalt* nature of linguistic activities.

Published materials designed as language assessment tools are usually classified as receptive or expressive tests, depending on the nature of the task presented to the child. Receptive tests require the examinee to listen, to read, or otherwise observe stimulus presentations and respond to them nonverbally. Responses may consist of pointing to a picture, manipulating objects, or choosing from an array of objects, pictures, or words. Responses are then scored as correct versus incorrect and tallied to produce a score on the test.

Expressive tests require the child to speak or write responses to various stimuli. These utterances are recorded by the examiner and analyzed according to their structure and content. Stimuli for expressive tests may consist of sentences to be repeated or completed by the child, or pictures or objects to be discussed or about which a story must be developed. A large number of utterances is necessary if the language sample is to be considered representative of the child's language knowledge and usage.

Language tests are also classified as to the type of language under investigation. Tests of syntax and vocabulary are most common, and the majority of language tests on the market assess both of these language components.

Choice of the tests to be used in assessing the language skills of a particular child should be based on several factors. First, a single test should never be used as the basis on conclusions about a child's language status. A battery of tests will be necessary if an unbiased estimate of linguistic status is to be obtained. Even so, a child's performance under test conditions may be biased by unfamiliarity of the situation and the nature of the test items. These factors cannot always be controlled by the examiner, nor their influence estimated accurately. They can be minimized, however, by use of a variety of test stimuli and response modes. In addition, using several tests provides a broader array of items and allows a comparison of performance on similar items for purposes of validity and reliability estimates.

Second, tests should be chosen on the basis of their usefulness in planning for the child in question. Language tests should be chosen that are relevant to the child's communicative needs and that can be administered and scored as efficiently as possible. The problem is to obtain the maximum amount of information in the minimum amount of time. Experienced clinicians usually depend on a group of tests that can be given in various combinations depending upon the needs of the children to be tested. Tests that involve limited, common vocabulary and basic, simple sentence or phrase structure will be more appropriate for very young children or children who exhibit severely reduced verbal skills. The same tests will yield little information about older or more verbally skilled children, and their administration will be a waste of time.

Third, the decisions to be made as a result of the language assessment may also influence the choice of tests. If the problem is to decide whether or not a child's language skills are within the norm, then tests based on developmental norms for various structures should be given, and age equivalency scores may be helpful. If the question to be answered is whether or not to enroll the child in therapy, tests should concentrate on the daily language *needs* of the child as they relate to developmental norms. If the decision to be made is one of academic placement, then tests should be given that include items known to be relevant to academic achievement, such as vocabulary associated with curriculum materials to be used, the language of instructions, and similar factors.

Fourth, the battery of tests administered should include more than one type of response, if possible, and as many types of stimulus presentations as feasible for a given child. Young children may be limited to a point-to-the-picture response to stimuli that are presented orally (with or without sign), while older children may be able to respond to written materials in a variety of ways. Comparison of performance under different testing procedures can be helpful in planning optimal remediation programs. If a child recognizes the name of an item, but cannot produce the name spontaneously, the focus of remediation for that particular item is obvious.

Finally, the examiner must be careful to choose tests that yield valid and reliable measures of the language behavior of interest. For example, a test that purports to evaluate reception of syntax must be designed so that each item actually requires comprehension of the syntactic form expressed in order for a correct answer to be given more often than by chance alone. If the child can answer the item correctly on the basis of one or two lexical items within the utterance, the test item is not a valid one for investigation of the syntactic form involved. It may be a test of vocabulary knowledge instead. Validity of receptive items is often a function of the foils included for them, which must be controlled carefully. Figure 7.1 shows a receptive test item that requires understanding of the form used in order for a correct answer to be chosen. Figure 7.2 shows an item in which the foils do not require sufficient discrimination among alternatives in order for the correct answer to be chosen.

The test must also be a reliable tool, one which can be repeated with similar results, either on the same children or on a similar group of children. The reliability of a test may be questioned if successive administrations of the test result in widely different scores or if many items answered correctly on one administration of the exam are answered differently on the next administration. When choosing a test for use in language assessment, examiners should review critically the reliability and validity data provided in the test manual.

The following are examples of available language tests and suggestions for their use with hearing-impaired children. This discussion is not meant to be all inclusive; the number of tests on the market precludes a discussion of each. There may be other tests that are equally as appropriate as the ones discussed as follows, but these have been found to be useful in the ways suggested.

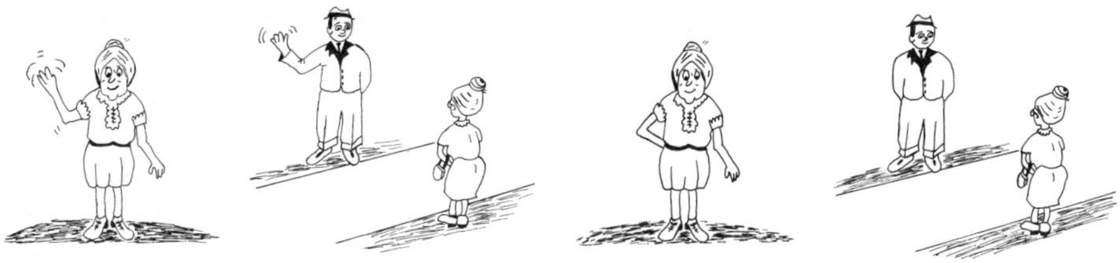

THE WOMAN IS WAVING

Figure 7.1. An example of receptive test foil items that require comprehension of the entire utterance for the correct choice of picture. The "woman" appears in all foils, but "is waving" in only one. Furthermore, the only other figure depicted is also waving in one foil.

Vocabulary Tests.

1. *Peabody Picture Vocabulary Test (PPVT)* (Dunn, 1965). By far the most widely used test of receptive vocabulary, the *PPVT's* major advantage is the testing procedure employed: the child points to pictures of the words spoken that increase in difficulty as the test progresses. Items can be presented in written form to children whose lipreading and auditory skills are poor. This test offers a general overview of vocabulary development but does not tap important factors such as knowledge of the multiple meaning of words or ability to determine word meaning by context. The validity of the test for all populations is questionable. It was standardized on white, middle-class children from the southeast region of the country, and it may not be an adequate representation of expected vocabulary knowledge of children whose race, region, or culture are not represented in the normative group. Slight variations in scores frequently result in large shifts in percentile rankings or age equivalency scores. Nevertheless, the *PPVT* is the most comprehensive and easily used vocabulary test available.

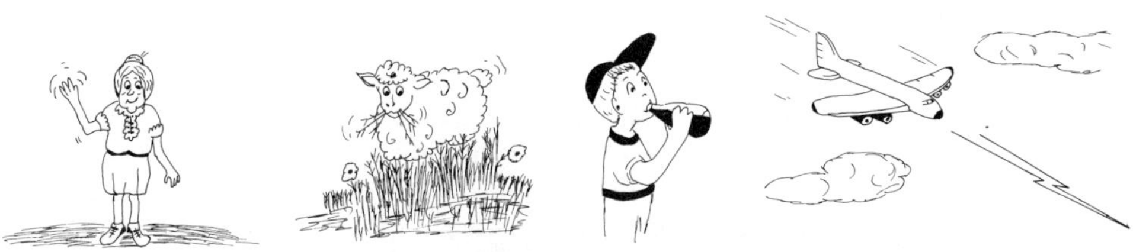

THE WOMAN IS WAVING

Figure 7.2. An example of receptive test foil items that require comprehension of only part of the utterance for a correct choice of picture. Only one "woman" is shown and only one figure "is waving." Comprehension of either lexical item results in a correct response.

The PPVT is designed for use with persons ages 3 to 21. The test is terminated when the examinee has responded incorrectly to six of the last eight items administered. The last item given is the *ceiling* score, from which the number of incorrect responses is subtracted to obtain the *raw* score. The latter can be converted into a percentile ranking for the examinee's age or a so-called "mental age." Use of the term mental age and its conversion into an IQ score is based on the assumption that vocabulary knowledge is closely related to intelligence. Although this may or may not be true for normally hearing persons, it is certainly not the case for hearing-impaired persons, whose verbal skills (including vocabulary knowledge) may have been seriously affcted by the hearing impairment. Therefore, results of the *PPVT* should *never* be reported for hearing-impaired children in terms of mental age or IQ. At the same time, results are meaningless when reported as a numerical raw score (57, 72, or 36). To make the results of the *PPVT* useful or meaningful to parents or professionals they may be reported as approximate age equivalencies. Statements such as, "Johnny's performance on the *PPVT* is similar to that associated with children aged 6 years, 6 months," or "Johnny's receptive vocabulary is similar to that expected of children about two years younger than he is," provide a reference point for Johnny's performance based on vocabulary knowledge without suggesting a direct relationship with mental ability. Because the test norms extend to age 21, age-equivalency statements are appropriate and their estimates are not seriously influenced by a ceiling effect.

In addition to reporting scores relative to age norms, it is helpful to analyze results according to the type of items missed. This is a time-consuming task with the *PPVT*, because items are not identified as to their word class and must be classified individually by the clinician. For children with severely reduced vocabularies the task is minimal due to the small number of items to be analyzed and may yield information regarding the type or types of vocabulary items known to the child. Because experience has shown that hearing-impaired children learn concrete and common vocabulary items more quickly than abstract ones, it should be possible to predict some of the errors that will be made by them. In fact, experience has shown that hearing-impaired children exhibit great scatter in their responses on the *PPVT*. They do not reach a ceiling item as quickly as normally hearing children with comparable vocabularies. It is not uncommon for hearing-impaired children to answer one item correctly, miss the next five, then answer two more correctly, and so on, teetering on the edge of reaching a ceiling for a large number of items. This unsystematic pattern of responses may be related to the nature of the items (word class, concretism), or it may reflect teaching strategies that have been employed.

Characteristic performance by hearing impaired children on the *PPVT* includes scores below those expected for children of comparable age. Increases in vocabulary knowledge occur with age, but at a slower rate than that of normally hearing children. The gap between the norms and a hearing-impaired child's score tends to widen with age, so that a child whose score represented a delay in vocabulary development of 12 months at age 5 will usually exhibit a greater discrepancy at age 7 and a greater one still at age 10. Figure 7.3 shows a typical vocabulary growth curve for a severely hearing-impaired child as it compares to normal vocabulary growth. Unless unusual attention is given to vocabulary development and extraordinary progress is made, hearing-imparied children do not "catch up" in vocabulary knowledge. The *PPVT* provides a means whereby vocabulary growth can be charted, however, as long as the limitations of the test are understood and considered during test intepretation.

The *PPVT* is difficult to sign, as many of the items are not represented by separate signs in most manual systems. Items can be fingerspelled or written for older children who cannot hear or read lips well enough to "understand" the test

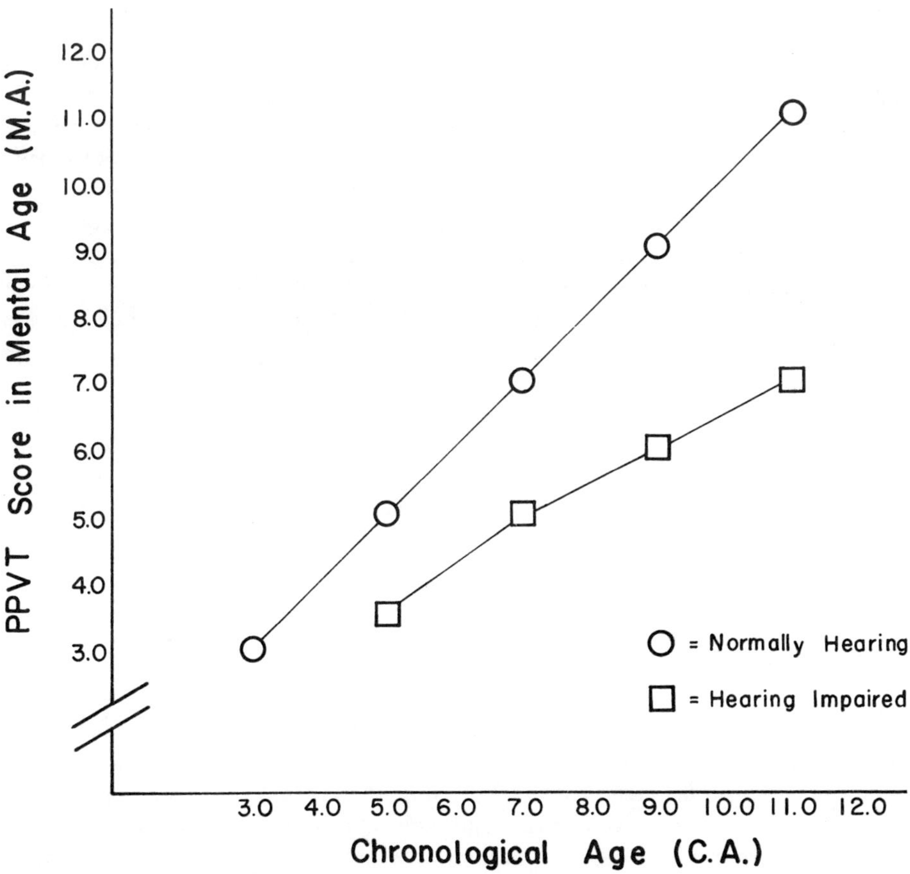

Figure 7.3. Example of a vocabulary growth curve exhibited by a hearing impaired child compared to normal vocabulary development.

items, but the test is most appropriate for hard-of-hearing children who communicate via the spoken word.

2. *Boehm Test of Basic Concepts (BTBC)* (Boehm, 1970). Strictly speaking, the *BTBC* is not a vocabulary test. It consists of 50 one- to three-word items considered to be necessary for understanding instructions and curriculum materials in the first three grades of school (kindergarten, first, and second grades). Items are graduated in difficulty and consist of time (before, beginning), quantity (more than, one-half), space (away from, next to), and miscellaneous concepts (matches, same). Test booklets allow the examinee to point to or make a mark on one of three picture foils for each item presented. The total number of correct responses is recorded and compared to one of nine sets of norms provided: high, middle, and low socioeconomic levels for each of the three grade levels. Percentile rankings are available for scores on each set of norms.

The *BTBC* is designed to be used as a group test in a regular classroom. Each child marks an individual booklet, and instructions include statements designed to insure that each child is looking at the proper row of pictures on the proper page. As a result, the instructions are wordy and may be confusing to children with hearing impairment. It is recommended that the test be administered individually to these children. The examiner should turn the pages and indicate the picture array to be considered for a given item. For highly distractible children, test pages can be cut up and presented to the child in segments related to the item under test. Either way, individual testing allows for reduction in the quantity of verbal instructions without changing the essential nature of the test item. An example of simplified instructions is given below.

Group instructions:

> Look for the gray box like this one on your page. Put your finger on the gray box with the book in it. Now take your finger off the box and pick up your pencil. Look at the flags on the poles. Mark the pole with the flag at the top. . . Mark the pole with the flag at the top.

Individual instructions:

> Look at these pictures. Show me the pole with the flag at the top.

Although test instructions do not suggest it, errors may be analyzed according to the type of concept (time, quantity, space, or miscellaneous) on which they occurred. Because the concepts tested are important to comprehension of much of the language used in early primary classrooms, results of this test can provide valuable information to teachers regarding a child's linguistic basis for many classroom activities. Failure to comprehend a task or follow directions may be related to a lack of knowledge of the vocabulary involved and not to a basic inability to perform the task. The distinction seems obvious, but is not always so, particularly to personnel who have little or no training or experience with children who have language dificits.

Results of the *BTBC* are also useful in making educational placement decisions, particularly when mainstreaming is an option to be considered. An estimate of the child's knowledge of the vocabulary necessary for comprehension of instructions and daily activities will contribute to predictions regarding probable success within a given grade. If Sally's first-grade classmates are from a high socioeconomic background and highly verbal, and her score on the *BTBC* and resulting percentile ranking are low, these factors may suggest a low probability of success in the classroom under consideration. If the decision to mainstream is made under these circumstances, *BTBC* scores at least provide guidelines for the focus of remedial and resource assistance in the form of preteaching or adjunct instruction.

The relationship between performance on the *BTBC* and academic achievement is not clear in spite of the assumptions inherent in construction of the test. It is possible that *BTBC* scores underestimate children's knowledge. Nevertheless, experience with hearing-impaired children's performance on the test has revealed that they exhibit spotty knowledge of the concepts tested, similar to that associated with the *PPVT*. Unlike normally hearing children whose knowledge of the 50 concepts increases with age in a systematic progression from items 1 through 50, hearing-impaired children show no systematic pattern of learning, even among the first 25 items. When compared to their normally hearing classmates, they exhibit shockingly poor knowledge of these basic concepts. Although their scores improve slightly with age (at least from 6 to 8 years), the percentile rankings associated with their scores decrease with age and grade level, indicating a widening gap between hearing-impaired children's knowledge of the concepts involved and that of their hearing classmates (Davis, 1974).

3. *IQ Tests*. Intelligence tests such as the Stanford-Binet and the Wechsler Intelligence Scale for Children include word definition tasks as part of their verbal sections. Performance on these portions of the tests can be used to estimate the vocabulary or word meaning level at which the examinee is functioning. Scores are related to age norms for the knowledge tested and are usually expressed as mental ages. For children with language deficits, including hearing-impaired children, reporting of scores in terms of mental age or IQ is misleading, for the reasons mentioned in the discussion of the *PPVT*. Performance on the verbal portion of IQ scales can be used, however, to chart vocabulary growth and to provide an estimate of expressive vocabulary. Unlike point-to-the-picture tasks like the *PPVT* or *BTBC*, intelligence test vocabulary measures require children to define words orally, using the vocabulary and language structures under their control. Because the identification of a picture represents a lower level of word knowledge than the formulation and expression of that word's definition, both types of vocabulary measures should be obtained for comparison purposes. Psychologists should be encouraged to provide vocabulary or verbal subtest scores when reporting intelligence test results for inclusion in the linguistic data bank to be compiled for a given child.

4. *Vocabulary portions of other language tests*. Many of the language tests currently available include brief vocabulary sections whose items form the core vocabulary of the remainder of that test. This procedure is sound, because a child's responses to syntactic or morphological items may be influenced by knowledge of the content or function words involved in the longer structures. Two examples of vocabulary presentation in tests designed for assessment of other aspects of language are the Assessment of Children's Language Comprehension (ACLC) and the Test for the Auditory Comprehension of Language (*TACL*). Other aspects of these tests will be discussed in detail below, but each begins with a series of vocabulary items. The *ACLC* presents 50 vocabulary items, consisting of 30 common nouns, 10 verbs, 5 prepositions, and 5 adjectives. Because these items occur frequently in spoken language and represent a cross section of word classes, the first 50 items of the *ACLC* provide an excellent vocabulary test for very young, low-verbal children. The point-to-the-picture response requires no verbalization on the child's part and allows a comparison of the child's relative knowledge of the four word classes presented. Results can be used as a basis for early therapy and preparation for further testing. The child who cannot identify the basic vocabulary of the *ACLC* is unlikely to be able to participate in more advanced language testing.

The *TACL* contains 41 vocabulary items, including 12 nouns, 18 adjectives, 8 verbs, and 3 adverbs. As in the *ACLC,* these words form the basis for the remainder of the test, but they represent a somewhat more advanced level of word knowledge. For example, in addition to the type of descriptive adjectives found in the *ACLC* (dirty and broken), the *TACL* presents adjectives of quantity (many, some, more) that represent less concrete modifiers. The *TACL,* therefore, is less useful as a vocabulary measure with very low-verbal children, but may yield more information for children whose language delay is not so severe. Examiners should not overlook performance on vocabulary items of tests such as the two examples given. They furnish an additional vocabulary measure at the same time that other facets of language are being investigated. Although no true norms for these subscores can be ascertained, the *TACL* provides information regarding the ages at which 75 percent and 90 percent of normal children have developed mastery of the words tested, and the *ACLC* vocabulary is assumed to be within the repertory of children aged 3 to 6 years. The important information to be gleaned from performance on the vocabulary portions of tests such as the *ACLC* and *TACL* is not the establishment of an age equivalency or percentile rank, but an estimate of the child's strengths and weaknesses concerning the several word classes involved. Analysis of errors, their comparison to errors on other vocabulary measures, and their relation to the communicative demands faced by a given child provide much more useful information to clinicians, teachers, and parents than a single score or an age-related norm or percentile ranking. The latter are important for establishing baseline data and charting growth, but they must be used in conjunction with error analysis data if they are to have any practical usefulness to the child or professional personnel responsible for remediation.

5. *Type-Token Ratio*. An estimate of the number of different word classes and the number of examples of each used by a child can be obtained by analysis of written or spoken language samples. Such an analysis provides an indirect measure of vocabulary size and complexity.

Tests of Morphology and Syntax. The morphology and syntax of a language is made up of several components. Word order, noun-verb agreement, verb tense, plurals, possessives, and clause structure are just a few of the categories included under the general heading of syntax. Because of the complexities of English, attempts to devise tests of its comprehension and usage are under constant revision and modification. Certain invariants of the language have become the focus of existing tests, most of which are labeled "screening" tests of syntax or morphology. The establishment of norms is a complex procedure and many so-called "tests" are marketed and used without the collection of adequate normative data. Persons who have constructed the tests defend them on the basis of their practical usefulness to clinicians, and their widespread use suggests that this may be a reasonable defense. Certainly clinicians feel more comfortable about language assessment now than they did 20 years ago, before most of the currently available tests of language structure were available for use. It is obvious that knowledge of some structures can be assessed more readily than that of others. This fact is reflected in the overlap of the content of many language tests on the market, with additional ones being developed frequently.

In choosing tests of syntax for clinical use, it is helpful for the clinician to reflect on the purpose of the assessment in general and the knowledge sought about a given child in particular. Establishment of a precise estimate of the chronological age level associated with certain language behaviors would demand use of a test for which normative data have been carefully and extensively compiled. On the other hand, understanding a child's strengths and weaknesses in comprehension and expression of certain useful and common language structures could be accomplished by administering any test or series of tests that provide several varied opportunities for a child to demonstrate the desired knowledge. For clinicians whose purposes correspond to the latter statement, there are several useful syntax assessment tools on the market.

1. *Northwestern Syntax Screening Test (NSST)* (Lee, 1969). This test consists of two portions, a receptive test and an expressive test. The receptive test uses 20 test arrays of four pictures each. Sentences representing two of the pictures are spoken by the examiner without identifying them with their respective pictures. Each of the sentences is repeated separately with the request that the child point to the picture of the sentence spoken. For example, for the array shown in Figure 7.4,

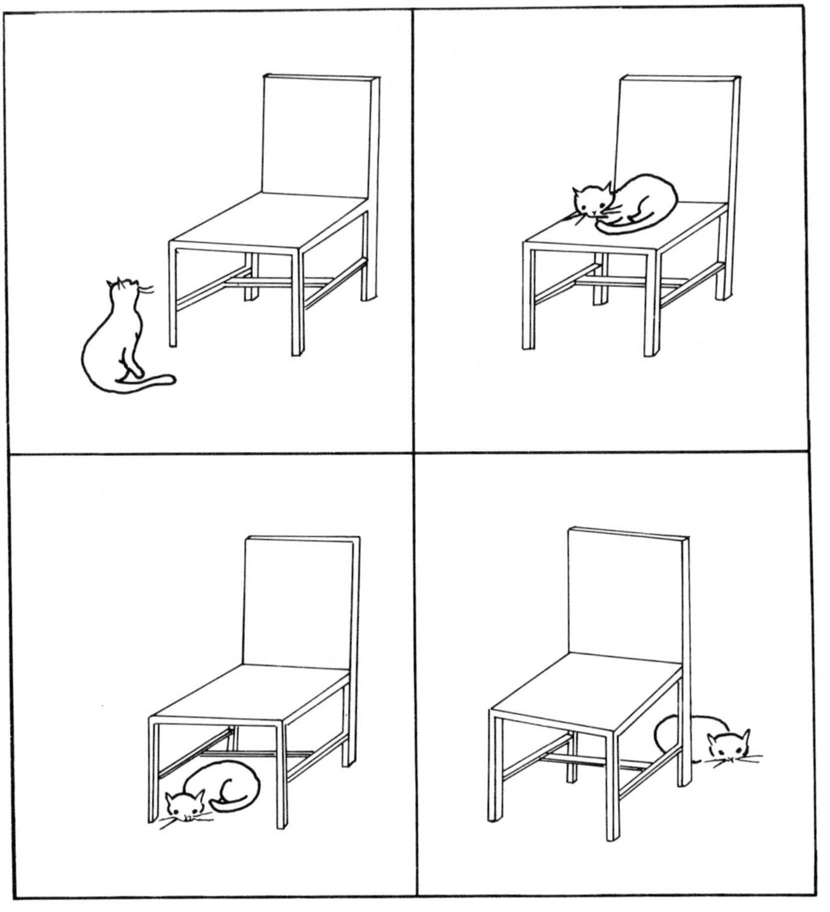

Figure 7.4. Picture array from the receptive portion of the *Northwestern Syntax Screening Test.* The stimulus items are, "The cat is behind the chair; the cat is under the chair." (Reprinted with permission from the *Northwestern Syntax Screening Test.* Copyright © 1969, 1971 by Northwestern University Press.)

the examiner would say, "The cat is under the chair. The cat is behind the chair. Show me 'the cat is under the chair.' Show me 'the cat is behind the chair.'"

The child receives one point for each picture correctly identified, for a possible receptive score of 40 (two pictures for each of 20 arrays). Test sentences for both the receptive and expressive subtests represent several sentence forms and seek to test knowledge of pronouns, verb inflection, plurals, prepositions, negative transformation, direct and indirect objects, question forms, and possessives. Many of these forms appear only once in the test. It is important to remember that the *NSST* is a screening test that yields only a gross estimate of the child's comprehension of the structures tested.

The expressive portion of the *NSST* consists of a delayed sentence imitation task. Twenty arrays of two pictures each are presented singly to the child being tested. The examiner points to each picture and produces the sentence associated with it. After providing the correct sentence for each of the two pictures, the examiner asks the child to produce the sentence associated with them individually. For the array shown in Figure 7.5 the examiner would point to the appropriate picture and say, "The baby is sleeping." Pointing to the second picture the examiner would then say, "The baby is not sleeping." (pause) "Tell me about this

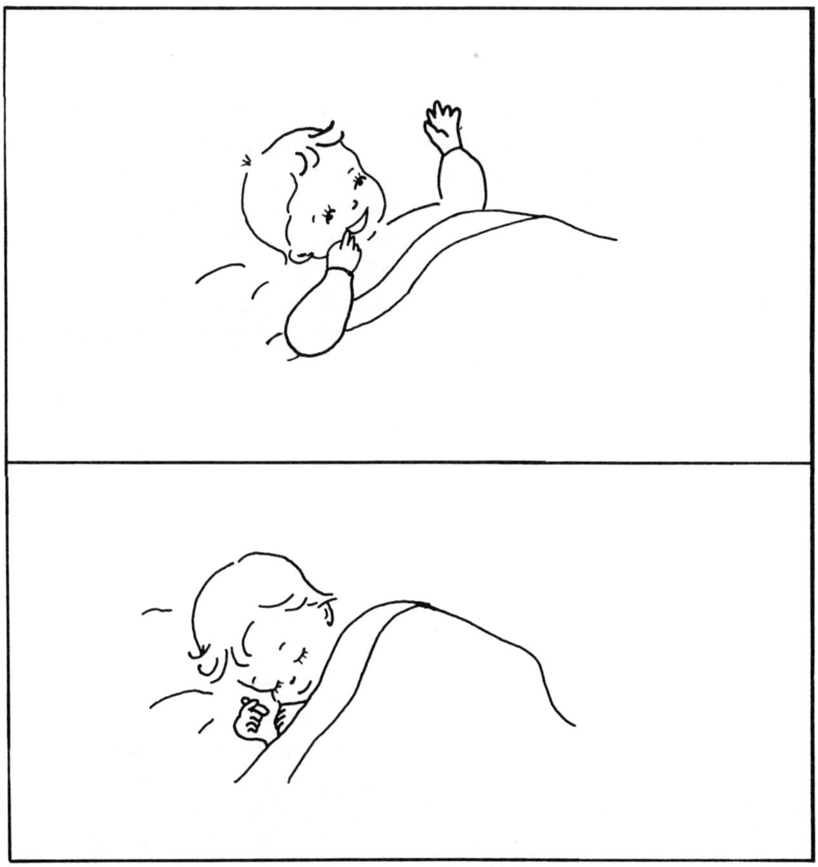

Figure 7.5. Picture array from the expressive portion of the *Northwestern Syntax Screening Test* designed to elicit the sentence, "The baby is not sleeping." (From L. Lee, *Northwestern Syntax Screening Test,* Northwestern University Press, © 1971.)

picture'' (pointing to the ''The baby is sleeping,'' then repeating the request for the second picture). The total possible score for the expressive subtest is 40 points, two per picture array. For both the receptive and expressive subtests, scoring is binary: either the answer is correct and worth 1 point, or it is incorrect and worth zero points. This probably affects the expressive subtest more than the receptive, because the child is required to repeat the sentence correctly in order to receive credit as opposed to a pointing response in the receptive portion. There is simply more margin for error. In fact, because the test is designed to screen for the ability to comprehend and produce certain structures, a semantically correct response of ''The baby is awake'' for the picture shown in Figure 7.5 must be scored as incorrect, because it does not contain the negative form, ''not sleeping.''

There are several difficulties involved in the use of the *NSST* with hearing-impaired children. Much of the vocabulary involved in the test is not visibly distinctive on the lips and several items rely on perception and comprehension of the placement of the morpheme **s,** for example, ''The boy writes; the boys write,'' and ''The girl sees the dog; the girl sees the dogs.'' Differentiation between such acoustically and visually similar items may be impossible for some hearing-impaired children with the result that the receptive portion may be testing speech discrimination or lipreading skills rather than language knowledge. The expressive subtest may be influenced by the child's ability to *hear* the sentence to be repeated and to produce word endings such as **s** and **ed,** and phonemes such as **sh** (she versus he). Misarticulations on the part of the child make scoring difficult and inconsistent. Every effort should be made to maximize the child's chances of perceiving the test items accurately, and effort should be made to determine the child's articulation errors as they relate to the test items. Scores on the *NSST* should always be interpreted in light of the peripheral deficit. To do this, test responses should be analyzed according to the errors made, and less emphasis should be placed on the overall score (receptive or expressive) as a measure of language knowledge.

Indeed, interpretation of test scores by hearing-impaired children is a major problem with the *NSST*. Norms for the test were established on young hearing children and scores are interpreted by comparison to their percentile rankings for ages 3-0 to 7-11. Assuming these norms are accurate, most hearing-impaired children whose language skills are sufficiently developed to enable them to participate in the *NSST* without severe frustration are beyond the ages for which norms are established. It is meaningless to describe a 9-year-old hearing-impaired child's score on the *NSST* as ''falling below the 1st percentile for seven year olds.'' Such statements are not helpful in planning for remediation, a primary purpose of language assessment. A much more meaningful description can be obtained by noting the child's score on each subtest, entering the normative data, and identifying the age for which that score represents the 50th percentile. For example, suppose 9-year-old Nancy obtained a receptive score of 28 and an expressive score of 19 on the *NSST*. According to the normative tables provided her scores represent the 50th percentile for children from 4-6 to 4-11 years (receptive) and children from ages 3-6 to 3-11 (expressive). Results could then be described as follows: "Nancy's performance on the receptive subtest was similar to that of the average 4-year-old hearing child; her performance on the expressive subtest was most like that of a 3-year-old normally hearing child. These results indicate a severe delay in Nancy's ability to understand and produce the type of sentence structures represented on the *NSST*." If the examiner goes on to report the type of sentence structures Nancy could and could not handle accurately, a picture of her ability to process sentences begins to emerge. This information, coupled with descriptions of other language behavior, can be used to determine an appropriate starting place for remediation.

Compared to other language tests designed for young children, the *NSST* is a difficult test because it consists entirely of sentences. Hearing-impaired children show their greatest language deficits when attempting to comprehend or produce grammatical and acceptable sentences. Even the relatively simple structures of the *NSST* involve complexities of form that must be taught to many hearing-impaired children, usually at an age well beyond that associated with the form's acquisition by normally hearing children. Therefore, the *NSST* is seldom the test of choice during an initial evaluation unless the child shows evidence of understanding and producing a variety of sentences. It can provide valuable information in conjunction with other measures and often provides dramatic documentation of the difference between comprehension of words or short phrases (red ball; big, black car) and understanding common English sentences.

Hearing-impaired children score well below their normally hearing peers on the *NSST*, and they usually socre significantly higher on the receptive than on the expressive subtests. The test can be signed, using a sign system that represents English. A concept system such as *ASL* does not provide necessary information for comprehension of the word endings, pronoun usage, and possessives that make up a large portion of the test.

2. *Assessment of Children's Language Comprehension (ACLC).* The *ACLC* (Foster, Giddan, and Stark, 1972) consists of 50 vocabulary items and 30 items designed to test comprehension of short phrases composed of what the test's authors refer to as *critical elements*. According to the authors, the *ACLC* assesses "how many word classes in different combinations of length and complexity" a child can understand. The 50-item vocabulary was chosen because the words were easily pictured, commonly used, and consisted of two syllables or less. These 50 words constitute the entire test vocabulary and consist of 30 nouns, 10 verbs, 5 prepositions, and 5 adjectives. Phrases representing the semantic relationships most commonly expressed by young children developing language consititute the 30 critical element test items.

As language develops, the number of syntactic units that children are able to process increases. These units constitute the critical elements included in the test. Ten items each represent phrases consisting of two, three, and four critical elements. The task involves a point-to-picture response by the child after each item is presented orally by the examiner. Test plates consist of black-and-white drawings representing the spoken phrase and three foils. The foils are carefully designed so that the child must comprehend the relationship among the critical elements in order to choose the correct answer. Recognition of the individual words spoken does not provide enough information on which to base an accurate choice. Figure 7.6 shows the stimulus plate for the two critical element test items, "horse standing." As can be seen, only one of the drawings represents the meaning of the phrase; comprehension of either word alone may result in an incorrect response.

The *ACLC* is scored according to the percentage of items correctly identified within each critical-element category. Within a given category, phrase structure varies considerably. Two element stimuli include agent-action (man sitting), attribute-object (big shoe), and attribute-agent (happy lady). Three critical element items include attribute-agent-action (happy lady sleeping) and agent-action-object (boy blowing the horn), among others. Examples of four critical element items are noun-verb-preposition-nouns (boy standing in house) and modifier-noun-preposition-noun (broken boat on table).

For low-verbal children, the vocabulary section of the *ACLC* is a more useful vocabulary screening tool than standardized vocabulary tests because it presents basic words commonly used by young children who are just developing language. It is not unusual for young, severely hearing-impaired children to be unable to respond to standard vocabulary tests well enough to establish a baseline score. This type of child frequently recognizes nouns and few, if any, words from other word classes. The *ACLC* provides a screening tool with which to ascertain a child's recognition of words from four basic word classes that are necessary for expressing early semantic relationships. If the child in question does not recognize the vocabulary items, the test cannot be completed.

Performance on the *ACLC* allows the examiner to determine the point of breakdown in a child's ability to process from one to four syntactic units. Percentage scores for vocabulary and two, three, and four critical element subtests are obtained. Performance may also be analyzed according to the consistency of the pattern of words missed (which sequential element was incorrect in the response chosen by the child). The authors of the *ACLC* suggest that auditory memory problems can be detected by such an analysis, but this is probably less true for hearing-impaired children than for others because of the peripheral hearing loss and its possible contamination of measures of auditory memory.

Normative data for the *ACLC* were collected on 365 nursery and kindergarten children, including a number of minority group children. Mean scores for ages 3-0 to 6-5 are provided in the manual, but no real norms are available. Results yielded by a child on the *ACLC* should be analyzed according to the child's strengths and weaknesses. How many of the 50 vocabulary items were correct and which word classes did they represent? Are there word classes that the child did not com-

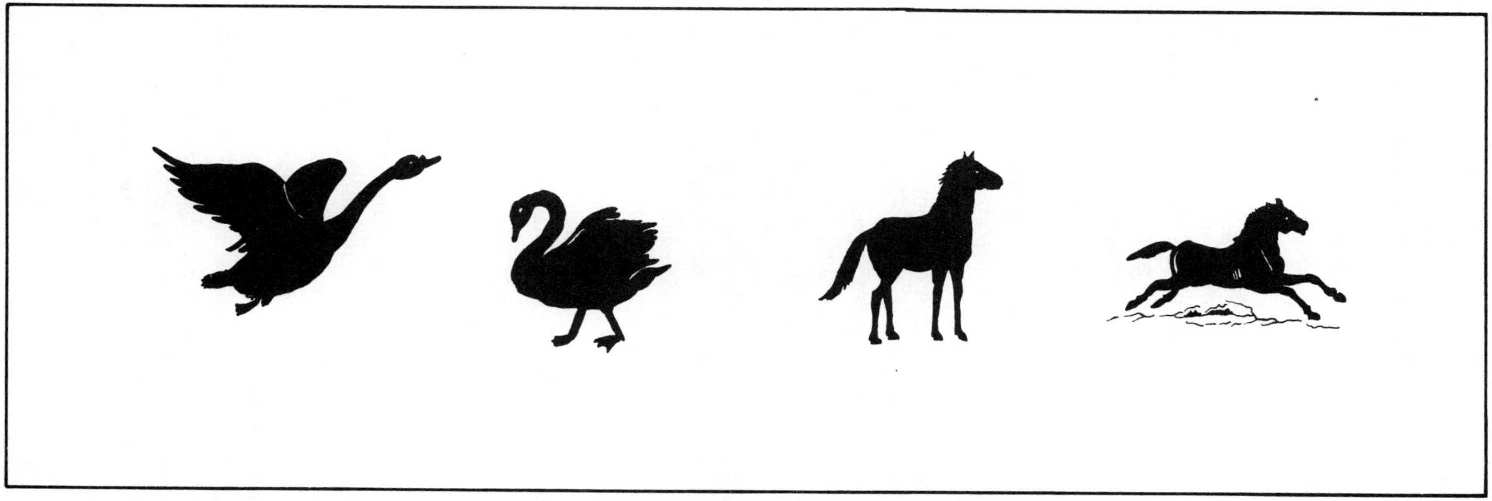

Figure 7.6. Picture array from the *Assessment of Children's Language Comprehension Test* for the stimulus item, "horse standing." (Reproduced by special permission from the *Assessment of Children's Language Comprehension Test* by Rochana Foster, Jane Giddan, and Joel Stark. Copyright 1972, published by Consulting Psychologists' Press, Inc.)

prehend? How many critical elements can the child process accurately? When performance breaks down, which word classes create the greatest difficulty? Is there a consistent pattern of word class usage or confusion? Are there certain semantic relations that are consistently misunderstood? The authors of the *ACLC* give suggestions for use of the test results in planning therapy.

For children whose knowledge of syntax is well advanced, the *ACLC* is too simple and yields too little information to be valuable. For young children struggling to develop syntactic skills, the ACLC is a useful tool, particularly for use with children who perform poorly on tests using adult grammar. It is made even more useful by its brevity; the test can be completed in about 10 minutes. Test items may be signed and spoken simultaneously with ease, because of the restricted and simple nature of the vocabulary included.

3. *Test for Auditory Comprehension of Language (TACL).* This test, published by Carrow in 1973, consists of 101 point-to-the-picture items in three categories: vocabulary (41 items), morphology (48 items), and syntax (12 items). Three picture stimuli are provided for each test item. The vocabulary items at the beginning are used throughout the remainder of the test to assess various morphological or grammatical forms. A child's responses can be analyzed according to the categories listed above, used to obtain a raw score that yields a "language equivalency age" and a percentile ranking by score and age, or compared individually to the established ages at which 75 percent and 90 percent of normally developing children demonstrate understanding of a given item.

The *TACL* is perhaps the simplest to administer of the receptive language tests currently in vogue. Items are short, except for a few relatively complex sentences, a fact that contributes to its usefulness with hearing-impaired children. Test items do not overwhelm the child with verbiage in order to test a given form; the form is presented in an abbreviated way (e.g., "has eaten" or "fattest"). It is possible, however, that elimination of the context for syntactic forms influences their comprehension in an undetermined way.

Norms for the *TACL* extend from age 3-0 to 7-0. The test was standardized on 200 children and reliability estimates have been obtained for several groups of children. Davis (1977) investigated reliability of *TACL* scores for two groups of hearing-impaired children: (1) children whose training and communication were oral-aural and (2) children who used total communication at home and at school. Both groups exhibited reliable responses to repeated administrations of the test (an r of .96 was obtained for the oral group and .90 for the total group). The test also appears to be a valid measure of language comprehension for hearing-impaired children, and, along with other test scores and observation, provides a reasonable estimate of a child's general level of language comprehension. The age-equivalency score should be used with caution, much the same way in which the *NSST* 50th percentile age estimate is described in the preceding discussion. Many hearing-impaired children will exhibit language comprehension skills within the range tested by the *TACL* even though their chronological ages are well beyond those associated with the test norms. Nevertheless, the age-equivalency score and the subtest results provide evidence concerning a given child's level of language comprehension compared to a developmental model that can be useful for educational and remedial planning.

Because of the direct way that language forms are tested by the *TACL,* the test is easy to sign using a system that represents English morphology. Davis (1977) reported no significant difference between reliability or validity measures for the *TACL* when it was signed and spoken versus when it was only spoken. Thus, it can be a useful tool in the assessment of young children who are accustomed to communicating via an English-based sign system.

4. *Test of Syntactic Abilities (TSA).* The only test of syntax designed for use in the assessment of the hearing impaired is the *TSA* (Quigley *et al.,* 1978). It is based on a generative grammar model. The purpose of the *TSA* is to provide an opportunity for children to demonstrate knowledge of a variety of syntactic structures that form the basis of English grammar, but which are difficult to elicit in spontaneous language samples. The absence of these structures in written language samples is not always due to the fact that the structure is unknown; it may be due to other factors related to the task at hand or its interpretation by the examiner and the examinee. Many important English structures (such as reflexive pronouns) rarely appear in children's written language samples, but it is impossible to know whether this is due to an inability to use the structure or the inappropriateness of the structure to the task at hand.

The original form of the *TSA* was used in a series of research studies by Quigley and his associates at the University of Illinois (Quigley, Wilbur, Power, Montanelli, and Steinkamp, 1976). Responses on the research edition of the test included multiple-choice, true-false, sentence completion, and sentence rewriting. The commercial form of the test (1978) consists of 20 subtests of complex sentence structures, each containing 70 items, and a screening test of 120 items that samples each of the subtest structures. Results of the screening subtest can be used as a general estimate of syntactic knowledge. Each subtest provides an in-depth view of the child's knowledge of a given structure. The major disadvantage of the *TSA* is the time required to administer it (about 30 to 45 minutes per subtest). It should be used when a detailed analysis of syntactic knowledge is desired.

Unlike most other tests of syntax, the *TSA* goes beyond the simple forms of English sentence structure and evaluates common, but more complicated, syntactic and semantic relationships among words. As a result, the test offers a unique means of assessing sophisticated language usage among older children, adolescents, and young adults, populations largely ignored by the constructors of language tests. The common use of these structures in oral and written communication among adults is evident. The surprising fact is that they also appear in curriculum materials associated with first- and second-grade reading series. The ability to use the structures represented on the *TSA* is important to academic achievement at an earlier age than previously assumed. Data from the *TSA* experiments were used to design a reading series for use with deaf children (Quigley and King, 1980).

Norms on the *TSA* have been established for 450 deaf children, aged 10 to 18, and 66 normally hearing children, aged 8 to 10. Norms are presently being established for children with mild to severe hearing losses. It should be a useful language assessment tool for each of these groups. Because the test is in written form, children must be able to read in order to participate. The test vocabulary was chosen by experienced teachers of the deaf and is designed to be within the knowledge of the average 10-year-old deaf child. As a result, the test is most appropriate for older deaf children, but could probably be used with somewhat younger children whose hearing losses are less severe. Because there are numerous language tests, although of a different nature, for younger children, the fact that the *TSA* is designed for older age groups in an advantage, rather than a disadvantage. It represents a badly needed addition to the clinician's battery of language assessment tests.

5. *Callier-Azuza Scale.* Designed specifically to assess deaf-blind and other multiply handicapped children, the *Callier-Azuza Scale* (Stillman, 1976) has five subtests: motor development, perceptual development, daily living skills, language development, and socialization. This is a developmentally based measure that allows assessment of children who cannot respond to other test materials because of the limitations imposed by their multiple impairments. It is heavily weighted on low-level skills in each area of development and its "norms" extend from 0 to 108 months. The scale is designed to be used by teachers in the classroom or by others who have extended contact with a child over a period of time. The authors recommend that a child be observed for at least two weeks, preferably in a classroom setting, before the scale is administered to the observer. The measure is most accurate when the scale is completed by several observers who can agree on the child's performance.

The language subtest of the *Callier-Azuza Scale* includes 13 receptive items, 17 expressive items, and 9 measures of speech development. Many of the items have several subcomponents, which represent behaviors that are expected to develop simultaneously, rather than sequentially. Receptive items range from changes in behavior upon stimulation by sound to following two-stage unrelated commands and identifying objects by their function ("Which one do you drink from"?). Expressive items range from differentiated cries for hunger and pain to requests for specific explanations ("How does it work"?) and correct use of possessives, past tense, and six- to eight-word sentences. Speech items range from the production of non-crying vocalization to exhibiting a vocabulary of 800 or more intelligible words. Examples are given for most items, enabling the observer to interpret test items more accurately.

The child's habitual performance on the scale items may be compared to age equivalencies from 0 to 18 months that are based on normal children's development of the skills measured. Less important than the age equivalency, however, is the description of the child's development through sequential stages of language usage that can be derived from the test results. The scale can be used to assess a child's developmental level, chart progress, and identify a sequence of skills that are appropriate targets for habilitation.

Analysis of Language Samples. There are two approaches to the analysis of the expressive language skills of children: sentence imitation tasks and collection and analysis of spoken or written language samples.

Sentence Imitation Tasks. The rationale underlying sentence imitation is that children will be able to repeat sentence structures over which they have expressive control but will not be able to repeat sentences representing rules they cannot yet employ. Questions regarding the validity of sentence imitation tasks and the factors that influence performance on them remain to be answered, but such measures of expressive language are widely used. The expressive portion of the *NSST* (discussed earlier) involves the delayed imitation of a variety of sentence structures, but responses are simply scored right or wrong. The *Carrow Elicited Language Test (CELI)* (Carrow, 1974) is another example of a sentence imitation task. This test employs sentences representing simple and complex transformations of kernel sentences. They are spoken to a child whose task is to repeat each sentence immediately. Scoring involves an analysis of the sentences produced by the child, in which points are assigned to the various sentence constituents used. The *CELI* involves an analysis of a controlled language sample. The child produces only the syntactic structures that are part of the test. Although limited in number, productions of a variety of different structures are obtained whether the child would normally attempt to produce them or not.

Language Samples. Spoken or written language samples may be *spontaneous* or *elicited*. A spontaneous sample occurs when the child is engaged in some free activity during which language is produced spontaneously. This does not usually occur in assessment situations, making it necessary to elicit a language sample. Pictures, stories, toys, games, and play activities can all be used to stimulate a child to produce a language sample, which may be scored in several ways. The simplest analyses involve counting certain aspects of the sample.

Mean Length of Utterance. A mean length of utterance (MLU) may be computed from any language sample by counting the number of words or morphemes in the sample, then dividing by the number of sentences produced. The result describes the average sentence length produced by the child. MLU appears to be descriptive of stages of language development through which children move as they develop linguistic skills (Brown, 1973). Many investigators have found MLU to be a better predictor of language behavior than age, and many studies of language acquisition have used MLU measures to group children for investigation of language skills.

Developmental Sentence Analysis (*DSA*). A more sophisticated analysis of the utterances of children is desirable, however, if specific information about expressive abilities is needed. The most widely used procedure is the *Developmental Sentence Analysis (DSA)* system developed by Lee (1974). The *DSA* is a classification system that involves a detailed analysis of a child's use of grammatical forms of standard English. Scoring procedures provide quantitative and qualitative measures of language usage.

1. Obtaining a language sample. The first step in the *DSA* is to collect a language sample that is representative of the child's use of language. To be considered representative of the child's ability to produce grammatical structures, the language sample should consist of at least 100 separate utterances, produced contiguously. According to Lee, *DSA* is not an appropriate procedure for use with children who cannot produce 100 utterances in an hour's clinical session. She describes in detail the taking of a language sample for analysis (Lee, 1974, pp. 57–81), and the procedures suggested are appropriate for hearing-impaired children with some modifications. Because of the peripheral impairment to speech comprehension, care must be taken to insure that the hearing-impaired child understands the clinician's comments and questions. The more severely impaired the child's understanding of the spoken word, the less spontaneous speech is likely to be produced, especially in a clinical situation. For this reason it is often difficult to obtain a language sample large enough for complete analysis. Nevertheless, an estimate of the child's use of grammatical structure can be obtained with fewer than 100 utterances even though *DSA* scoring cannot be completed.

While any tape recording of language produced by a child with language delay may be characterized by poor intelligibility, samples obtained from hearing-impaired children are likely to be even more difficult to understand and transcribe. In addition to the articulation errors typical of many language-delayed children, hearing-impaired children may also exhibit unusual vocal quality and deviant prosodic features, such as in the use of stress, intonation, and pause. These suprasegmental features of speech are helpful in determining the differences between statements and questions (in here too? not here, right? Daddy go? Mommy sit.) and the boundaries that separate utterances (Baby, go sleep, or Baby go sleep, or There, doggie versus There doggie). The interpretation of the sentence forms spoken will influence analysis and scoring. Therefore, the unusual qualities associated with the speech of many hearing-impaired children are likely to interfere with transcription of tape recordings of language samples. Some, but not all, of the extra difficulties can be minimized by the use of videotaped language samples. The visual clues associated with speech production, facial expressions, and body language or gestures may allow for a more accurate interpretation of spoken utterances when intelligibility is poor. Of course, the presence of a camera can be distracting; wall-mounted cameras in a familiar room will minimize the influence of these fascinating objects. Filming through an observation window is also a possibility.

If the child in question usually communicates by means of manual communication, video taping the language sample will be the only means of preserving it for later analysis. Neither Lee nor other clinicians who advocate systematic analysis of spontaneous utterances discuss the possibility of collecting language samples that are signed rather than spoken or written. This seems to be a logical procedure in view of the availability of videotape equipment and the increasingly widespread use of sign language by young hearing-impaired children. Use of only spoken and written language samples imposes some unfortunate limitations on language analysis. For one thing, intelligible language samples can seldom be obtained in spoken form for very young children because of slow development of intelligible speech. If written samples are collected, the children must be at least 10 years old if an adequate sample is to be obtained. Indeed, most of the information available about hearing-impaired children's language output has been obtained from written samples of older deaf children. Little is known about the early utterances of these children and how closely they parallel those of normally hearing children at similar developmental stages. The language sampled through writing often represents well-established patterns of grammatical form usage rather than emerging rule development such as that usually assessed in much younger children. Therefore, the picture of language development that results is incomplete, with the most interesting parts (at least from the standpoint of psycholinguistics) absent or badly blurred.

The language sample collected from children should allow them to use their most natural means of communication if it is to reflect reasonably accurately the status of their language knowledge. In the case of many severely hearing-impaired children this means that the examiner must be able to communicate in the mode used by the child being tested. Videotape recordings can be analyzed later by the examiner or other persons familiar with the communicative mode used by the child. Procedures such as these can best be carried out within the program in which the child is being educated or habilitated, for obvious reasons. Children will be more comfortable in familiar surroundings and thus more likely to produce a representative language sample. There is also a greater likelihood that the examiner will be able to communicate in the child's accustomed code.

2. Analyzing the language sample. Once the language sample is obtained and transcribed it can be subjected to *DSA*. This procedure actually consists of two types of analysis: the classification of presentence utterances (known as *Developmental Sentence Types* or *DST* analysis) and the scoring of sentences according to the grammatical constituents they contain (called *Developmental Sentence Scoring* or *DSS*).

Lee distinguishes between presentence and sentence utterances on the basis of the semantic relations expressed. Simply put, a sentence contains a subject and a predicate (a noun phrase and a verb phrase). Presentence utterances may contain one, two, or multiple words, but they do not express a subject-verb relationship. *DST* involves tallying the number of single words, two-word combinations, multiword constructions, and complete sentences produced by a child in a corpus of 100 utterances. Successive analyses can chart the child's progress as the number of single-word utterances decreases and the number of complete sentences increases. Lee (1974) suggests several ways of analyzing the presentence utterances obtained (pp. 119–130). When 50 percent of the child's utterances are complete sentences, the *DST* analysis is discontinued and the *DSS* analysis replaces it.

The *DSS* requires a corpus of 50 sentences for analysis, although there is some evidence that a larger sample will result in an analysis that is more representative of a child's daily language usage (Johnson and Tomblin, 1975). The *DSS* scoring procedure assigns a weighting factor to items that fall into eight grammatical categories: indefinite pronouns, personal pronouns, main verbs, secondary verbs, negatives, conjunctions, interrogatives, and wh-questions. These categories represent important grammatical structures whose developmental progression can be demonstrated and quantified. Weighted scores range from 1 to 8 within a category. For example, in the pronoun category, first- and second-person pronouns (I, me, my, mine, you, your) count 1 point when used in a sentence; plurals (we, us, they, them, their, our) count 3 points; reflexives (myself, yourself) count 5 points; and pronouns such as *whichever* or *whoever* count 7 points. A similar weighting system is used for items within each of the eight categories. Using *DS*, the examiner can assign a score to each sentence, then obtain a mean sentence score for the 50-sentence corpus. The latter is given as the child's *DSS,* which can be compared to the norms established by Lee and her associates. Because of the variability exhibited by normal children in the use of the word class categories, there is a wide range of scores that falls within the normal range. In using the norms and percentiles furnished by Lee, it is important to remember that the allowable margin of delay between the norms and a score that falls within the normal range increases with age. A delay of 10 months may be significant at age 3-0 to 3-6 whereas a delay of 20 months may not be significant at age 4-0 to 4-6.

Aside from providing a means of quantifying the language usage of children and its growth over time, the *DSA* is designed to assist clinicians in selecting appropriate goals for language teaching, based on developmental norms. Details concerning the use of DSA results in remediation can be found in Lee (1974).

There are many language tests available that have not been discussed here. The examples given are meant to be exactly that—examples of the tests available and examples of the modifications sometimes necessary for their use. Some tests that are widely used in the assessment of language disorders whose etiology is less well-defined than hearing loss, have not been found to be particularly useful with hearing-impaired children. An example would be the *Illinois Test of Psycholinguistic Abilities (ITPA)* (Kirk, McCarthy, and Kirk, 1968). The *ITPA* is designed to compare performance on a number of skills through the two primary modalities of vision and audition. The typical profile of a hearing-impaired child reveals better than average visual skills and poor auditory skills. There is nothing wrong with verifying such an obvious pattern, especially if the child is suspected of having language processing problems other than those caused by hearing loss. However, if the assessment procedures and tools to be employed are chosen on the basis of how much new information they will yield in a reasonable amount of time, tests such as the *ITPA* will occupy a low priority for administration. The actual tests and procedures chosen should depend on factors such as the age of the child, degree of the hearing loss, preferred communication mode, educational status, known language behavior, primary questions to be answered, and the time available for assessment.

ASSESSMENT OF SPEECH

The systematic evaluation of the speech production of hearing-impaired children has been a neglected aspect of their speech development. Procedures for assessing the types of speech problems described in the preceding chapter have not been standardized in the way that they have for other types of speech disorders, such as stuttering or articulation disorders. Within the last 10 years attempts to quantify the speech skills of hearing-impaired speakers have been reported by personnel at the National Technical Institute for the Deaf (NTID) (Subtelny, 1975), who reported a series of scales for rating intelligibility, voice, and rhythm. Subtelny and her associates at NTID also have collected samples of speech and compiled them into a series of training tapes designed to give clinicians experience judging speech produced by hearing-impaired (including deaf) speakers.

Ling (1976) stressed the need to evaluate systematically the speech skills of children before attempting to remediate them. He suggested assessing two aspects of speech development, the phonetic (articulatory) and phonologic (linguistic) use of speech sounds.

A complete description of a given child's ability to speak is necessary if remedial efforts are to be appropriate and effective. Therefore each aspect of speech known to be affected by hearing loss must be assessed.

Assessment of the Speech Mechanism

Ling (1976) estimated that approximately 5 percent of hearing-impaired children exhibit abnormalities of the oral-peripheral structures. Because of the possible negative effects of physical abnormalities, the oral speech mechanism should be examined carefully. Movement of the lips, tongue, jaw, and soft palate should be observed. The examiner may demonstrate movements such as lip rounding and flattening, raising of the tongue tip, and sideways movements of the jaw and tongue. Older children will usually imitate such movements, but young children respond best when the movements are introduced as gamelike activities. Blowing a candle flame or a ping-pong ball, licking a lollipop, removing a drop of syrup, chocolate, or peanut butter from the corners of the mouth or the alveolar ridge allow the examiner to observe a variety of movements. Guidelines for conducting an oral-peripheral examination can be found in Darley and Spriestersbach (1978). These procedures are appropriate for hearing-impaired children if special effort is made to insure understanding of the instructions.

Assessment of Voice Production

Hearing-impaired children produce normal voicing under certain circumstances. Laughter, throat clearing, coughing, and spontaneous sounds made during play are more indicative of the actual voicing capabilities of these children than sounds made in deliberate attempts to communicate. Therefore, vocal characteristics observed during play should be noted, including a description of pitch and quality. A second set of observations of the voice should be made while the child is attempting to produce speech sounds. How well does the child control breath flow? How many syllables are produced on one breath? Does pitch vary during production of syllables? If so, what is the nature of the variation? Is it under the child's control? Is pitch appropriate for age and sex? Can various pitches be imitated? Does the voice seem hoarse, strained, breathy? Is loudness appropriate? Can it be varied at will? Questions such as these provide a framework for descriptions of the adequacy of the voice as it is used habitually. It is difficult to quantify any deviations in phonation that occur, although it is easy to decide whether the voice ''sounds'' appropriate or not. Attempts to quantify various aspects of the speech produced by hearing impaired people have included rating scales for pitch, loudness, rate, breath control, and voice quality. A rating system suggested by Subtelny (1975) is shown in Appendix A.

Ling (1976) included judgments of pitch, loudness, and the ability to sustain phonation in his protocol for both phonetic and phonologic speech evaluation. Instead of a rating scale, he suggested binary judgments of normal-faulty, present-absent, or consistent-inconsistent. The exact nature of the judgment made is not important as long as systematic observations are reported that can be used as guides for developing a speech training program. Being able to produce voice at will and to control it during speech is an important contribution to intelligibility.

Assessment of Articulation

Many speech sounds are difficult for hearing-impaired children to learn to produce, and their attempt can provide important information for speech training. Tests of articulation may be administered to hearing-impaired children who are familiar with the vocabulary involved. However, most word tests do not provide for an adequate sampling of a child's skill in producing sounds in a variety of phonetic contexts. The severely hearing-impaired child must often learn speech sounds under unnatural conditions, and the strategy employed for production of an acceptable sound in one context may not be generalized to others. In addition, most tests of articulation involve only consonants. Because hearing-impaired children frequently misarticulate vowels as well, some measure of their production is necessary. For these reasons a complete picture of the child's phonetic skills requires an analytical approach that goes beyond the usual test of articulation.

For assessment of speech sound usage, children should imitate a series of vowels and diphthongs, varying pitch, intensity, and duration. Consonants should be produced in conjunction with front, mid, and back vowels in initial and final positions. Ling (1976) described a comprehensive protocol for the evaluation of speech sound production by hearing impaired children on two levels, phonetic and phonologic. The phonetic level evaluation consists of several procedures, as follows:

1. The nonsegmental features of vocalization, vocal duration, vocal intensity, and vocal pitch are judged as being produced consistently, inconsistently, or not at all.
2. Attempts to imitate or initiate productions of vowels and diphthongs are judged as consistent, inconsistent, or not produced. Each vowel must be produced, sustained, repeated at a rate of three per second, and alternated accurately with another vowel before mastery is complete. Vowels should be produced at different loudness and pitch levels as well.
3. Simple consonants are evaluated in three vowel contexts (**a**, **ee**, and **oo**) under the same conditions as vowels; that is, simple production, repetitions and alternations while varying loudness and pitch.
4. Word-initial and word-final blends are evaluated in the same manner as simple consonants.

The phonetic level evaluation can be carried out with any child who will attempt to imitate speech productions. Children who have been exposed to phonetic or orthographic symbol systems may be stimulated by them to initiate production of phonemes and syllables.

The phonologic level evaluation requires that the child produce an oral language sample which can be analyzed according to the following:

1. Nonsegmental aspects such as pitch control, intonation, duration, and stress.
2. Production of vowels, diphthongs, consonants, and blends.
3. Linguistic structure.
4. Intelligibility.
5. Common faults.

The phonologic level evaluation cannot be completed until a child can produce oral language beyond single words.

Ling's speech evaluation procedures constitute the most systematic and thorough approach available for hearing-impaired children. Furthermore, the evaluation procedures are directly related to his training procedures, which are also the most detailed to be found in the literature on speech of the hearing impaired.

Assessment of Speech Rhythm

Speech that is articulated accurately in a voice that is appropriately pitched may still be largely unintelligible if its rhythm, rate, and inflectional patterns are very different from normal. The slow rate described earlier, the failure to differentiate between stressed and unstressed syllables, the inability to use pitch, loudness, and duration shifts to signal stress, and the lack of a variety of intonation contours can alter the rhythm of speech until the message is unrecognizable. The resulting speech is difficult to describe with accuracy, but remediation depends on identifying and quantifying its components. Subtelny (1975) provided rating scales for rate, stress, and inflections that allow a general description of these components of speech rhythm (see Appendix A).

Aspects of rhythm and intonation are more easily judged during production of connected discourse than from single words. A connected speech sample can be obtained by having the child read a passage, describe a picture, or engage in a conversation. If the sample is obtained through reading, measures of speaking rate can be made, because the length and content of the utterance will be known to the examiner. A reading sample can be analyzed according to articulation as well, because the intended phonemes will also be known.

Speech samples elicited in response to pictures, stories, events, or conversation can be used for linguistic as well as speech analysis. If the content of the child's utterance can be understood, it will be easier to judge whether or not shifts in intonation and stress occur appropriately.

Several questions about the rhythm of the speech sample should be answered during the evaluation. How does speaking rate compare to normal speech? Can the type of sentence (declarative, question, imperative) be identified by stress or intonation patterns? When stress occurs is it related to the content of the utterance? Which contributes more significantly to the perception of stress: pitch, durational, or intensity characteristics? Do pitch breaks interfere with perceptions of stress or rhythm?

In addition to the analysis of spontaneously produced or read speech samples, the child should be asked to imitate productions of common sentence patterns. All of these samples may differ from each other because of the cues that are available to the child under each set of circumstances. When reading, visual representations of the phonemes to be uttered should be available. Many children depend on orthographic symbols when learning to produce speech sounds; seeing them may remind the children to produce sounds they would not remember to produce spontaneously. An imitation task may provide auditory and lipreading clues, which may elicit different speaking behavior than either reading or talking spontaneously. The child's ability to approximate the patterns presented by the examiner or to modify habitual rate or stress patterns when imitating someone else's speech will provide useful information for planning remediation. Successful attempts to imitate pitch, loudness, or stress are usually indicative of useful residual hearing, because these components of speech cannot be observed visually unless some special code is used, such as a hand signal for raising or lowering pitch or loudness. Specific procedures to be used for teaching or remediating speech may be indicated by the differences or lack of them among speech samples obtained in different ways.

REFERENCES

Boehm, A., *Boehm Test of Basic Concepts*. New York: The Psychological Corporation, 1970.

Brown, R., *A First Language—The Early Stages*. Cambridge: Harvard University Press, 1973.

Caccamise, F. and Blasdell, R., Reception of sentences under oral-manual interpreted and simultaneous test conditions, *Amer. Ann. Deaf,* 122, 414–421, 1977.

Carrow, E., *Test for Auditory Comprehension of Language*. Austin. TX: Learning Concepts, 1973.

Carrow, E., *Carrow Elicited Language Inventory*. Austin, TX: Learning Concepts, 1974.

Darley, F. and Spriestersbach, D., *Diagnostic Methods in Speech Pathology*. New York: Harper & Row, 1978.

Davis, J., Performance of young hearing impaired children on a test of basic concepts, *J. Speech Hearing Res.,* 17, 342–351, 1974.

Davis, J., Reliability of hearing-impaired children's responses to oral and total presentations of the Test of Auditory Comprehension of Language, *J. Speech Hearing Dis.,* 42, 520–527, 1977.

Dunn, L., *Peabody Picture Vocabulary Test*. Circle Pines, MN: American Guidance Service, Inc., 1965.

Foster, C., Giddan, J., and Stark, J., *ACLA: Assessment of Children's Language Comprehension*. Palo Alto, CA: Consulting Psychologists Press, Inc., 1972.

Johnson, M. and Tomblin, J., The reliability of developmental sentence scoring as a function of sample size, *J. Speech Hearing Res.,* 18, 372–380, 1975.

Kirk, A., McCarthy, J., and Kirk, W., *The Illinois Test of Psycholinguistic Abilities, Revised Edition*. Champaign-Urbana: University of Illinois Press, 1968.

Lee, L., *Northwestern Syntax Screening Test*. Evanston, IL: Northwestern University Press, 1969.

Lee, L., *Developmental Sentence Analysis: A Grammatical Assessment Procedure for Speech and Language Clinicians*. Evanston, IL: Northwestern University Press, 1974.

Ling, D., *Speech and the Hearing Impaired Child.* Washington, D. C.: A. G. Bell Association, 1976.

Public Law 94–142: The Education for All Handicapped Children Act, Federal Register, August 23, 1975, Part II.

Quigley, S., Wilbur, R., Power, D., Montanelli, D., and Steinkamp, H., *Syntactic Struc-*

tures in the Language of Deaf Children. Champaign-Urbana: University of Illinois Press, 1976.

Quigley, S. and King, C., *Reading Milestones*. Beaverton, OR: Dormac, Inc., 1980.

Quigley, S., Steinkamp, M., Power, D. and Jones, B., *Test of Syntactic Abilities*. Beaverton, OR: Dormac Inc., 1978.

Stillman, R. (Ed.), *The Callier-Azuza Scale*. Dallas: Callier Center for Communication Disorders, University of Texas at Dallas, 1976.

Subtelny, J., *Speech and Voice Characteristics of the Deaf,* an auditory training package published by the National Technical Institute for the Deaf, Rochester, NY, 1975.

National Technical Institute for the Deaf Speech and Voice Diagnostic Form

INTELLIGIBILITY

1. Speech is completely unintelligible.
2. Speech is very difficult to understand—only isolated words or phrases are intelligible.
3. With difficulty the listener can understand about half the content of the message (intelligibility may improve after a listening period).
4. Speech is intelligible with the exception of a few words or phrases.
5. Speech is completely intelligible.

PITCH REGISTER

If pitch register is judged to be below optimal, mark rating with a (-).

1. Cannot sustain phonation.
2. Much above or below optimal level.
3. Moderately above or below optimal level.
4. Slightly above or below optimal level.
5. Appropriate for age and sex.

PITCH CONTROL

1. Cannot sustain phonation.
2. Noticeable breaks or fluctuations of large magnitude.
3. Noticeable breaks or fluctuations of small magnitude.
4. Flat within limited speaking range.
5. Normal—satisfactory modulation of pitch.

LOUDNESS

If loudness is judged to be below an appropriate level, mark rating with a (-).

1. Cannot sustain audible tone.
2. Much above or below appropriate level.
3. Moderately above or below appropriate level.
4. Slightly above or below appropriate level.
5. Normal intensity level.

LOUDNESS CONTROL

1. Cannot sustain audible tone.
2. Noticeable breaks or fluctuations of large magnitude.
3. Noticeable breaks or fluctuations of small magnitude.
4. Flat within limited speaking range.
5. Normal—satisfactory modulation of intensity.

RATE

If rate is too rapid for efficient communication, mark rating with a (+).

1. Cannot control rate of syllable articulation.
2. Much too slow—labored single syllable utterances. Rate definitely interferes with content of communication.
3. Moderately below optimal rate for efficient communication.
4. Slightly below optimal rate, but monitored well for clarity.
5. Normal.

CONTROL OF AIR EXPENDITURE DURING SPEECH

1. Severe problem—cannot coordinate respiration and phonation to sustain tone.
2. Marked excess or deficiency in air expenditure.
3. Moderate excess or deficiency in air expenditure.
4. Slight excess or deficiency in air expenditure.
5. Normal.

BREATH CONTROL

(Record average of three trials)

1. Maximum duration of sustained /s/______seconds.
2. Maximum duration of sustained vowel ______seconds.
3. Counts on one breath, number______. (Provide count model three digits per second.) "Count as far as you can in one breath."
4. Number of words per minute in reading______. (Record data from second trial.)

PROSODIC FEATURES—BLENDING, STRESS AND INFLECTION

1. Cannot evaluate.

2. Severe problem.
3. Moderate problem.
4. Mild problem.
5. Normal.

VOICE QUALITY

Breathy, Weak, Lacking Clarity

1. Voice quality varies or is too weak to judge.
2. Severe breathiness.
3. Moderate breathiness.
4. Mild breathiness.
5. Normal quality.

Tense, Harsh

1. Vocal tension too great to sustain tone.
2. Severe tenseness.
3. Moderate tenseness.
4. Mild tenseness.
5. Normal quality.

Nasal Resonance

1. Resonance varies and cannot be judged.
2. Severe denasality or hypernasality.
3. Moderate denasality or nasality.
4. Mild denasality or nasality.
5. Normal resonance.

Pharyngeal Resonance

1. Resonance varies and cannot be judged.
2. Marked pharyngeal resonance.
3. Moderate pharyngeal resonance.
4. Mild pharyngeal resonance.
5. Normal resonance.

MODE OF COMMUNICATION

1. Uses writing instead of speech or manual communication.
2. Signs, fingerspells, and gestures without voice.
3. Signs and fingerspells frequently with voice.
4. Resorts to signs and fingerspelling occasionally during speech.
5. Uses oral communication habitually.

CHAPTER 8

Remediation of Language and Speech

Attempts to devise methods of teaching language to hearing-impaired children have resulted in a variety of remediation programs. The purpose of each is to increase language skills for communication and as a basis for further learning. The dual nature of the task contributes to the variety of programs that have been divised or modified for the hearing-impaired population. The complexity of language and the many factors entering into its natural use have also influenced the type of training programs developed. Not only must children learn the phonological rules of language, they must learn its grammatical rules and how to use them to comprehend and produce utterances of infinite variety. Furthermore, language comes in several forms, each of which contributes to communication and learning. The spoken form enables us to communicate easily with others; the written form allows us to learn about facts and events that do not occur within the confines of our daily lives. Becoming an educated and literate person depends on becoming a user of language in several forms.

THE LANGUAGE LEARNING TASK

Baron (1975) delineated five domains of linguistic consciousness that are prerequisite to the objective knowledge and use of language, both for speaking and listening and for reading and writing. Her discussion of these prerequisites to sophisticated, adult use of language is helpful in clarifying the language learning task faced by children and the language teaching task faced by clinicians. The first domain is an awareness that human language consists of an identifiable and consistent system of noises that can be used for a variety of functions. It is important that the child be able to discriminate language noises from nonlinguistic noises and to associate them with human communication. Because studies show that human infants respond differentially to speech and nonspeech sounds soon after birth (Condon and Sander, 1974), this linguistic domain appears to develop immediately as a part of the language acquisition device innate to humans. Children who fail to acquire this domain of linguistic consciousness are relatively rare, consisting of children who cannot *hear* the sounds of language and those who cannot *process* the sounds, such as autistic children. Under ordinary circumstances recognition of the sounds of language occurs before any other linguistic knowledge. The hearing-impaired child who cannot make this early distinction may experience a significant language delay almost from birth. Children who must be taught the task of this domain are almost always seriously language delayed by the time the necessity for teaching it is recognized.

The second domain is an awareness of the structure and function of the speech sounds that have been recognized. Because language takes many structures and functions, children learn them gradually over time. Early knowledge of these factors includes the understanding that language can be used to refer to people, objects, activities and relationships. The structure of language that functions in these ways is quite complex. Knowledge about it includes some understanding of fundamental semantic relations and how to express them through basic sentence types. It is this domain in which much early language training of hearing-impaired children is concentrated, for awareness of the factors given above is learned normally through the auditory system. Failure to learn them precludes the development of the remaining domains.

The third domain involves several important linguistic distinctions. One is the ability to make judgments about the grammaticality of utterances encountered. Surprisingly enough, children as young as age 3 can recognize which of several utterances is "better" and these judgements are in the direction of more correct grammar (de Villiers and de Villiers, 1972). Older children can identify the reasons why ungrammatical sentences are not correct (Gleitman, Gleitman, and Shipley, 1972). The ability to make such judgments is based on previous knowledge of the structure and function of language, knowledge that is developed in early childhood.

Included in Baron's third domain is the perception of ambiguity, including the comprehension that a given word may have several meanings. The multiple meanings of words, such as *bark* or *get,* often involve a change in the grammatical class to which the word belongs within a given utterance. *Bark* has different meanings when used as a noun and a verb, and it has been estimated that the word *get* has as many as 20 different meanings, depending upon the context in which it occurs. It means *move* (get back), *become* (get sick), *acquire* (get one), *fetch* (get the book), and so on. Less obvious semantic changes occur in sentences such as "They gave her baby food." The word baby has the same general meaning, but alters the meaning of the sentence when intended as an adjective versus a noun functioning as an indirect object.

The third domain also includes an understanding of the appropriateness of certain language under certain conditions. Social restraints operate on the use of language, and children must learn the differences among situations that may dictate the language that is acceptable. For example, asking the age of adults is considered rude in our society; repetition of parental comments to others ("he's a jerk") is not always met with acceptance, especially by the parents; baby talk may be employed with animals but is not productive when used with teachers.

This domain marks a level of language knowledge that goes well beyond the simple learning of words and the not-so-simple learning of rules by which words are strung together. Successful mastering of the third domain moves the child into a sophisticated level of language usage that is very difficult to teach. The rules shift in ways that are difficult to describe. How does one explain, for example, that the telephone conversation in which mother expressed obvious delight over the shocking behavior of a neighbor is okay to have in the home, over the telephone, with a friend, but that the delight must be masked when the topic is introduced elsewhere. "Well, yes, dear; it's true that I *sounded* pleased, but. . ." The consciousness of language usage that is involved in the third domain is easily learned but difficult to teach, and language training for the hearing impaired, for the most part, has not attempted to do so.

The fourth and fifth domains involve levels of linguistic consciousness that are essential to learning to read and write. The fourth domain includes recognition of the fact that words and sentences may be represented in a form other than the spoken. Spoken language can be written but the correspondence between what is written and what is spoken may not be perfect, at least in English. Orthographic symbols are not always synonymous with the phonemic ones. Children must learn to recognize when vowels are long or short (cat versus cake) and to learn exceptions to pronunciation rules (**gh** = f in laugh but **g** in ghoul). Sounding out words by dividing them into sounds and syllables is important to the reading process, and children must now recognize boundaries between words that may not have been obvious before. Utterances from early childhood often appear to be single units although they may consist of several words, as in "let me go" or "I don't want to." Karpova (1955) has shown that preschool children cannot identify the first word of a sentence upon request. It is not unusual for preschool children to respond "Jack and Jill" when asked "Who came tumbling down first?" "Jack and Jill" are often understood as an entity. Learning to read and write depends on the child's ability to segment utterances successfully, and to recognize the parts as separate items.

Under certain circumstances hearing-impaired children may have an advantage over normally hearing children in mastering the fourth domain. Children who have been exposed to fingerspelling, cued speech, or sign comprehend earlier than the average child that language can be represented in several forms. Children whose parents have labeled items within the house with printed words for reinforcement of vocabulary development may also realize that spoken language takes alternate forms.

The fifth domain involves a high level of language usage associated with adult literacy. Older children, adolescents, and adults continue to learn vocabulary, to develop their abilities to verbalize with imagery, and to distinguish between descriptive, argumentative, or expository styles. The use of humor, sarcasm, and satire are advanced stages of linguistic development. Most language training programs never address the more subtle, complex and sophisticated use of language, even though adolescent children are faced with academic tasks requiring the fifth domain of linguistic consciousness. Indeed, the task of *teaching* this type of language skill is overwhelming and may explain why there are almost no language programs designed for use with older children. The ease with language that is necessary for mastery of the fifth domain may also explain the frustration felt by many clinicians who are faced with the task of "working with" older hearing-impaired children whose language skills and knowledge are not sufficient for the academic and communicative tasks they face.

LANGUAGE REMEDIATION MODELS

Language intervention models fall into two general categories: natural and grammatical approaches. The natural models attempt to parallel natural language development by increasing a child's exposure to the type of language known to emerge early in the normal child's development. The content and sequencing of material are determined by the child, the environment, communicative needs, and baseline language skills. The functional aspects of language are stressed, and lessons center around activities of interest to young children.

Grammatical approaches focus on the structural aspects of language, concentrating on the recognition and appropriate use of parts of speech, syntactic rules, and basic sentence structures. Lessons involve much formal instruction and drill, although generalization to spontaneous conversation and activities is the desired end product.

Although the two models appear to be at odds, at least with regard to the method of instruction, features of each are often combined in actual treatment situations. The natural environment is used as much as possible, but the structure of utterances may be stressed as a goal.

Regardless of the model employed, adult utterances during early language therapy fall into several categories that have been shown to be effective in modifying children's language behavior.

1. *Expansion* of a child's utterances occur when the adult corrects the child's grammar in a nonpunitive, conversational manner. If the child says "Dog bite me," the adult replies "The dog bit you."
2. *Modeling* is a technique in which the adult converses with the child, commenting on the child's utterances, but not correcting them. Using the same example, "Dog bite me," the adult might say "He's only playing," or "Be careful. Maybe you shouldn't play with him."
3. *Echoing* occurs when the child's utterance is not entirely intelligible. In an attempt to clarify the utterance, the adult repeats it and fills in the unintelligible portion with a question word. Responding to the sentence, "I ate the ______," the adult would say, "You ate the what?"
4. *Imitation* is a procedure in which the adult requires the child to repeat the adult's production. This can be used for words or sentences. "Dog bite me" would be responded to by a request that the child repeat "The dog bit me" after the adult until correct production is achieved or the adult terminated the repetitions.

Obviously, there are other types of responses that adults may make to children, such as simple requests for repetition or instructions for producing utterances. These four basic responses are widely used, however, and are referred to in descriptions of the various models. Once a child has moved beyond a basic level of language knowledge, as represented by linguistic domains one and two as described earlier, the remediation methods become more complex and more difficult to define. It is essential that the clinician understand the goals of remediation for the particular child involved and the improbability of meeting those goals through a rigidly employed language training program. Procedures and materials must be matched to the individual goals and the individual child if they are to result in improved language skill. The following description of language remediation programs is intended as an overview and not as a series of prescriptions.

Natural Language Intervention Approaches

Environmental Language Intervention (ELI). The purpose of this approach is to expand the length of a child's utterances and increase the number and complexity of the semantic relations that can be expressed (MacDonald, 1976). The approach is intended for use with children whose expressive skills are limited to one- and two-word utterances. The procedures involve playing with the child in a comfortable environment and using toys and activities chosen by the child. Conversation during play is the major remedial activity.

ELI is based on the semantic relations that have been identified as central to children's early attempts to communicate. They represent the relationships among people, objects, and events within the child's world and include the following:

1. Agent-action (Daddy go).
2. Action-object (drink milk).
3. Agent-object (Daddy car).
4. Action-locative (go school).
5. Entity-locative (Daddy home).
6. Possessor-possession (Daddy's coat).
7. Entity-attribute (big book).
8. Demonstrative-entity (that dress).

Bloom (1970) demonstrated that a single utterance may represent more than one semantic relation, depending on the environment and what is occurring in it at the time. For example, the utterance *Daddy car* may represent agent-object (Daddy is in the car) or possessor-possession (Daddy's car). Thus, environmental factors influence the utterances used to stimulate the various semantic relations in the clinical situation. Using the *ELI,* the clinician chooses the relations to be emphasized according to a developmental model based on studies of early acquisition of language by normal children. The chosen relation is expressed repeatedly by the clinician during play (Mommy throw, teacher go, baby sit, Sally hit, doggie run) and the child's and clinician's utterances are gradually expanded into adult grammatical form. Users of this model usually provide intensive therapy for a short period of time (a few weeks or months). Parents are required to observe and participate in therapy, preparatory to continuing the same type of stimulation in the home, both during and following the treatment period by professionals. It is essential that the utterances used by the adult be related to the environment and based on the child's interests. Introduction of pictures designed to teach certain vocabulary would not be a part of the initial *ELI* treatment. Use of a favorite picture-book would be acceptable, because it would represent an interest of the child. *ELI* is partially based on the observation that children learn most quickly and easily those things of importance to them. For a toddler, food, play, and important people are of interest; shapes, colors, and selected verbs may not be of concern and their use in therapy will result in slower learning.

This model can be adapted easily for use with the hearing impaired. It stresses the fundamental elements necessary to communicate a message and builds them slowly into grammatical utterances. Because hearing-impaired children appear to develop language in a sequence similar to that of normally hearing children, it seems reasonable to encourage them to move through stages of sentence production similar to those associated with early language acquisition. Insistence on the production of adult grammar by a child whose expressive skills are at the two-word level is inadvisable. Another advantage of the *ELI* approach is the concentrated presentation of the language needed to express certain important relations, especially those involved in discovering the functions of language (Baron's domain number two). Systematic stimulation with utterance after utterance expressing the same function provides the sort of redundancy that is ordinarily missing for hearing-impaired children.

Finally, *ELI* procedures can be used to provide repeated auditory stimulation in an interesting environment. They can also be accompanied by sign or other manual forms of language. Because of the reduced utterance length, parents and clinicians who are just learning to use alternate forms of communication can easily manage simultaneous speech and sign or cues during therapy.

"Natural" Approach. A number of slightly varied approaches to language remediation of the hearing impaired have borne this label. It is used to designate procedures that are structured around some activity or topic, but which evolve naturally as a result of conversation and comments. The natural approach usually does not stress semantic relations or certain basic sentence structures. Instead the clinician uses language that is appropriate to the task at hand without limiting its structure in well-defined ways. In actuality, the complexity of the utterances varies according to the child's language status, and the clinician must keep pace with the language growth exhibited by the child or children involved.

A typical remedial session of the natural approach involves the setting up of an activity, such as making a cake. The clinician guides the activity, producing language that describes each step of the process. Children are encouraged to comment on the activities and the clinician models or expands their utterances. The clinician explains actions and the reasons underlying them, asks questions, and repeats often. When the activity is completed, a story may be written, usually on large newsprint or tablets. Children are encouraged to produce the sentences for the story, which are expanded by the clinician, placed in the proper sequence, and written down. Later, or on succeeding days, the story can be read again and again so that the language involved is reinforced frequently. Group activities are particularly good ones for use with the natural method, as children stimulate each other. If the activity is interesting enough to them, they tend to converse with each other, and their output can be used as a basis for modeling, expansion, echoing, or imitation. When children exhibit different language levels, the clinician must be skillful at drawing from each child the most advanced language possible. The clinician's response to one child might entail expansion into adult grammar, while the response to another might involve requiring imitation of a basic semantic relation.

Although the natural language lesson looks deceptively easy when conducted by an experienced clinician, it requires careful planning and execution. The clinician must decide on the language to be taught, the vocabulary and general sentence structures must be determined in advance. During the activity, the clinican must listen carefully for the children's comments and respond to them differentially. The major difficulty exhibited by inexperienced clinicians is the tendency to talk too much or too little, either prattling on and on without giving the children a chance to make comments, or simply performing activities with little language stimulation provided. The former is by far the most common mistake made by the clinician, the latter by parents.

The following is a sample of probable conversation from the activity described above.

Clinician. We are making a chocolate cake. When we finish, we will eat it.
First child. Eat cake.
Clinician. Yes, we will eat the cake. Do you like cake?
Second child. I like cake.
Clinician. Good, I like cake too.
(To another child) Do you like chocolate cake?
Third child. (nods head)
Clinician. I like chocolate cake.
Third child. Like chocolate.
Clinician. Let's make the cake now. Who knows what to do? First, we pour the mix into the bowl.
First child. Me pour mix.
Clinician. Do you want to pour the mix?
First child. Me want pour mix.
Clinician. Good, you pour the mix. Where did you pour it?

The story resulting from the activity might begin as follows: We made a chocolate cake. Sally poured the mix in a bowl. Tom broke two eggs. Anne poured a cup of water.

Obviously, the variety of sentence structure and vocabulary can vary considerably within the same activity and should be under loose control by the clinician.

The natural approach is appropriate for children with a wide variety of verbal skills. The sophistication of the language used by the clinician and elicited from the children will depend on their previous language development. It is essential that the clinician know the approximate level of language functioning of children within the group before planning the lesson, because the purpose of the activities is to improve and expand each child's language usage. This can only be accomplished by stimulating the child with new forms of language and expecting progress beyond the current language usage level. Activities and topics must be chosen with the children's age and interests in mind, because older children are no more inclined to learn maximally from dull activities than young ones.

Cognitive-Developmental Approach. Recently there has been renewed interest in approaching language development on a cognitive basis. The role of language in the development of cognition has been the subject of much study in both normal and hearing-impaired populations (Piaget, 1962; Furth, 1966). Unfortunately, it is still unknown to what extent the one depends on the other. Much of the recent interest in the development of curricula designed to teach thinking skills concurrently with language has stemmed from the less than satisfactory educational status of most hearing-impaired children (see Chapter 9). Descriptions of hearing-impaired persons often include references to "rigid" thinking, failure to use abstractions, and the inability to generalize information. At least one explanation for the behavior that leads to such descriptions is that hearing-impaired children are presented with facts, right and wrong answers, and concrete, labeled examples of concepts to be learned through their educational experiences. Because hearing-impaired children tend to be delayed in knowledge of language and of the world, educators have often used teaching time to present as many facts as possible, with little emphasis on development of the thinking skills that would enable an individual to deduce facts independently.

The cognitive approaches to language teaching are based on certain of Piaget's principles regarding the cognitive stages through which individuals must move in order to reach the highest level of mental operations. Piaget's theories are complex and will not be discussed in detail here. Generally, his research has indicated that children progress through four stages of mental development:

1. The sensorimotor stage (0 to 2 years), in which information is gathered and stored on the basis of the child's sensory experiences with stimuli.
2. The preoperational stage (18 months to 7 years), in which children begin to function in a conceptual-symbolic mode, no longer requiring the physical presence of stimuli that they have learned to represent internally by use of symbols, such as language.
3. The concrete operations stage, (7 to 11 years), in which children learn to apply logical operations for the purpose of solving concrete problems.
4. The formal operations stage, (11 to 15 years), in which children have developed the ability to apply logical operations to any logical situation or problem.

It is during the preoperational stage that language development is its most rapid.

According to Piaget, a child must possess the mental operation associated with a given linguistic concept before learning the language involved. For example, a child who does not yet understand the mental operation of reoccurrence, the knowledge that things that disappear from sight are not lost forever but may reoccur, will not learn the language concept "more." The vocabulary items may be learned, but the concept will not be generalized for use in such utterances as "more milk," "more swing," "more sleep," "more Grandmother." Furthermore, young children learn the properties of concepts by involvement, usually action, with them. The baby bottle may represent a feeding device to adults, but an infant may associate the bottle with feelings of satisfaction, with the person who provides it, with its contents, with the sensations involved in drinking from it. Consequently, when the mother says, "bottle" she may be referring to a container, whereas the child may have a different connotation altogether. Because of the strong influence of action on learning, children should be given ample opportunity to explore objects or places to be used in teaching language.

Development of Abstract Thinking Skills. The cognitive approach is designed to foster independent thinking and problem solving. According to Taba (1962), abstract thinking results from the mastery of three cognitive tasks. The first of these is the absorption of data leading to formation of concepts. This is achieved by presenting information to the child and requiring the child to manipulate the stimuli by grouping, classifying, and identifying common and disparate elements among items. Children are required to organize and reorganize groups of objects or pictures or words, explaining the basis on which they are classified each time. In this way, similarities and differences among items may be identified and relationships established conceptually. An example of such concept formation is provided by Eccarius (1978). Using pieces of fruit, she presented each with an explanatory statement, such as "Here is a red apple. You can eat it. I like apples. Do you like apples? Here is a green apple. They are both apples, but different colors. Apples grow on trees. Let's cut one open; it's white inside. We can see the seeds. If you plant this seed. . ." Other fruits are also introduced with comments and questions. Children are then asked to group the fruits according to any criteria they wish. The following groupings may occur:

apple	banana
pear	orange
grapes	lemon
lime	plum

Such a grouping could occur on the basis of green and not-green fruits. If the child can explain why the fruits were grouped in a given way, it is accepted and a different grouping is requested. Other possibilities of groupings include texture of peel, sweet versus sour, edible or no seeds versus inedible seeds, and so on.

Children are encouraged to use the information they have (knowledge of the appearances of the cut apple) to make inferences about information they do not yet have (the appearance of the inside of the uncut apple). They are encouraged to guess, reason, decide, and explain. A very important aspect of the cognitive approach is the acceptance of each child's classification and reasons for them. The object is not to teach correct answers, but to provide an opportunity to learn thinking skills that will enable the child to arrive at solutions and answers that reflect fact.

The second task in the development of abstract thinking involves the use of the data obtained in the preceding activities. In this task children are required to answer questions about the information presented. "If we cut open the green apple, what color will the fruit inside be?" "How are these two apples different?" "If we plant an orange seed, what will happen?" "Do orange trees grow in our town?" "How can we make the green and red apples look alike?" Children are also encouraged to compare and contrast items. Same-different charts can be developed in which the similarities and differences of items are listed and discussed. Stories can be written using the information obtained.

The third task is that of applying the principles distilled in the previous tasks and of generalizing the knowledge obtained to novel situations. In the case of the fruits, children may generalize the following knowledge:

1. Many fruits regenerate through seeds.
2. Most fruits consist of edible and inedible parts.

Opportunities to apply new concepts should be provided. A strange fruit can be introduced and discussed. Although questions can be used, the real purpose of this stage is for the child to hypothesize about the new fruit, support the hypothesis with reasoning, and then test the hypothesis to verify the reasoning. Hypotheses about the new fruit may include statements about the edibility of its skin or the presence of seeds. Reasons are given for the hypotheses (thick skins don't usually taste good, thin skins do) and the hypothesis is then verified (by cutting, looking, and tasting).

Grammatico and Miller (1974) have described a preschool curriculum based on Taba's (1962) objectives and principles. The tasks of absorbing data, using data, and applying the principles learned can be used with an infinite variety of materials and concepts, ranging from vocabulary training to sex education. The objective is to teach critical thinking skills, not facts, in an open environment. Children are urged to be creative and inquisitive. They are presented with sequencing, cause and effect, and other problems to solve. Their efforts to deduce answers to problems are reinforced. Clinicians find this approach a complex one to plan and implement. They often fall into the habit of giving answers instead of allowing the children to deduce them. With practice, however, clinicians tend to be enthusiastic about the cognitive approach. When a child, after reading the sentence, "The boy wailed, 'I can't find my mother,' " announced, "I don't know what 'wailed' means, but it told me how he talked because it went where 'said' usually is. And the boy is unhappy, so I think the word means 'cried,' " it is obvious that the effort involved in cognitive teaching has paid off.

Linguistic—Educational Abilities to Be Developed. The cognitive approach is classified as a natural approach, because it uses environmental factors as a focus of teaching and because sentence structure is not stressed as a teaching goal. Teachers or clinicians encourage the use of sentences by expanding and modelling children's utterances, but parts of speech and linguistic forms are not the focus of instruction. Proponents of the cognitive approach suggest that it is more important for a child to develop skills of analysis, classification, and deduction than to learn facts, including grammatical ones. Because normally hearing children use exposure to language as a means of deriving rules about its structure, it seems reasonable to assume that hearing-impaired children will be better equipped to deduce linguistic rules if they have developed the skills described above. Accordingly, early therapy activities center around development of abilities such as the following examples described by Eccarius (1978):

1. Ability to list under differing conditions. How many words can you think of that:
   have double letters
   tell things you do outside in the rain
   need capital letters
2. Ability to predict more than one outcome to a situation.
   A girl smells smoke and no one else is home. What can she do? Very good, what else can she do? Great, and if that doesn't work, what else?
3. Ability to visualize situations contrary to present fact.
   If you were a baby. . .
   If you had a lot of money. . .
   If you lived on the moon. . .
4. Ability to vary one part of a sentence to match a change in another part.
   On rainy days I like to . . .
   On sunny days I like to . . .
   On sunny days I don't like to . . .
   On cold nights I like to . . .
5. Ability to tell how two words/things are the same and different.
   Washington and Lincoln

same	*different*
both men	different times
both presidents	different names
both dead	one shot, one died in bed

Grammatical Language Intervention Approaches

Vocabulary Approach. The procedures involved in this approach are most useful for children who exhibit little or no receptive or expressive language. Vocabulary is taught to provide a basis for further language development. Initially, a 50-word noun vocabulary is taught. The nouns are then combined in adjective/article/noun groupings for further teaching. Verbs are introduced next in the imperative and present progressive (is V ing) forms. Complete sentences are then taught in present tense (The cat is sleeping. Jane drops the ball.) When these are mastered, sentences using other verb tenses are introduced, and finally, sentences representing more complex structures are presented.

This approach uses drill activities involving pictures, objects and actions. As a result the vocabulary consists primarily of nouns, verbs, and adjectives that can be pictured easily. Vocabulary cards, such as those found in *Peabody Language Kits* and *Developmental Learning Materials* are popular stimuli. *The Newby Visual Language Series* (Newby, 1969) is appropriate for use with the vocabulary approach; it consists of line drawings depicting nouns, adjectives, and verbs. Each verb picture depicts three tenses of the verb: present, past and future. *The Visual Language Series* was developed for use with deaf children at the Pennsylvania School for the Deaf.

The vocabulary approach is a structured one, usually based on suggested lists of vocabulary for preschool deaf children. As such it may minimize the actual environment and interests of the child that are central to the natural methods. Teaching of vocabulary by rote also tends to ignore the multiple meanings of words. Vocabulary items are taught as nouns, verbs or adjectives and the possibility of a word's being used as two or more of these is not addressed. For example, swimming is almost always taught as a verb, almost never as an adjective. Generalizing usage of a word in a variety of ways is difficult for hearing-impaired children, and the vocabulary approach does little to foster that skill.

Slot-Filler Grammatical Models. The attempt to present language in a structured, logical form to children who cannot hear has been the focus of educators for centuries. Although the goal of natural language development under natural conditions is recognized as laudable and preferable, the realities of providing language instruction to hearing-impaired children have resulted in the development of many schemes for the analysis and presentation of English. Examples of a variety of these systems can be found in Moores (1978). The most popular of the slot-filler systems in use in this country is the *Fitzgerald Key* (Fitzgerald, 1929). The *Key* consists of six columns or charts of grammatical headings, under which vocabulary words are listed as they are taught. Teaching begins with vocabulary items for a who/what chart that differentiates person nouns or pronouns from other nouns. This is the subject chart for use in developing sentences. Names of common classroom objects and of students and teachers are entered on this chart. Pronouns such as *you, I,* and *we* also are recorded here.

Table 8.1 The Six Columns (Charts) that Form the Basis of the Fitzgerald Key

Who/What (Subject)	*Verb (Verb)*	*What (Object)*	*Where Phrase (Prepositional Phrase)*	*Modifiers (How, How Many, With, From, For)*	*When Phrase (Adverbial Phrase)*
Mrs. Jones	Run	Book	On the table	Five	Tomorrow
Desk	Sit	Me	In the car	Pretty	After awhile
Teacher	Stand	Table	Under the book	Hard	Later
I	Cry	Paper	There	Bad	In the morning
John	Write	Us	Here	Happy	At night
Puppy	Yell	John	Outside	For	Yesterday
Pencil	Jump	Teacher		With	Before
Chair	Ride			Several	
You	Fall			All	
Sally	Drop				
Bob	Play				
Floor	Cut				
Car					
Blocks					
We					

The boy went home.

The second chart contains verbs; initially these are action verbs that can be demonstrated or called attention to in class. On the right of the verb chart is another noun-pronoun list containing words that can be used as direct and indirect objects of verbs. Three more charts are developed for *where* phrases, modifiers telling *how* and *how much,* and words such as *for, from,* and *with;* and for phrases telling *when*. Table 8.1 shows the six columns used in the *Fitzgerald Key*.

To enhance memory and provide visual clues as to the function of a word in a sentence, symbols were devised to represent each category of words included in the *Key*. Figure 8.1 shows the Fitzgerald symbols and examples of their use in sentences. To further aid young children in their attempts to build sentences, the

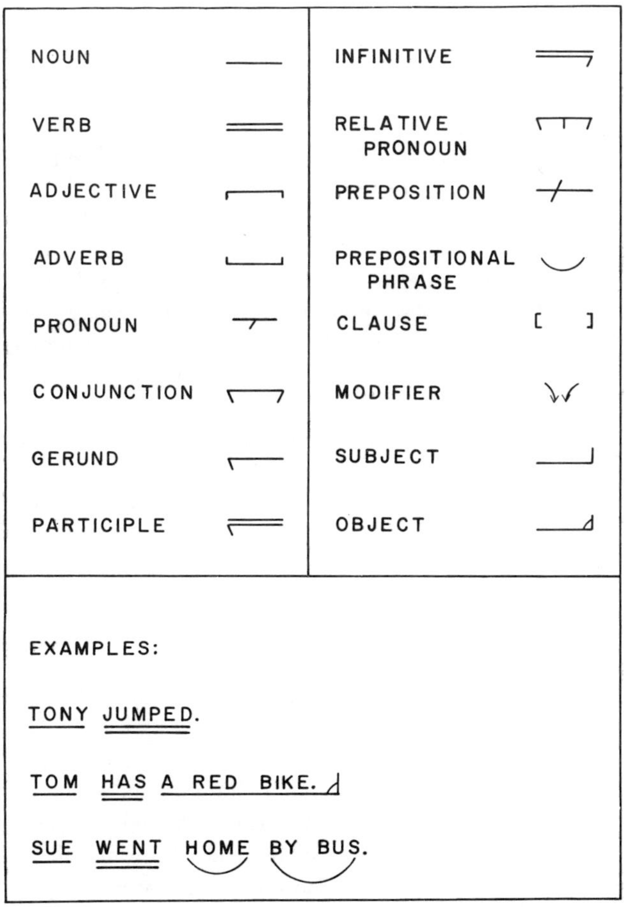

Figure 8.1. Symbols used in the *Fitzgerald Key* and three examples of their use in sentences. The symbol is always placed under the word or phrase it represents.

symbols were color coded. Young children associated a symbol and a color with each different word class, such as red double lines for verbs, a blue curved line for where phrases, and a yellow single line for the subject of the sentence.

When several words on the first two charts are known, the first sentences are presented. They consist of descriptions of actions that are demonstrated in class. Someone jumps or sits or walks or runs and the children identify *who* performed the action, producing their first sentences (John runs. Sally sits.). The sentences are written and symbols are provided to designate the function of each word in the utterance. Verbs in past tense form are presented at this point (Mary cried. The teacher wrote.). Gradually, sentences are lengthened and their complexity is increased to include transitive verbs, objects, prepositions, phrases of place and time, and other verb tenses.

In time, children are able to use the entire *Key* and to fit their utterances into its structure. Incomplete or incorrect sentences are often pointed out by providing the symbol for the missing grammatical constituent. Theoretically, the child can then recognize the rule that has been violated in that sentence's construction. In some cases, children are presented with *Key* symbols and required to produce sentences that represent the rule depicted. For example, when provided with the symbols ______ ══════ ______⌐ and a stimulus picture, a child who is proficient in use of the *Key* will produce subject-verb-object sentences that describe the picture.

The use of symbols as guides for sentence construction is the reason for the use of the term "slot filler" as a description of the *Key*, the Barry five slate, Wing's symbols, and other analytical systems. The number and type of symbols used varies from one system to the next, but the principles are the same. The symbols provide nonambiguous visual clues as guides to sentence construction.

Critics of the slot-filler methods point out the artificiality involved in them. The ability to use idiomatic language is not acquired by means of rule memorization. Simply telling an individual that the number of the subject influences the form of the verb in present tense is not enough, even when instructions include examples. ("Look, when you're talking about one person, you put an 's' on the end of the verb, ok? He sleeps. But when you're talking about more than one person, you don't add the 's'. They sleep. Got it? Ok, you do it now.") Language simply is not learned by the *teaching* of rules, and our understanding of how it is learned is not yet complete enough to allow for an analytical teaching strategy that results in normal language development.

Nevertheless, the slot-filler grammatical systems represent an ingenious attempt to present the complexities of sentence structure to children who are not adequately exposed to it under normal circumstances. The *Key* and similar systems are in widespread use in classes and schools for the deaf. They provide teachers with a structured approach to a difficult task. These systems are most appropriate for use with severely or profoundly hearing-impaired children. They are much less appropriate for moderately hearing-impaired children, who capacities for *hearing* spoken language and learning it through the auditory system are much greater. Slot-filler systems should not be the method of choice for children, unless it can be demonstrated that sentence rules must be provided in symbol form in order to be learned.

Generative Linguistic Models. Several systems have been developed based on the principles of generative-transformational grammar and recent psycholinguistic research. These models are predicated on the theory that sentences may be interpreted on two levels, the *deep* level and the *surface* level. The deep structure of a sentence determines its meaning, the relationships that are being expressed. Sentences representing only this base level would be dull and boring to listen to or to produce over long periods of time. For example, "This is a locket. The locket belongs to Jane. The locket is broken. Jane is crying." are deep level sentences that express the same meaning as the surface structure sentence, "Jane is crying because her locket is broken."

Surface level refers to how the meaning is expressed, and it is at this level that the variety and complexity of language is represented. Different surface structures may be employed to express the same meaning, as in the following: "John hit Bob." "Bob was hit by John," or "Jane failed to hit the ball," "Jane did not hit the ball." The basic component of any sentence is its deep structure, for this determines the meaning of what will be uttered. The variety of surface structures are produced by transformations of the base structure designed to convey the meaning in efficient and expressive ways. Once children acquire the ability to take basic relationships and apply transformational rules to them, they are able to generate sentences to express themselves in a variety of ways.

Several language training systems have been devised to encourage language development in the hearing impaired through a transformational grammar approach (Streng, 1972; Blackwell, Engen, Fischgrund, and Zarcadoolas, 1978; Caniglia, Cole, Howard, Krohn, and Rice, 1973). Two of them will be discussed here, APPLETREE (Caniglia et al. 1973) and the Rhode Island School for the Deaf curriculum (Blackwell et al. 1978). Both of these systems consist of a number of basic sentence types viewed as necessary for the development of English language skills.

Appletree. APPLETREE was developed at the Iowa School for the Deaf and includes 10 basic sentence types, the components of which are designated as nouns (N), verbs (V), adjective (Adj.) and so on. The APPLETREE sentence types are as follows:

1. $N_1 + V_{(be)} +$ adj. (The ball is red.)
2. $N_1 + V_{(be)} +$ where. (The ball is on the table.)
3. $N_1 + V_{(be)} + N_1$. (Mrs. Smith is a woman.)
4. $N_1 + V$. (Sally jumped. John can run.)
5. $N_1 + V +$ where. (John lives in town.)

6. $N_1 + V +$ where $+$ when. (John went to town yesterday.)
7. $N_1 + V + N_2$. (Mother washed her hair.)
8. $N_1 + V + N_2 +$ where. (Jerry took the book to the library.)
9. $N_1 + V + N_2 +$ where $+$ when. (Jerry took the book to the library yesterday.)
10. $N_1 + V + N_3 + N_2$. (Mother gave her book to John.)

Note that nouns are designated by the letter N and by a subscript denoting the function of the noun within the sentence. N_1 designates the subject or the predicate nominative, another noun representing the subject (see sentence type 3); N_2 represents the direct object (sentence type 7); and N_3 denotes the indirect object (sentence type 10). The 10 sentence types are taught sequentially.

APPLETREE curriculum materials are available that include teaching suggestions, language unit outlines, and procedures for use with children. Subgoals associated with each sentence pattern are explained. For example, in order to teach the $N_1 + V_{(be)} +$ where construction, prepostitions must be taught. Detailed instructions for their teaching are provided in the APPLETREE manual. Pictures are used extensively to stimulate the desired sentence type, which is written repeatedly using different vocabulary. For example, sentence type 1 would be elicited by a red ball, green car, large dog, white horse, little girl, and so on.

Rhode Island School for the Deaf Curriculum. This curriculum is based on five basic sentence patterns, as follows (NP = noun phrase, V = verb, LV = linking verb):

Pattern				
1	NP	V		The baby cries.
2	NP_1	V	NP_2	The baby drinks milk.
3	NP	LV	Adjective	The baby is cute.
4	NP	LV	NP	The baby is a boy.
5	NP	LV	Adverbial	The baby is in the crib.

Operating on the assumption that "big sentences are made up of little sentences," the objective of the Rhode Island curriculum is to help children acquire the ability to comprehend and produce simple sentences (Blackwell et al. 1978). The designations used in this system reflect the psycholinguistic orientation of its authors. Children are taught to represent sentences as tree diagrams for added comprehension of the relationship among words. Thus, designations of noun phrase (NP) and verb phrase (VP) are used, and children learn that complete sentences must contain these two components. Longer, more complex sentences can be diagrammed according to phrase structure rules and shown to be combinations of simple sentences. Figure 8.2 shows a tree diagram representing an analysis of the surface structure sentence, "The boy hit the girl who ate his ice cream." The two simple sentences involved ("The boy hit the girl." "The girl ate his ice cream.")

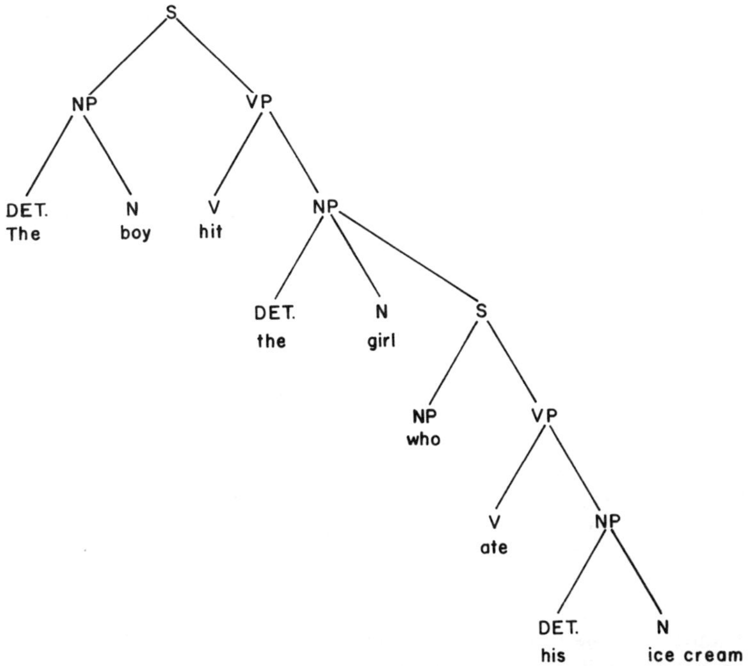

Figure 8.2. Tree diagram of the type used in the Rhode Island School for the Deaf curriculum. This diagram illustrates the combination of two sentences [the boy hit the girl; (the girl) ate his ice cream.] into one complex sentence containing a relative clause.

represent two sentence pattern 2 structures, joined together by relative clause construction.

By using tree diagrams children learn to fit the components of complex sentences into patterns they have used and understood in the past. They then examine and analyze those portions of the complex sentence that do not fit into simple diagram. In this way relationships among the sentence components are visualized and worked through, and new rules are absorbed by which sentences can be formed. The goal is for each child to be able to generate increasingly complex sentences spontaneously as representations of the surrounding world. The ability to analyze complex sentences and derive their meaning is invaluable to success in reading, and proponents of generative grammer approaches include improved reading comprehension as a major goal of the approach.

Recognizing the value of contrasts among sentences as a teaching device, the five Rhode Island sentence patterns are presented simultaneously, rather then in sequential order. This also allows for greater variety of expression early in the language training curriculum. According to Blackwell et al. (1978), children are able to begin sentence analysis as a formal activity by the age of 7.

Because the language taught should relate to the child's own experiences, *experience charts* are used to provide permanent records of the language that represents the events of the child's daily life. Later, sentences generated by classroom activities are grouped according to their structure and *structure charts* are used as visual reinforcers of the sentence types produced. Questions are asked about activities or persons that can be answered by use of the sentences previously produced ("Who dropped the chair?" "Sally dropped the chair.") and association between **wh** pronouns and other vocabulary items are made. Sentences can be written on paper, cut up, and rearranged to illustrate flexibility in surface structure. When children are knowledgeable about the five basic sentence patterns, complexity is introduced in the form of conjunctions, relative clauses, subordinate clauses, complementation, and other transformations.

Generative grammar approaches may be used with children within a broad age range. It is recommended that older children who have not developed basic sentence structures and word order be taken through the same steps as younger children. When they are thoroughly familiar with simple kernel sentences, complex ones may be introduced. This will entail the development of curriculum materials that are of high interest to older children, but which involve less complex sentence structures.

Association Method. The most analytical method proposed for use with hearing-impaired children was developed at Central Institute for the Deaf by McGinnis (1963). It is designed for use with children who exhibit severe language disorders in addition to hearing impairment. The children for whom the method was devised were labeled "aphasic," and were believed to have unusual difficulties in sequencing, memory, and perceptual motor skills. The *Association Method* reduces language to its most basic components and teaches phonemes in isolation, CV combinations, CVC combinations, nouns, article-noun combinations, then sample sentences involving S-V, S-V-N, or S-V-adjective combinations. Table 8.2 illustrates

Table 8.2 Examples of Teaching Stages Employed in the Association Method[a]

Isolated Phonemes	*CV Syllables*	*CVC Syllables*	*Nouns*	*Article-Noun*	*Sentences*
b	**b o-e**	**b o-e l**	Bowl	The bowl	The bowl is blue.
m	**m-a-**	**m-a-n**	Man	A man	A man has two legs.
o-e	**s o-e**	**s o-e p**	Soap	The soap	The soap is wet.
-a-	**k-a-**	**k-a-t**	Cat	A Cat	A cat has a tail.

[a] All phonemes must be learned in isolation before they are combined into syllables. After sequences of phonemes (**b o-e l**) can be remembered, recognized and produced, they are presented as words with referents. CV and CVC syllables are usually nonsense syllables, representing many of the possible combinations of phonemes in English.

the teaching sequence employed. The name of the method derives from its intent to teach an association among the visual, auditory, and motor representations of each language component. As each consonant is presented, for example, the child is required to recognize it in written or spoken form (through reading, lipreading, and listening) and to produce it accurately, before moving on to the next consonant or vowel. Obviously, this is a slow, painstaking approach toward language. McGinnis (1963) stated that the slow building of association is necessary because of the problems the target population has with sequencing and memory.

The majority of hearing-impaired children do not have unusual sequencing or memory problems and have no need for such an analytical approach. The artificiality of learning words as a string of phonemes and being required to pronounce them in the same manner is not beneficial to language learning in the average hearing-impaired child and may impede progress significantly.

Choosing a Therapy Approach

The choice of a remedial approach toward language will be influenced by many factors, and different approaches may be appropriate at different times in a child's life. The baseline language status of the children to be served must be known before remediation begins. The communicative style and language skills exhibited will influence the choice of teaching strategy.

Age is also a significant factor. *ELI* and the vocabulary approach are most appropriate for young children. A slot-filler approach assumes an understanding that language symbols can be used to represent concrete and abstract referents, a stage of linguistic development that many hearing-impaired children do not reach until they have been in school for several years. APPLETREE was designed for use with deaf children in the middle primary grades and the Rhode Island procedures are appropriate only after age 7.

The educational demands faced by the child are important determiners of teaching strategy. A mainstreamed child who encounters unfamiliar vocabulary and complex sentence structures in daily lessons may be served best when taught how to derive meaning from context or generalize rules or information learned previously. The cognitive approach provides this type of training in one way; the Rhode Island generative grammar approach provides it in another way.

The amount of time available for remedial work may also influence the choice of strategies. *ELI* and vocabulary work procedures may be taught to parents. The natural approach is best carried out in a natural environment, such as the home. These approaches can be used when therapy is not available in the home community. After a period of training and observation, parents in rural settings can carry out the programs in the home, checking periodically with the professionals involved. When special services are readily available, the slot-filler, generative grammar, and cognitive approaches can be provided on an ongoing basis. If children are grouped to make maximum use of the clinician's time, the approach employed should be one that makes use of interchanges among children, such as *ELI* or the natural approach.

The degree of hearing loss is sometimes pertinent to the choice of language program. Children who use residual hearing effectively will have less need for slot-filler approaches than children whose hearing losses are profound. For the most part, all of the other approaches are appropriate for children with any degree of hearing impairment.

No matter which approach is chosen, evaluation of its effectiveness is important. Some children respond well to any approach, while others have learning styles that make one set of procedures more effective than another. Periodic reevaluation will allow the charting of progress as language skills develop. If a child shows little progress, changes in programming should be considered. Using a different approach may be all that is necessary to stimulate greater language growth. For example, if a child experiences unusual difficulty with teaching strategies that employ adult grammar, shifting to one that involves more use of child grammar or basic semantic relations may be helpful.

The preceding discussion provided guidelines concerning the types of remedial programs in use and references to which the reader may go for further details concerning them. In actuality, few clinicians use a single approach as described above. Procedures, goals, and activities from a variety of approaches are often combined in an effort to meet the needs of the children served. The important thing is to assess language skills carefully, be familiar with the linguistic needs of the child, and establish objectives based on both. Any language teaching strategy that will meet those objectives and with which the clinician feels comfortable will be a good place to start. Careful reevaluation will provide feedback concerning the adequacy of the approach.

REMEDIATION OF SPEECH SKILLS

Speech has been advocated as the most effective means of communication by oral educators of the deaf for the last 200 or more years. In view of that fact, it is reasonable to expect that well-established remedial methods for teaching speech have been developed, tested for effectiveness, and taught widely. Such is not the case.

There is a startling absence of consensus regarding how, when, or under what conditions speech should be taught. Many books have been written on the subject, most of which describe the author's own teaching procedures. A few authors (Calvert and Silverman, 1975; Leshin, 1975) list what they describe as the most commonly used techniques of speech remediation. Unfortunately, the lists given by different authors bear little resemblance to each other. There appears to be agreement in only three areas. First, the quality of speech produced by severely hearing-impaired children is extremely poor, *but could be improved by systematic use of the proposed techniques*. Second, there are three general aspects of speech that must be treated in hearing-impaired speakers: voice, articulation, and prosodic features, such as rhythm, rate, and intonation. Third, effective use of residual hearing is the key to the development of intelligible speech. After reviewing the lack of agreement mentioned above, Moores (1978) characterized the current status of knowledge about the speech of the deaf as being in "sad disarray."

Importance of Audition to Speech Development

The establishment of an effective auditory feedback loop is the most important prerequisite to development of good speech skills. Responding to the success of a few unusual children, some authors (Ling, 1976; Whetnall and Fry, 1964) use the term "natural" or "normal" speech to describe the goal of speech remediation with the deaf. Certainly "natural" speech is to be desired but most clinicians would settle for intelligible speech, even though it is not always "natural" sounding. Completely normal speech is unusual in children with profound hearing losses. Recognizing this fact will reduce frustration in beginning clinicians and allow them to establish reasonable objectives for these children.

Children with moderate-to-severe hearing losses are capable of developing excellent speech skills, however, and natural speech is a feasible goal for them. For many children with useful residual hearing across a wide band of frequencies, there is no need to concentrate on the development of coordinated respiration and phonation, appropriate pitch, or adequate rhythm. These aspects of speech will develop without special training as a result of extensive auditory experience with the spoken word, if appropriate amplification is provided early. Auditory stimulation, such as that described in Chapter 2, results in improved production as well as reception of speech. For most children who receive and discriminate speech effectively through the auditory system, speech remediation may consist primarily of articulation therapy. Many of the techniques used with normally hearing children are appropriate for use with them. They are able to match their own productions with those they hear, especially with the addition of some simple placement guides and visual clues that are available through observation of other speakers. For sounds such as **r, s, ch,** and **z,** attention may be called to the tactile or kinesthetic characteristics of these sounds during production. Guided practice in the observation and use of these cues as feedback can substantially improve the production of speech sounds whose acoustic properties preclude auditory reception by the hearing impaired.

Symbol Systems for Teaching Speech

Children whose hearing losses are severe or profound require structured remediation if they are to develop good speech skills. Because of their limited hearing, these children benefit from symbol systems that serve as visual reminders of the sounds to be produced. A variety of symbols have been used with hearing-impaired children.

Northampton Chart. Sometimes referred to as the Yale chart, this set of symbols was devised at Clarke School for the Deaf in 1885 and revised in 1925. The chart consists of orthographic symbols using the letters of the English alphabet rather than special phonetic symbols. One advantage to the use of the Northampton symbols is that they correspond to written English and do not require the learning of special symbols that will not appear in ordinary curriculum materials. Primary symbols are provided for all English letters and secondary symbols are provided for those letters that may be pronounced differently depending upon the word in which they appear. For example, the letter **c** may be pronounced as **s** (in city) or as **k** (in cake) and is used as a secondary symbol for both **s** and **k**. Similar distinctions must be made between the **s** that is pronounced as a voiceless **s** and that pronounced as **z**. These are distinguished by the symbols $\overset{1}{\text{s}}$ (as in $\overset{1}{\text{s}}$ink) and $\overset{2}{\text{s}}$ (as in car$\overset{2}{\text{s}}$). The Northampton consonant and vowel charts are arranged systematically according to certain characteristics of the phonemes. Figure 8.3 shows the consonant chart. The first column includes primary and secondary symbols for most voiceless consonants, the second for voiced consonants, and the remainder for nasal, liquid, and sound combinations

h									
wh		w-							
p		b		m					
t		d		n		l	r		
					kn			**wr**	
k		$\overset{1}{\text{g}}$		ng					
	c				n(k)				
	ck								
f		v							
	ph								
$\overset{1}{\text{th}}$		$\overset{2}{\text{th}}$							
$\overset{1}{\text{s}}$		$\overset{2}{\text{s}}$				y-			
	c(e)		(z)						
	c(i)								
	cy								
sh		zh							
ch		j							
	tch		$\overset{2}{\text{g}}$						
			-ge						
			-dge						
						X=k$\overset{1}{\text{s}}$		qu	= kwh
									kw

Figure 8.3. The Northampton consonant chart.

$\overset{1}{\text{oo}}$	$\overset{2}{\text{oo}}$	aw law	-o- not	
b$\overset{1}{\text{o}}$ot	b$\overset{2}{\text{o}}$ok	ball		
		au caught		
		o(r)		
ee beet	-i- sit	-e- bed	-a- cat	
-e me	$\overset{1}{\text{-y}}$	$\overset{2}{\text{ea}}$ bread		
be				
$\overset{1}{\text{ea}}$ m$\overset{1}{\text{e}}$at				
		a(r) (**ah**)	-u- cup	ur
			butter	er
				ir
			a	
a-e cake	i-e pie	oi toy	o-e coke	
ai rain	igh kite	oy boy	oa coat	
ay day	bike			
	$\overset{2}{\text{-y}}$ fight		$\overset{2}{\text{ow}}$ b$\overset{2}{\text{o}}$w	
	sky		so	
		ou mouse	u-e mute	
			blue	
		$\overset{1}{\text{ow}}$ c$\overset{1}{\text{o}}$w	ew few	

Figure 8.4. The Northampton vowel chart.

represented by alphabet letters, such as x and q. Each row consists of phonemes representing a defferent place of articulation.

Figure 8.4 shows the Northampton vowel chart. Vowels are arranged in three groups: back round vowels, front vowels, and diphthongs. The presence of a dash (-) indicates another phoneme and its effect on the one represented. For example, in the consonant chart, **h**- means that **h** is always an initial consonant. In the vowel chart, -**i**- symbolizes a short **i** sound, since the two dashes mean that the **i** occurs in a CVC context. The symbol **i-e** indicates a diphthong such as that occurring in the word *ice*. The dash represents the missing consonant.

This complex system is necessary in order to account for the pronunciation rules of English. In many languages, a given phoneme carries only one pronunciation (e.g., Spanish). In English, however, rules of pronunciation are so complex that alphabet letters alone are insufficient guides for the hearing-impaired speaker. The Northampton chart symbols do not provide a completely accurate representation of English, but they constitute a helpful pronunciation guide that is widely used with hearing-impaired children.

The chart is presented to children as a guide to articulation. Symbols are presented along with oral productions of the sound to be learned. Sounds are taught in isolation by some clinicians, in syllables or words by others. Because the production of a given phoneme varies according to the phonetic context in which it appears, consonants should be learned in association with various vowels. When using the Northampton chart, clinicians should be sure to present the symbols for the *entire* utterance to be produced by clinician and child. Production of "buh," for example, should be represented by the symbols **bu-**, not **b**.

The Northampton chart may be used as a pronunciation guide after speech has been learned by another technique. It simply offers a visual monitoring system by which the child can evaluate and correct pronunciation of known words or "sound out" unfamiliar ones.

Diacritical Markings. Most dictionaries use pronunciation symbols called diacritical markings. Many clinicians and teachers prefer to use diacritical symbols as pronunciation guides with hearing-impaired children from the beginning, rather than teaching from one symbol system, then switching to another. A child's use of the dictionary is enhanced by prior knowledge of the markings and their meaning. Shifting from use of the Northampton chart to diacritical symbols is probably not as confusing as a shift from the International Phonetic Alphabet (IPA), whose symbols do not correspond to the Roman alphabet used in written English. Examples of common diacritical markings may be seen in Figure 8.5. They may be used during speech instruction in the same way as the Northampton chart.

Symbol	**Key Word**
s͜h	ship
t͜h	think
~~th~~	bother
oo	boot
o͝o	book
ô	saw
ē	me
i	sit
e	bet
a	cat
â(r)	father
u	cup
ə	sofa
er	bird
ā	cake
ī	pie
ō	no
oi	oil
yo͞o	cute

Figure 8.5. Common dictionary diacritical markings.

Alcorn Symbols. In a rough way these symbols constitute visual representations of the shape of the mouth during the production of vowels. They can be used alone or superimposed on a simple face drawn by the teacher. The purpose is to help the child associate the oral movement with the written symbol. Because only vowels are represented in the Alcorn system, it must be used in conjunction with another orthographic system that allows for representation of consonants. Figure 8.6 shows the Alcorn symbols (Streng, 1955). These symbols are usually used with very young children and can be drawn on round paper plate "faces" and used as flashcards or as reminders during speech activities. When combined with alphabet letters, words may be written as follows:

m—t (meet)
bok (book)
fo□m (farm)

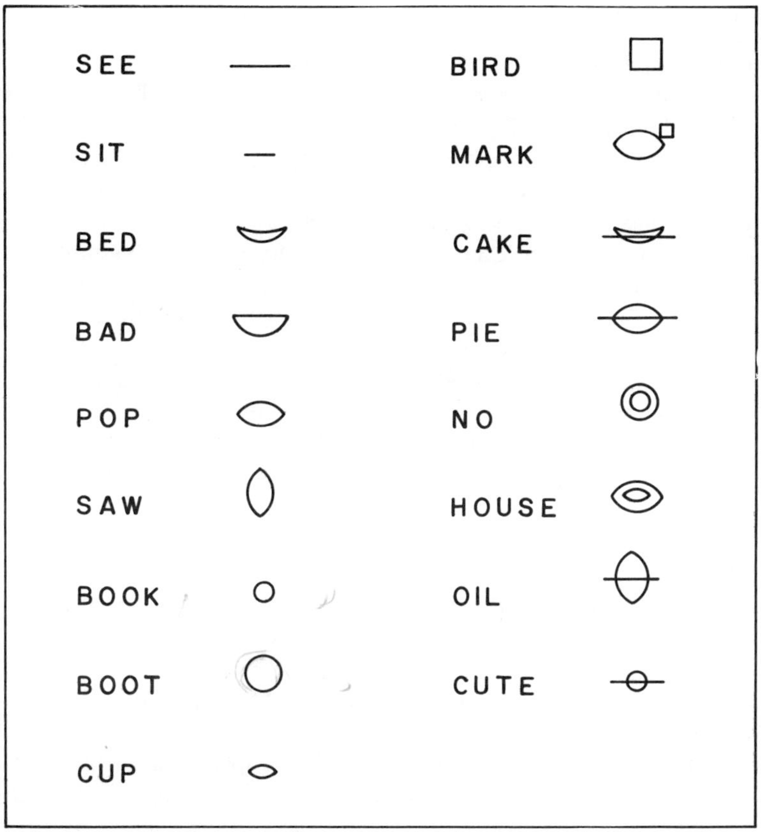

Figure 8.6. The Alcorn vowel symbols and key words illustrating the vowels for each symbol.

To be most successful, the symbol system chosen must be taught thoroughly. Unless association of the symbol with the speech sound it represents is automatic, the systems may only confuse the child. For this reason, many teachers and clinicians concentrate early speech work on the articulation of phonemes and syllables before children have learned to control other components of speech production, such as phonation.

Methods for Teaching Speech

There appear to be two major methods for teaching speech to hearing-impaired children, although the procedures used within each are widely different and often overlapping. For lack of systematic terminology they are referred to as the *traditional* and the *auditory stimulation* methods.

Traditional Method. The outstanding characteristic of this method is its concentration on the development of speech sounds in syllables.

Teaching Phonemes. At least 90 percent of the books and articles written about speech and hearing impairment describe procedures designed to teach the phonemes of English. Many books (e.g., Haycock, 1933; Leshin, 1975; and Calvert and Silverman, 1975) present analyses of phonemes with regard to how they are produced by the vocal mechanism, suggestions for teaching production, and descriptions of common errors and how to avoid them. Phonemes are taught in a predetermined sequence, which varies from teacher to teacher. Most teachers begin with bilabial consonants (p, b, and m) and mid and back vowels (such as those in c**u**p, b**oo**t, and f**a**rm). The more difficult consonants, such as **ch, r, s, ng,** and vowels such as **-i-, -e-,** and **oo** are not taught until the child can produce many other sounds. Procedures such as these dictate that sounds be taught in some sort of sequence, rather than expecting development of all or most phonemes simultaneously. This being the case, speech work is necessarily done at prescribed times during the day or week as an activity somewhat separate from language or academic instruction. A visual symbol system is chosen and taught systematically. When the child can produce certain phonemes accurately, they are monitored during spontaneous speech by teachers and clinicians. Poor productions are not accepted without comment and good productions are reinforced positively. This method requires specific teaching of each phoneme in a variety of vowel contexts and much practice under structured conditions.

Calvert and Silverman (1975) refer to the traditional method as the Multisensory Syllable Unit method because the auditory, visual, tactile, and kinesthetic features of the various sounds are presented and emphasized during instruction. Attention is called to the visual components of bilabial consonants, the tactile and kinesthetic sensations that accompany voiced sounds, and the auditory information available in vowels. All sensory clues are emphasized through mirror work, simultaneous presentations by clinician and child, and use of the child's hand to feel vibrations of the throat, nose, or stream of air during sound productions by both adult and child. Auditory training equipment or other amplification is used to call attention to the audible components of speech available to each individual child.

Once phonemes have been demonstrated and taught in isolation or in CV or VC syllables, they are presented in a variety of syllable contexts. This procedure insures that children learn to produce phonemes in various ways depending upon the phonetic context in which they appear. Concentrating on a few productions of a given sound will deter generalization of the sound to other situations and other contexts and may result in speech that is less natural sounding than is possible. The use of various contexts in teaching speech is illustrated by Calvert and Silverman (1975, p. 163):

> Since the syllable is the recommended unit of speech, drills should generally be in a syllabic pattern and proceed as the child gains in skills from simple CVC patterns to more complex ones. The order could be CVC (tot), CCVC (street), CVCCC (desks). Even within a pattern, varying combinations should be appropriately employed. For example, if the t is the phoneme being drilled on, the CVC could include the following patterns, each representing a class of drill:
>
> tVt—vowel changed, initial and final t included
> tVp—place changed in final consonant
> pVt—place changed in initial consonant
> tVd—same place but final voicing
> dVt—same place but initial voicing
> tVn—same place but final nasal
> tVs—place and manner changed in final consonant

Lists of words according to their phonetic structure are available that can serve as stimulus material for drill on phonemes in varying contexts (Rockey, 1973).

Teaching Phonation. Although the traditional method emphasizes the articulation of speech sounds, its proponents must also be concerned with the development of a pleasant voice and its coordination with articulation. An adequate voice depends on adequate breath support. Because they do not hear normally, hearing-impaired children may not associate the breath stream with production of speech. It is not uncommon for these children to attempt to speak while inhaling or fail to fill their lungs with air prior to speaking. The result is often breathiness, inadequate vowel intensity, inappropriate pitch, and the production of one or two syllables per breath. All of these problems affect the general quality of the speech produced. As a result, speech training includes teaching the child to control the breath stream, producing, prolonging, and interrupting it at will. Blowing bubbles, ping pong balls across a table, candle flames, paper strips, or pinwheels will improve control over the breath supply.

Production of a voice that is clear and pleasant to listen to is a difficult task for severely hearing-impaired children. The traditional approach toward developing good vocal quality involves the use of babbling. The child is reinforced for producing voice and encouraged to use the tactile sense to monitor voice production. When voice can be produced at will, exercises are introduced that result in loudness, pitch and duration variations. Visual and tactile clues are provided to help the child monitor the desired voice patterns. A hand placed on the child's or teacher's throat, use of a balloon held by the child next to the mouth, and placing a finger on the nose are all techniques to call attention to the presence of vibration and its characteristics. Visual clues to duration can be provided by activities such as moving a crayon along a piece of paper as long as voice is produced and allowing the child to monitor duration by the length of the crayon mark. When available, oscilloscopes or other electronic display equipment can be used to provide a visual display of the frequency and durational characteristics of vocal utterances. Because tension is so detrimental to the production of a pleasant voice, this type of therapy is usually accomplished during brief periods, several times a day. Tension often results in high pitch and strained vocal quality and should be avoided by making speech training as pleasant as possible. The clinician must arrange for the child to experience success as quickly and as often as possible. This may mean that difficult tasks are alternated with easily performed ones in order to increase self-confidence.

Hypernasality represents a particularly prevalent and difficult problem for hearing-impaired children. Hearing children learn automatically to close the velopharyngeal port when producing nonnasal sounds as a result of auditory monitoring of their speech production. Hearing-impaired children must learn through painstaking effort to avoid nasalization of most speech sounds. Velopharyngeal closure is an *active* speech movement; the soft palate, tongue, and pharyngeal walls must move deliberately to avoid nasal emission of the breath stream. If the requisite movements are not made, closure is not achieved and hypernasality results. Failure of the velum to raise, as during the production of the nasals **m, n,** and **ng,** is detrimental to clear, nonnasal voice quality. If, during early teaching, vowels are learned and produced habitually with the velum raised, hypernasality is less likely to develop. Thus, the teaching of vowels has an important effect on eventual voice quality and should not be rushed or slighted.

Teaching Speech Rhythm. Proponents of the traditional approach toward speech training recognize the need to develop appropriate speech rhythm. Far less is written by them concerning this essential aspect of speech, however, than about articulation of speech sounds. Rhythm exercises are proposed in which a piano or other musical instrument is used to emphasize accent and number of beats. Once attention has been drawn to rhythmic patterns of sound, the child is required to imitate the patterns with motor movements of various parts of the body. Marching, clapping, and swinging the arms are examples. Sometimes the child is asked to reproduce the pattern observed by tapping, drawing on a blackboard, or vocalizing. The latter is

Table 8.3 Examples of Visual Symbols to Indicate Accent, Phrasing, and Pauses in Connected Speech

Accent Marks:
I don't thínk he wánts to gó.

Phrase Markers:
I don't think he wants to go.

Pause Indicators:
In other words // I don't think he wants to go.

most directly related to speech production, but may be the most difficult to achieve initially.

Most speech rhythm work is done after the child has learned considerable expressive language. Nursery rhymes or poems ("Mary Had a Little Lamb"), finger plays (the eentsy, teensy spider climbed up the water spout), and words and sentences representing various accent, phrasing, and intonation patterns (Where are you going? I don't want to.) are presented for imitation. Visual symbols, such as accent marks, phrase markers, and pause indicators are provided in written form. Examples are shown in Table 8.3. When used creatively, these symbols provide clues regarding breathing patterns that are appropriate for the utterances involved.

Auditory Stimulation Method. The principles and techniques underlying this method of teaching speech to the hearing impaired are synonymous with those of the educational methods labeled acoupedic, oral-aural, acoustic, and unisensory. They stress the role of audition in the normal development of language and speech skills. If auditory skills are to be developed to their fullest potential, use of other sensory systems must not be encouraged. Therefore, the multisensory clues described above are not used.

The first step toward speech development is in the early selection of appropriate amplification. Most proponents of the auditory method strongly advocate the use of binaural amplification. Hearing aids should be monitored closely; a daily hearing aid check is recommended, either by the teacher, clinician, or parent.

The major component of this method is auditory stimulation with speech. An environment must be established in which the child is constantly stimulated with language appropriate to ongoing activities. Utterances are reinforced immediately, usually by social responses (smiling, touching, or hand clapping), but sometimes by tangible rewards (cereal, use of special toy, fruit drink).

Importance of Imitation. Imitation of sounds produced by others is an integral part of the auditory stimulation method. In the beginning babbling is encouraged, along with the imitation of sounds made by adults. The latter may be the sounds made by animals, toys, or household appliances and utilities (vacuum cleaner, water running). The purpose of imitation is to call attention to the variety of sounds in the environment and to establish an auditory feedback loop that will enable the child to interpret sounds and engage in self-monitoring. Imitation of pitch change, intonation and rhythm are important as well as imitation of articulation. An utterance such as "uh oh," with its rising, then falling intonation can be used in games to call attention to nonsegmental aspects of speech. Because they are learned and practiced by normally hearing children before the first words are used, the prosodic features of speech are among the first targets for imitation by hearing-impaired children.

Connected Speech as the Major Stimuli. The auditory stimulation method stresses the use of connected speech in phrases and sentences. This allows the child to become familiar with the rhythmic patterns of the language. Children are encouraged to listen; visual and tactile clues are not provided. Specific techniques for teaching the production of various sounds are not suggested by proponents of this method. Constant bombardment of speech by the adults and children in the home, school, or playground are felt to be the essential components to the development of speech. Pollack (1974) gives examples of games and activities that can be used to stimulate utterances and imitations by young children. Most other authors simply describe the philosophy of the method without providing practical guidelines. Proponents of the auditory stimulation method draw distinctions between it and *auditory training* (Pollack, 1970), but the techniques associated with both are similar. The major distinction appears to be that auditory training is accomplished at specific times for specific purposes, whereas the auditory stimulation method involves a constant, ongoing effort by everyone in the child's environment.

The development of good articulation is not a major concern in the auditory stimulation method, probably because it is used primarily with preschool children. One of the goals of the method is the complete integration of hearing-impaired children into regular educational settings. Therefore, using the method with older children has not been reported. In effect, children who have developed some speech using the auditory stimulation method are taught fine articulation skills by the traditional methods described above. If the earlier method has been successful, the task of teaching good articulation should be greatly enhanced by the child's use of good voice quality and speech rhythm.

Developmental Approach ("The Ling Thing"). If the reader is feeling frustrated regarding the lack of specifics regarding teaching speech to the hearing impaired, it is not surprising. Available descriptions of the methods in current use are vague and open to many interpretations. This fact has contributed to the lack of consensus among educators and clinicians and, probably, to the poor speech skills of hearing-impaired children. In an effort to clarify and specify techniques for speech development in this population, Ling (1976) developed and reported a developmental model of speech. He described two levels of speech acquisition: the *phonetic* level, which involves the production of the sounds of the language and the *phonologic* level, which involves the use of speech sounds within a meaningful utterance. According to Ling, it is necessary for deaf children to master both levels of speech production by progressing through five broad stages of development. The stages described are largely sequential but may overlap to some extent.

Stage 1 consists of undifferentiated vocalizations. These include laughing, crying, sounds accompanying physical effort, and babbling. The child is encouraged to vocalize, to produce voice at will. Until this can be done, refinement of the voice into speech patterns is not possible.

Stage 2 consists of nonsegmental voice patterns. The loudness, pitch, and duration of the voice can be varied intentionally.

Stage 3 involves the use of a range of different vowel sounds. Ling suggests teaching at least three vowels that are quite distinct from each other, such as the high front vowel **ee,** the high back vowel **oo,** and the neutral vowel **a(r).** Because deaf children tend to neutralize and nasalize all vowels, use of high vowels in the beginning will encourage maximum tongue movement and provide a means of contrasting these with low vowels taught later.

Stage 4 consists of simple consonants produced in the initial, medial, and final positions within syllables. Teaching order is usually stops, nasals, semivowels, liquids, fricatives, and affricates. CV, VC, and CVC syllables are practiced and produced with ease at this stage.

Stage 5 involves consonant blends. Ling describes blends as those made by using two articulatory organs sequentially (sm, sp), one organ sequentially (sn, thr), two organs simultaneously (pl, br), one organ simultaneously (tr, gl), and complex blends (skr, spr).

Ling recommends the systematic training of speech, following the stages described. The child is first taught to vocalize, to vary suprasegmental patterns, to produce vowels and diphthongs, to produce consonants by manner, place, and voicing in combination with vowels, and finally, to produce consonant blends with vowels. There are subskills within each stage that must be mastered. The secret to the successful development of speech skills, according to Ling, is to master each subskill before moving on to the next step. The subskills are similar for each aspect of speech to be taught and the goal of each is to achieve automaticity. Children move from one subskill to another only when production is automatic and completely under control.

An example of the thoroughness of the subskill teaching required can be seen in the following description of the subskills for teaching the phoneme ***b***:

1. Production in a single syllable with the vowels **ee, a(r),** and **oo.**
2. Production in a series of repeated syllables using a single vowel (boo, boo, boo).
3. Production in a series of repeated syllables using different vowels (bee, ba, boo).

4. Alternation of syllables released with another consonant (boomooboomoo).
5. Production of **b** in syllables varying in intensity.
6. Production of **b** in an intervocalic position with one syllable stressed (bába, beeboó).
7. Production in repeated or alternated syllables varying over eight semitones in pitch.

Ling's model and procedures represent a combination of elements of the traditional and the auditory stimulation methods of teaching speech. He advocates the use of auditory stimulation and the imitation of the nonsegmental aspects of speech. At the same time his procedures include drill on syllables rather than connected speech. Ling's procedures are most appropriate for children who have useful residual hearing and are least effective with children whose auditory systems are severely limited. In describing specific teaching techniques, Ling depends heavily on the child's ability to *hear* the contrasts to be produced. When audition is not sufficient, he recommends the use of tactile and kinesthetic clues. Ling does not recommend the use of visual aids, primarily because they are not very useful to the child in developing the orosensory feedback he considers essential to speech production. Only by learning to use the natural receptors of touch, vibration, and movement sensations that are present in the chest, throat, tongue, and other articulators, will severely hearing-impaired children learn to monitor their speech effectively.

Ling's procedures constitute the most systematic and well thought out outline for teaching speech skills that is currently available. He does not present data to support his claims of ''natural'' speech, so clinicians will have to evaluate the effectiveness of the procedures themselves. Specific instructions for teaching various phonemes or other aspects of speech can be found in Ling (1976), Calvert and Silverman (1975), Haycock (1933), and Leshin (1975).

REFERENCES

Baron, N., Linguistic consciousness: Prerequisites for learning to read and write. Address delivered to the Summer Institute on Applied Linguistics, Rhode Island School for the Deaf, 1975.

Blackwell, P., Engen, E., Fischgrund, J., and Zarcadoolas, C., *Sentences and Other Systems*. Washington, D. C.: A. G. Bell Association, 1978.

Bloom, L., *Language Development: Form and Function in Emergency Grammars*. Boston: M.I.T. Press, 1970.

Calvert, D. and Silverman, S., *Speech and Deafness*. Washington, D. C.: A. G. Bell Association, 1975.

Caniglia, J., Cole, N., Howard, W., Krohn, E., and Rice, M., *APPLETREE: A Developmental Language Program*. Beaverton, OR: Dormac Inc., 1973.

Condon, W. and Sander, L., Synchrony demonstrated between movements of the enonate and adult speech, *Child Development*, 45, 456–462, 1974.

Eccarius, M., Language habilitation for hearing-impaired children. Address delivered to the Summer Residential Program staff at the University of Iowa, 1978.

Fitzgerald, E., *Straight Language for the Deaf*. Staunton, VA: McClure Company, 1929.

Furth, H., *Thinking Without Language*. New York: The Free Press, 1966.

Gleitman, L., Gleitman, H., and Shipley, E., The emergence of the child as grammarian, *Cognition*, 1, 137–164, 1972.

Grammatico, L. and Miller, S., Curriculum for the preschool deaf child, *Volta Rev.*, 76, 280–289, 1974.

Haycock, G., *The Teaching of Speech*. Washington, D. C.: Volta Bureau, 1933.

Karpova, S., Awareness of the word composition of speech in the preschool child, *Voprosy Psikhologii*, 1, 43–55, 1955.

Leshin, G., *Speech for the Hearing-Impaired Child*. Tucson: University of Arizona Press, 1975.

Ling, D., *Speech and the Hearing Impaired Child*. Washington, D.C.: A. G. Bell Association, 1976.

MacDonald, J., Environmental language intervention. In F. Withrow and C. Nygren (Eds.), *Language, Materials, and Curriculum Management for the Handicapped Learner*. Columbus, OH: Charles E. Merrill Publishing Corp., 1976.

McGinnis, M., *Aphasic Children: Identification and Education by the Association Method*. Washington, D.C.: A. G. Bell Association, 1963.

Moores, D., *Educating the Deaf: Psychology, Principles, and Practices*. Boston: Houghton Mifflin, 1978.

Newby, R., *Visual Language Series*. Eagleville, PA: Newby Visual Language, Inc., 1969.

Piaget, J., *The Language and Thought of the Child*. New York: World, 1962.

Pollack, D., *Educational Audiology for the Limited Hearing Infant*. Springfield, Il: Charles C Thomas, 1970.

Pollack, D., Remedial practices with the hearing-impaired. In S. Dickson (Ed.), *Communication Disorders—Remedial Principles and Practices*. Glenview, IL: Scott, Foresman and Co., 1974.

Rockey, D., *Phonetic Lexicon*. New York: Heyden, 1973.

Streng, A., *Hearing Therapy for Children*. New York: Grune and Stratton, 1955.

Streng, A., *Syntax, Speech and Hearing: Applied Linguistics for Teachers of Children with Language and Hearing Disabilities*. New York: Grune and Stratton, 1972.

Taba, H., *Curriculum Development: Theory and Practice*. New York: Harcourt, Brace, and World, Inc., 1962.

de Villiers, J. and de Villiers, P., Early judgments of semantic and syntactic acceptability by children. *J. Psycholing. Res.*, 1, 299–310, 1972.

Whetnall, E. and Fry, D., *The Deaf Child*. Springfield, IL: Charles C Thomas, 1964.

CHAPTER 9

Educational Deficits and Their Assessment

I. Academic Achievement
   A. Achievement by Severely Hearing-Impaired Children
   B. Achievement by Moderately Hearing-Impaired Children

II. Assessment
   A. Personnel Involved in Assessment
   B. Guidelines for Assessment
   C. Assessment Tools

The most obvious outcome of reduced language proficiency in children is retarded academic achievement. Although the relationship among hearing loss, language development and educational achievement is often poorly understood, it is difficult to ignore the latter once a child has entered school. The deficit in classroom performance for severely hearing-impaired children is profound and obvious. For children with mild to moderate hearing impairments, the educational delay may be slow in developing and is often attributed to other causes, such as poor attitudes, reduced intellect, or other conditions involving brain damage or emotional maladjustment. Although there may be a circular relationship among achievement, attitude, and self-confidence, the underlying cause of poor academic achievement is the language deficit incurred as a result of the hearing loss. It is important for speech-language pathologists, audiologists, and teachers of the deaf to understand the nature of the educational problems faced by hearing-impaired children, both for purposes of planning remediation and as a basis for intelligent consulting with other school personnel. This chapter describes the academic deficits associated with hearing loss, assessment of academic skills, and the types of remedial programs and educational placements currently in vogue.

ACADEMIC ACHIEVEMENT

Because of the pronounced differences between children who cannot learn well through the auditory system and those who can, the discussion that follows treats children with different degrees of hearing loss separately. The term *deaf* will appear as it was used by authors of the studies reported. A strong case can be made for a continuum of hearing impairment, at least with regard to hearing losses that do not exceed 80 to 90 dB (ANSI, 1969). Experience with hearing-impaired children reveals, however, that different procedures, techniques, and materials are necessary for children who are able to process information auditorily versus those whose primary input mode is visual. Unfortunately, this distinction has not been understood well by educators and clinicians who sometimes concentrate on stimulation of the wrong sensory system at the wrong time. As a result, moderately hearing-impaired children are often enrolled in lipreading therapy although their primary mode of message reception is, or could be, auditory. Conversely, many children with profound hearing losses spend hours in auditory stimulation activities beyond those that are appropriate and useful to them. The importance of auditory input to hearing-impaired children cannot be overemphasized. Professionals must evaluate its usefulness to each individual child and modify teaching strategies accordingly. Procedures used by teachers in self-contained classes for deaf children may not be appropriate for children who are seen for resource room assistance or by itinerant teachers.

Achievement by Severely Hearing-Impaired Children

Of all the deficits associated with hearing impairment, educational achievement is the one most studied and best understood. More than 90 percent of the studies conducted in the area of academic achievement have investigated progress of deaf children. Few data exist concerning the educational status of children with mild to moderate hearing losses, although they outnumber the others greatly. These children are not grouped easily for study, and the task of teaching children who are seriously deficient in language knowledge and usage is so difficult that educators have concentrated on the most severely impaired.

The educational data collected illustrates the devastating effects of severe congenital hearing impairment. Investigations have centered around measures of reading achievement, although some data exist for other academic areas. Reading and mathematics skills are easily measured by standardized tests because these skills are not curriculum bound. Whether the school uses the *Houghton-Mifflin* reading series or the *Wisconsin Design* series, the same general reading skills are taught. The same cannot be said for social studies or science curricula, however; the achievement tests in these areas must reflect a specific curriculum in order to provide a fair measure of knowledge in these academic disciplines.

Reading Achievement. It is disheartening to review the literature on reading skills among deaf children. Results of a number of studies are remarkably similar and reveal two major facts. First, reading levels fall far below the norms for normally hearing children regardless of the age of the subjects involved in the studies. Second, although reading skills slowly increase between the ages of 8 and 14 years, there is a leveling off of achievement in the early teens. Minimal growth in reading achievement occurs beyond age 13 or so. The eventual level of reading achievement is probably dictated by the level of language development achieved in early childhood.

Reading is a linguistic skill that is based on an auditory knowledge of language. The normal child approaches the reading task with well-developed language skills based on five or six years of auditory experience with linguistic codes. Reading for this child involves the pairing of visual stimuli with previously acquired auditory information. As Baron (1975) suggested, the child is now learning that language can be represented in more than one form. The learning of the new form is enhanced by thorough knowledge of another form, in this case, speech.

For hearing-impaired children the task of learning to read is a dual one. They are expected to learn *language* and *reading* simultaneously. Reading is the key to further language development and is essential to academic success. The fact that preschool hearing-impaired children are often taught reading readiness skills attests to their importance. Unfortunately, certain aspects of language are poorly taught through reading. Some lexical items, particularly nouns and verbs, may be taught with reasonable success in written form because they can be pictured, acted out, or otherwise represented easily. Other grammatical items are difficult to teach in any but the usual ''auditory-experience'' manner. Included in this category are auxiliaries, modals, and prepositions such as *of* and *for,* both of which have a variety of meanings not easily explained. Idiomatic language involves nonliteral usage of words that are learned best through repeated auditory experiences. Knowledge of the multiple meaning of words is important in learning to read but poorly taught in written form. Prosodic features of language, such as stress and timing patterns, cannot be taught in written form.

The development of good reading skills, therefore, depends on the development of good language skills. The two cannot be separated, and under optimal conditions they are sequentially learned. As a general rule, severely hearing-impaired children do not exhibit sufficient knowledge of language to insure a basis for the normal development of reading skills. They are expected to learn to read without extensive experience with basic psycholinguistic skills and to use reading as a means of increasing linguistic knowledge from the beginning. With these facts in mind, it would be foolish to expect these children to be able to read as well as their peers.

McClure (1966) reported the reading achievement scores of 93 percent of the deaf pupils in the United States who were leaving school after age 16. His data revealed that only 5 percent of these students achieved at the tenth-grade level or above, 60 percent of them achieved at or below the 5.3-grade level, and 30 percent of them were classified as "functionally illiterate."

Hester (1963) reported on 1104 students, aged 16 and older, from 55 residential and 9 day schools for the deaf. Of the 1104 students, 601 did not graduate and 503 did graduate from the school attended. Reading achievement levels were different for the two groups. The graduates had an average achievement level of grade 7.9; their scores ranged from grade levels 3.1 to 12.8. The students who did not graduate had an average reading achievement level of 4.7, with a range from 0.9 to 10.5. Unfortunately, more than half the students leaving school fell within the latter category.

Denton (1966) surveyed 28 large schools for the deaf in an effort to determine the academic skills of the top 10 percent of the students enrolled. His data revealed that the reading achievement level for this elite group of deaf students was at a sixth-grade level. Between the ages of 12 and 18 years, there was an increase of only 2.1 grade levels in reading achievement. Pugh (1946) obtained almost identical results on students from 54 schools for the deaf 20 years earlier. Pugh reported minimal improvement in reading scores from the seventh to the thirteenth year of schooling. Wrightstone, Aranow, and Moskowitz (1963) investigated reading achievement in more than 5000 deaf children in Canada and the United States. Their data revealed an average reading achievement score of fourth-grade level. The average score increased only 0.8 between ages 11 and 16.

More recent estimates of reading achievement are reported by Trybus and Karchmer (1977) for 1543 students from across the nation. They report data from 1971 to 1974 on Stanford Achievement Test scores of hearing-impaired children. The median reading score for students age 20 and above was grade 4.5. Highest reading achievement was obtained by 18-year-olds, but only 10 percent of them scored at or above the eighth-grade level. Data for hearing impaired were compared to those for normally hearing children; a disparity of about one and one-half grades at age 9 to more than five grades by age 14 was found. Improvement in reading achievement levels averaged only 0.3 of a grade per year, for a total of 0.8 grade equivalents over a three-year period. Trybus and Karchmer point out that no other minority groups appear to progress so slowly in reading achievement.

Other investigators (Myklebust, 1964; Goetzinger and Rousey, 1959) have also documented reduced reading achievement in hearing-impaired children and a tendency for their scores to plateau somewhere around ages 12 to 14.

Depressing as these findings are, there is evidence that reading achievement test scores *overestimate* the actual psycholinguistic functioning level of deaf children. Moores (1970) administered the *Metropolitan Reading Achievement Test* to two groups of children, one normally hearing and one deaf. The normally hearing children had an average age of 9 years 10 months and a reading achievement score of 4.84. The deaf group had an average age of 16 years 9 months and a reading score of 4.77. Using a cloze procedure, Moores presented reading materials to both groups in which every fifth word had been deleted. He instructed the subjects to fill in the missing words. Responses were analyzed according to verbatim reproduction (in which the subject filled in the exact word that was missing), form class reproduction (in which the word provided fell into the same grammatical class as the one deleted), and verbatim-given-form class (in which a ratio between the form class and verbatim responses was established). Results of the analyses revealed that deaf children performed significantly poorer than normally hearing children on the task regardless of the scoring procedure used. Deaf children often supplied words of a different grammatical form than the deleted word. When the word class was correct, responses revealed reduced vocabulary skills on the part of the deaf children. Moores concluded that standardized reading achievement test scores produce inflated estimates of the grammatical and semantic functioning of deaf children. He advised caution in the interpretation of achievement test scores.

Other Areas of Academic Achievement. Investigations of achievement in areas such as social studies, science, and mathematics have been relatively rare. The best source of this type of information are the reports of the Office of Demographic Studies, a federally funded project in which hearing-impaired children from preschool through college age are surveyed. The Office of Demographic Studies is located at Gallaudet College, and has collected achievement data on thousands of hearing-impaired students since 1968. In 1972 data on 16,908 students were reported for primary through advanced batteries of the Standford Achievement Test (Gentile, 1972). Although 14,000 of the children were ages 10 or older, almost 12,000 of them took the primary test batteries designed for children aged 9 or younger, indicating that hearing-impaired children are most frequently administered test batteries designed for younger children. Patterns of scores within test batteries revealed spelling and arithmetic computation scores to be the highest, paragraph and word meaning scores to be among the lowest, along with word study skills, science, and social studies. Arithmetic concepts and applications scores were considerably lower than computation scores. These data suggest that dependence on language as a basis for educational achievement is not limited to reading.

The data reported indicate the same general trends in achievement by deaf children as the studies reported eariler on reading. Seventeen-year-old deaf students showed an average achievement level of sixth grade in arithmetic computation, their highest area of achievement, and fourth grade in paragraph meaning. The rate of growth in achievement for arithmetic computation was approximately 0.5 grade levels per year. For paragraph meaning, the growth rate is only half as fast; scores improved only 2.12 grades over nine years of school, a growth of only 0.25 grades per year (Gentile, 1972).

Persons not associated with education of the deaf are startled, to say the least, by these facts. The data reported are based on children from a variety of programs that employ a variety of teaching strategies. It would be comforting to believe that recent advances in hearing aid technology and changes in teaching strategies could be expected to lead to higher academic achievement levels in the future. Indeed, Balow and Brill (1975) have reported data that suggest a slight trend toward improved academic achievement from 1956 to 1971 in graduates of one school for the deaf. Their data show an increase in paragraph meaning scores of almost a full grade over 16 years' time. Balow and Brill attempted to identify those factors associated with higher achievement and reported the following facts:

1. Students entering the school for the deaf during the primary years scored higher academically than those who entered during their high school years.
2. Deaf children who have at least one deaf parent scored significantly higher on academic achievement tests than children whose parents were both normally hearing.
3. Children who attended the John Tracy Clinic nursery school scored higher academically than those who did not, with the exception of children having at least one deaf parent.

Balow and Brill suggest that the superior achievement by the children of deaf parents and those who attended the John Tracy nursery school was the result of early development of communication skills. They reasoned that the John Tracy children were systematically exposed to language at school and from their parents who were trained in language stimulation activities. Children of deaf parents were exposed to manual communication in the home from infancy. The early development of communication skills resulted in higher academic achievement levels.

The superior achievement of children who entered the residential school during the primary years was interpreted as evidence of the positive influence of special educational procedures when they are instituted early in a child's educational experience.

Achievement by Moderately Hearing-Impaired Children

Although there are probably 20 times as many children with mild to moderate hearing impairments as there are those with severe hearing losses, a search of the literature reveals little precise information regarding their academic status. Unless otherwise noted, the investigators whose studies are reviewed as follows did not define the type or duration of hearing loss exhibited by the children studied. Therefore, the data probably reflect achievement by children having both sensorineural and conductive hearing losses of indeterminate duration. Sprunt and Finger (1949) attempted to determine the incidence of hearing loss among school children and its effect on their academic achievement. They tested school children in rural Virginia and identified 6.6 percent of them as hearing impaired. Hearing losses ranged from 11 dB (the reference level is not given) to "more than 45 dB." Only four of the children included in the study had hearing losses greater than 45 dB; the majority had hearing losses of less than 30 dB. The average grade placement for a control group of hearing children was retarded by 0.77 grades; the hearing-impaired group was retarded in placement by 0.95 grades. Fifty-nine percent of the hearing impaired group had repeated one or more grades. Using matched pairs, it was determined that only eight of the hearing-impaired children scored higher than their controls in academic achievement approximately 0.5 years below their grade placement. Because more than half of these children had failed one or more grades, the academic achievement levels are probably overestimates of performance relative to norms for the children's ages.

In 1955 Reynolds reported the results of a study primarily designed to investigate "school adjustment" of hearing-impaired students. His data included estimates of spelling, arithmetic, and overall academic achievement by 36 mildly hearing-impaired children and their normally hearing controls. The mean hearing loss was 21 dB. The students were enrolled in junior high school; the average duration of their hearing losses was 4.29 years. None of the children wore hearing aids, but all had been enrolled in lipreading therapy since the hearing loss was identified. Comparison of academic scores of the two groups revealed no significant differences between them, but control group scores were higher on all measures except spelling. The hearing losses of the experimental group either were not congenital or were not identified as being present in very early childhood.

Kodman (1963) investigated the academic achievement of 100 hearing-impaired children ranging in age from 7 to 17 years. His subjects exhibited a mean hearing loss of 40 dB (no reference provided), with a range of 20 to 65 dB. Using a 30 dB criterion, Kodman estimated that 65 percent of the children were candidates for hearing aids, but only 35 percent of them wore them. Only 24 percent of the 100 students were receiving support services of any kind in the schools they attended. The mean academic achievement of the group was 3.84; mean grade placement was 4.84. By considering age 6 as the school entrance age, Kodman determined that the predicted grade placement of the group should have been grade 6.08. A total of 57 grades had been repeated by the hearing-impaired pupils, and 10 of them had repeated two grades. Seventy percent of the children who repeated grades had done so in either the first or third grades. Kodman concluded that his subjects were retarded in academic achievement from 1.0 to 2.24 grades.

Quigley and Thomure (1968) reported the differences between expected grade level performance and actual grade level performance of 116 hearing-impaired children in Illinois public schools. Hearing losses of the subjects ranged from less than 15 dB (59 children) to 56-70 dB (ASA, 1951). *Stanford Achievement Test* subtests of word meaning, paragraph meaning, and language were administered. The total group showed a delay of 1.12 in grade placement, 1.66 on word meaning, 0.90 in paragraph meaning, and 1.30 in language subtest scores. The difference between expected and actual achievement on the three subtests ranged from 1.73 grades for children whose losses were less than 15 dB to 2.87 grades for children whose losses fell between 56 and 70 dB. These data suggest that mildly hearing-impaired children may experience serious retardation of academic achievement in language related areas. Children whose hearing levels are often considered to be within normal limits experienced some delay in educational achievement.

Peterson (1972) investigated the level and rate of academic achievement of 60 children whose hearing losses ranged from mild to severe (16 dB to 66+ dB, ANSI, 1969). Forty of them had hearing losses between 16 and 55 dB. Peterson obtained scores on the *Iowa Test of Basic Skills (ITBS)* from the children's records at both the fourth- and sixth-grade levels and compared them to national and local school norms. As a group, the hearing-impaired children exhibited significantly delayed academic achievement at both grade levels; they functioned at the third-grade level when enrolled in the fourth grade and at the fourth-grade level when in the sixth grade. On the average, their rate of achievement was two-thirds that of their normally hearing classmates. The greatest deficits occurred in verbal skills.

In an effort to determine factors contributing to achievement, Peterson administered additional tests and conducted personal interviews with 15 of the poorer and 15 of the better achievers. She found no significant differences between speech discrimination or lipreading scores for the two groups, nor in age, grade placement (eighth grade at the time of the study), average hearing loss, use of hearing aids or support services received. On the *Wide Range Achievement Test (WRAT)* the better achievers were performing 1.5 grades below the national average in reading and 3 years below the national average in arithmetic, while the poorer achievers were performing 3½ years and 4½ years below the national averages in reading and arithmetic, respectively. Although these data seem to indicate greater deficiencies in arithmetic than in reading, the *WRAT* reading score is based on word recognition rather than reading comprehension and reading scores tend to be inflated as a result.

The sparse data on educational achievement by moderately hearing-imparied children can be supplemented by a few studies that bear indirectly on the topic. Young and McConnell (1957) investigated vocabulary development in 20 hearing-impaired children and their matched controls as an indicator of educational achievement. Hearing losses of the experimental group ranged from 32 to 75 dB (no reference given), with a mean hearing loss of 51 dB for the group. The *Ammons Full Range Picture Vocabulary Test* was administered; stimulus words were presented in spoken and written form to both groups. The mean raw score for the hearing-impaired group was 31.45 compared to a mean of 49.20 for the normally hearing children, a difference that was significant beyond the .01 level. Not only was the mean for the normally hearing group higher, but every hearing child scored higher on the test than the hearing-impaired match. Comparison of IQ scores to performance on the vocabulary test revealed that every hearing-impaired child scored lower than would have been predicted by IQ. Young and McConnell concluded that hearing-impaired children will experience problems with school achievement because of their low verbal abilities.

Davis (1974) administered the *Boehm Test of Basic Concepts (BTBC)* to 24 hearing-impaired children in public schools and compared their performance to 24 normally hearing children from the same classrooms. The children in the study were 6 to 8 years old, enrolled in regular classrooms from kindergarten to second grade. The purpose of the study was to compare the status of hearing-impaired children's knowledge of the *BTBC* concepts to that of their normally hearing classmates. The hearing-impaired children scored significantly poorer on the task than the normally hearing children. Children whose hearing losses ranged from 51 to 70 dB (ANSI, 1969) showed significantly poorer knowledge of the concepts than children whose hearing losses ranged from 35 to 50 dB. Although the number of concepts identified correctly increased slightly with age (about three concepts per year), the gap between the hearing-impaired children's performance and that of their classmates widened over the age range studied. Half of the hearing-impaired children scored below the 1st percentile on the task. Davis stated that hearing-impaired children with hearing losses greater than 50 dB, "appear to lack enough knowledge of specific basic concepts to compete satisfactorily with their hearing peers." Her concerns are further justified by the fact that all the children included in the study wore hearing aids and received support services from speech-language pathologists, audiologists, and special teachers.

Effects of Fluctuating Hearing Loss. The adverse effects of fluctuating hearing levels during the early years of life have been stressed by Downs (1977), Ling (1969), and others but few data exist to support their logical contentions. This type of hearing impairment is usually associated with chronic or recurrent otitis media. Attempts to study the effects of this disease on development have been complicated by several factors. Most studies have been retrospective, with no measure of hearing loss during earlier stages of the disease. Otitis media is more prevalent among disadvantaged children and the effects of middle ear disease cannot be separated easily from those of other factors affecting families whose economic status is low, such as diet, breadth of educational experiences, availability of stimulating materials in the home, parental support, motivation to achieve, and others. The methodological problems involved in the study of the effects of otitis media on language and academic achievement are discussed extensively by Ventry (1980).

Holm and Kunze (1969) studied articulation, vocabulary, and visual, auditory, and motor skills represented on the *Illinois Test of Psycholinguistic Abilities* in two groups of children: children with mild hearing losses secondary to otitis media and a control group of children with no history of otitis media. The children in both groups were between 5½ and 9 years of age. The experimental group exhibited significantly poorer language and auditory processing skills than the control group. Visual processing was unimpaired in the children with a history of recurrent otitis media.

Ling (1969) studied academic achievement of hearing-impaired and normally hearing children in England by comparing achievement test scores of two matched groups. Hearing losses of the experimental group ranged from 15 to 45 dB; children included in this group had histories of otitis media. Comparison of test scores for the two groups revealed a delay for the group with otitis media of 15 months in word recognition reading skills, 16 months in arithmetic computation, and 19 months in arithmetic problem solving. The degree of academic retardation was related to degree of hearing loss. Ling's most disturbing finding was that delays that occurred in early childhood were "not generally overcome without special teaching" (p. 250).

Kaplan, Fleshman, Bender, Baum, and Clark (1973) reported an extensive survey of Eskimo children. In a blind experiment they correlated audiological, psychological, and achievement test results with presence or history of otitis media in more than 300 children. Their findings indicated that 80 percent of the children determined to be retarded academically had histories of otitis media. Sixty-three percent had their first episode before age 2, and 17 percent had an onset of otitis media after age 2. Fifty-six percent of children with hearing losses greater than 26 dB ISO were behind their expected grade placement; 29 percent of the children with otitis media but no hearing loss were retarded in grade placement. Children with no history of otitis media or hearing loss were also delayed in academic achievement according to U.S. norms. Those with hearing losses, however, exhibited a greater delay in achievement than their classmates by two to five months. The delay for the otitis media group increased with age and grade. Kaplan et al. concluded that chronic otitis media can have a serious effect on language development and academic achievement.

Needleman (1977) investigated phonological skills in children aged 3 to 8 who had histories of severe otitis media with onset before 18 months. She found that children with recurrent otitis media exhibited problems with articulation, sound-blending, auditory discrimination, auditory closure, and use of word endings. Although linguistic and academic measures were not included in the study, Needleman hypothesized that children with otitis media would exhibit problems in these areas as well as those studied directly.

Downs (1977) interpreted the Kaplan et al., Holm and Kunze, and Ling studies as evidence that children with recurrent otitis media represent a syndrome referred to as Irreversible Auditory Learning Disaster (IALD). IALD is not further defined by Downs, but she intimates that learning skills, especially those based on audition, are irreversibly damaged by early otitis media and its accompanying mild hearing loss. Included in the syndrome is reduced intelligence. She bases this assumption on data (Paradise, 1976) indicating lower Stanford-Binet scores for children with chronic otitis media. Because the Stanford-Binet involves verbal measures of IQ, it is likely that the lower scores of children with otitis media reflect reduced language development rather than intellectual capacity per se.

Kessler (1978) investigated the auditory skills, educational achievement, and need for special support services of children with histories of early middle ear disease. Her subjects were third-grade students in a public school, 19 of whom had no history of middle ear disease (CONTROL) and 29 of whom had a history of middle ear disease before age 3, but whose hearing levels were normal at the time of the investigation. The children who experienced early middle ear disease (EMED) exhibited significantly poorer performance on four of nine measures of auditory skills than the control group. These skills included auditory memory, listening in noise, auditory closure, and sentence repetition tasks. In addition, the EMED children were delayed in word comprehension and word study skills. A significantly higher percentage of the EMED group were receiving special services, including reading, learning disability, and speech/language remediation. Even when significant differences between groups were not obtained, EMED children exhibited behavioral differences during auditory tasks. They responded more slowly, appeared anxious, sought visual cues, and expressed a lack of confidence in their judgments. Variability in performance was high among EMED children, low among CONTROL students. Kessler concluded that early, mild sensory deprivation may significantly affect auditory processing. If children are not successful in compensating for reduced auditory efficiency, they may have problems acquiring language and academic skills.

The preceding studies indicate that mild hearing losses of any origin interfere with the development of language skills, which, in turn, affect academic achievement. Additional data are needed before a clear picture of the extent of the deficits experienced by children having mild hearing losses of various origins will be available. It seems obvious, however, that mild hearing loss often results in delays in the development of language and academic skills to a measurable extent. If, as Ling suggests, these deficits are not overcome without special help, the implications are clear. Identification of children with mild hearing losses is important, and follow-up, including provision of remedial services, is essential if thousands of children are to reach their potential in educational achievement. The term *underachievers* seems appropriate as a description of mild to moderately hearing-impaired school children.

Ross (1977) has estimated that at least one hearing-impaired child can be found in every school building in the country. If this is the case, how can we explain the fact that these children are ignored and undereducated by educational systems?

There are several reasons for this state of affairs.

1. Hearing loss, especially mild hearing loss, is an invisible impairment. Children having moderately impaired hearing appear no different from their peers. They have enough residual hearing to respond to many auditory events, a fact that convinces educators that hearing loss is not the basis of any suspected problems. Often the children themselves do not realize they are hearing impaired, and they do not complain of difficulty hearing.
2. Hearing screening programs do not exist in many school systems. Testing may be done on referral only. If no one suspects hearing loss, hearing testing is not accomplished. Experience suggests that teachers and other observers are poor judges of mild impairments. When hearing screening is provided, test conditions are often so noisy that screening is done at high intensity levels under the mistaken assumption that presenting test tones at higher levels will overcome the effects of room noise without decreasing the accuracy of the screening results. In actuality, such a procedure is more likely to overlook children with mild hearing losses than to detect them.
3. No professional group has taken responsibility for children whose hearing losses are not severe. Other handicapped children (blind, cleft palate, cerebral palsied, deaf, mentally retarded, learning disabled) are represented by national organizations, parents' groups, and professional educators who engage in fundraising events and other activities designed to call attention to their needs. Moderately hearing-impaired children are represented by none of these organizations. Educators of the deaf are trained to serve children whose primary mode of language reception is visual. They receive little or no education in the differences between the learning patterns of children with severe to profound hearing losses and those with moderate impairments. Speech-language pathologists, although trained in language disorders, have not been encouraged to apply the principles of language remediation to hearing-impaired children. They have caseloads and waiting lists of children with a variety of speech disorders, for which they are specifically trained to provide treatment. Audiologists have been overly concerned with the identification and evaluation of hearing losses; as a result they have often ignored the larger problems of hearing-impaired children. Furthermore, few audiologists are employed in educational settings. Special education personnel have minimal, if any, training in the language and educational deficits associated with hearing loss.

These are the forgotten children of public school systems. They have traditionally been placed in regular classrooms or schools for the deaf, neither setting being conducive to their optimum achievement. Placement is seldom based on adequate assessment of their skills and deficiences, but is determined most often by factors such as age, degree of physical maturity, and the willingness of teachers or schools to accept them. Is there any wonder that our knowledge of their educational and linguistic status is incomplete and inadequate for the task of serving them appropriately?

ASSESSMENT

Many school systems require annual standardized academic testing of the children enrolled, especially after grade 3. This type of testing is done in groups using a paper-and-pencil task. Tests are usually timed, and instructions are either written or given orally by the teacher at the beginning of the testing period. Scoring is usually accomplished by the test publisher. Scores are obtained for several subtests such as paragraph meaning, use of dictionary and vocabulary. They are returned to the school in the form of standard scores and percentiles, based on local and/or national norms. Although the scores obtained by this type of testing are useful in estimating a given child's standing within the class or school, they do not furnish information that is helpful in planning remediation, and results of testing are seldom available immediately. Group tests may penalize hearing-impaired children because they are timed and because of the complexity of the instructions provided (Vernon and Brown, 1964) or they may result in inflated scores (Moores, 1970). Therefore, performance on group tests of academic achievement may not be representative of hearing-impaired children's capabilities. Individual testing is necessary for a complete description of their academic status.

Personnel Involved in Assessment

Theoretically, assessing academic achievement in hearing-impaired school children is within the professional responsibility of educational personnel such as school psychologists, resource teachers, and learning strategists, rather than speech, language, and hearing personnel. In actuality, however, much of the individual assessment of academic skills of hearing-impaired children is accomplished by audiologists and speech-language pathologists, if it is accomplished at all. There are several reasons for this.

1. Many school systems do not employ psychologists or educational strategists. Special support personnel may be limited to special education classroom teachers and/or speech-language pathologists.
2. Educational personnel within school systems may not be effective communicators with hearing-impaired children unless they can have frequenct contact with them. It is difficult for hearing-impaired children to lipread

and understand strangers, a fact that often affects their performance on tests. To avoid penalizing children, their assessment should be delegated to personnel with whom they are more familiar. In many cases, the professional who comes in most frequent contact with the hearing-impaired child is the speech-language pathologist or audiologist.

3. Time contraints on teachers and special personnel may dictate that assessment be accomplished early in the school year by someone whose schedule allows individual contact with children.

Coordination of speech-language management with classroom activities necessitates that clinicians have accurate knowledge of a child's classroom status. The academic difficulties of hearing-impaired children are based on their linguistic deficits, including reduced vocabulary, poor use of syntax, and limited knowledge of idomatic English. The clinician's task is to teach the language that is related to the child's other needs, as a relevant contribution to overall educational goals. The planning of this type of coordinated therapy is enhanced by precise knowledge of how the language deficit is affecting the child's performance in the classroom. Therefore, educational assessment data contribute to effective planning of language remediation. If they are not readily available, such data should be collected by the clinicians charged with the responsibility of planning and executing language therapy.

Guidelines for Assessment

The following guidelines are suggested for speech-language pathologists and audiologists involved in assessment of academic skills:

1. Tests should be individually administered, preferably be someone with whom the child is reasonably familiar.
2. Tests should provide specific information about academic skill areas that can be obtained within a reasonably short period of time. Inexperienced clinicians sometimes find themselves bogged down in assessment of problems to such an extent that they have little time remaining for remediation.
3. Tests should not be timed; the necessary time should be allowed for completion of tests and subtests. Testing may need to be done in more than one session, but the rules given for test administration should not be violated any more than necessary. Norms for some tests may be invalid when they are not timed. Instruction manuals should be reviewed for information about this aspect of test administration.
4. Instructions should be given by the tester in the child's customary communicative mode. If they must be reworded, the new form must be a complete and accurate representation of the original. Therefore, instructions must be straightforward and without unnecessary complicated detail.

Instructions for group testing, such as, "Turn to page 2 of the booklet; put your finger on the gray box with the telephone in it. When I give the signal, put an X on the picture of the words that begin with the same letter that is next to the gray box," can be abbreviated when the test is being given individually. The page is turned by the examiner, and the stimuli to be used in the test item indicated clearly by pointing. The instructions may then be limited to a description of the child's task: "Mark the picture of the words that begin with this letter."

5. In the case of diagnostic tests, the instrument should include measures that yield specific information about the strengths and weaknesses exhibited by the child. Each academic skill being tested should be broken down into the subskills necessary for its mastery. A single numerical reading or math score is useless, since it is impossible to ascertain the behavior that contributed to the score. Did the child get all the addition problems correct, but none of the division, or was performance equally good or poor across computation skills? Was computation accurate, but comprehension of arithmetic reading problems poor, or was computation inaccurate under any circumstances? Does the reading score represent word recognition or comprehension of paragraphs? Unless questions like these can be answered by analysis of test performance, the assessment tool is inadequate for purposes of planning language remediation.

Assessment Tools

Two types of education achievement tests are used widely in public school systems. They are *screening* tests, designed to sample a wide range of academic achievement across grade levels, and *diagnostic* tests, whose purpose is to delineate performance on specific academic skills according to some model of skill development. Results of the latter are used primarily by teachers in planning activities to achieve the objectives of a given curriculum. A wealth of information regarding the use of language in written form may be obtained from diagnostic tests. For older children, these tests are more accurate indicators of linguistic functioning than many of the language tests discussed in Chapter 7. For example, intermediate level reading tests involve more advanced vocabulary and language structure than that included in the usual tests of language comprehension, such as the *Test of Auditory Comprehension of Language* (Carrow, 1973) or the *Basic Concept Inventory* (Engelman, 1967).

Screening Tests of Academic Achievement. Although there are several screening tests available, only two will be reviewed here. The purpose of this discussion is to acquaint the reader with the nature of screening tools and their strengths and their limitations. Public school clinicians will probably have access to one or more screening tests used in the school district. Clinicians in other settings have to choose screening or diagnostic tests for their own use. The tests discussed in the next two sections are not presented as the "best" tests available, but simply as examples of those currently in use. The screening tests described below are used widely by psychologists, teachers, reading specialists, and other professionals. Results of these tests are likely to be included in the cumulative folders of children referred for speech and language remediation.

Wide Range Achievement Test (WRAT) (Jastak, Bijou and Jastak, 1965). The *WRAT* consists of three subtests (reading, spelling and arithmetic) at two levels (I for children from 5 years, 0 month to 11 years, 11 months and II for persons from 12 years, 0 months to adulthood). The *WRAT* is described by its authors as a diagnostic test of reading, spelling, and arithmetic for persons of all ages, but it does not provide sufficient assessment of these academic areas to serve as a basis for remediation. Therefore, it is included here as a screening test.

The reading test consists of naming and identifying letters and pronouncing 75 words from their written form. In essence, this is a word recognition reading task, and it does not test reading comprehension. It is important to remember this fact when interpreting *WRAT* scores, whether they are provided by others or obtained personally. Recognizing and sounding out words is only one aspect of reading and requires very different skills from those involved in comprehension of sentences or paragraphs. Most hearing-impaired children learn to recognize and sound out words with relative ease; thus the *WRAT* overestimates their reading ability if it is interpreted as a general measure of reading. Hearing-impaired children often score two or three grade levels higher on the *WRAT* reading subtests than on a test of reading comprehension.

The spelling subtest consists of copying symbols, printing the subject's name, and writing words to dictation. The spelling test is given orally with the instructor pronouncing the words and using them in sentences.

The arithmetic subtest consists of an oral and a written part. The oral test involves counting, reading digits, following instructions involving numbers, and solving a few addition and subtraction problems. The written part consists of computation of a variety of arithmetic problems, ranging from addition to the computation of square roots.

Scoring is achieved by converting raw scores into grade equivalents, percentiles, and standard scores. Norms for each are provided in the manual.

The *WRAT* was designed as a group test, with the oral subtests to be given individually, but the entire test can be given individually without biasing the results. The test is timed, although extra time is suggested for persons whose motor skills do not allow them to write answers within the time limit. No modifications are suggested for hearing-impaired children. The major modification suggested for handicapped children is to allow oral responses for blind, cerebral palsied and other children for whom rapid writing is difficult.

Peabody Individual Achievement Test (PIAT) (Dunn and Markwardt, 1970). The *PIAT* is a screening tool of achievement in the areas of mathematics, reading, spelling, and general information. A child's scores can be used to determine the general level of scholastic achievement and whether or not further diagnostic evaluation is indicated in any area. The PIAT consists of five subtests:

1. Mathematics (including tasks ranging from recognizing numerals to understanding concepts of geometry and trigonometry).
2. Reading recognition (letters and words).
3. Reading comprehension (multiple-choice task involving four illustrations of test sentences).
4. Spelling (recognizing alphabet letters, identifying spoken phonemes, and spelling words from dictation).
5. General information (involving oral responses to questions about science, social studies, fine arts and sports).

The test is designed for use with children from kindergarten through twelfth grade. Four scores can be derived from the results: grade equivalent, age equivalent, percentile rank, and standard score. Results can be compared to the child's IQ in order to estimate whether functioning is at, above, or below native capacity. Norms for each measure are provided in the test manual.

The *PIAT* is especially useful with hearing-impaired children because its materials are clear, attractive, and uncluttered and it is designed to be administered individually. Test items representing a wide range of academic skills are arranged in order of difficulty. Rules are provided for determining starting points and ceiling items for a given child, who completes only those items within a critical range determined individually. For this reason, the test can usually be administered within 30 to 40 minutes. The *PIAT* is not timed, an advantage for hearing-impaired children. The format of the test allows for a pointing response to be used throughout, even for spelling words, so that intelligibility of speech is not a factor in judging responses. The *PIAT* was standardized nationally and is designed to be administered by a variety of different professionals. Formal training in its use is not necessary.

Diagnostic Tests of Academic Achievement. The two areas of academic achievement of major concern to clinicians for coordination of language remediation and classroom activity are reading and math. Two diagnostic reading tests and one math test will be discussed as examples of those currently available.

Reading Achievement. There are numerous reading assessment tools available at present, a fact that reflects the importance of this academic skill to children's overall achievement. Most reading curricula include their own assessment measures, which are based on the skills and objectives to be accomplished by the curriculum materials, rather than on the content of the reading program. The tests reviewed here are taken from reading curricula. They have been chosen because they illustrate clearly the characteristics of good diagnostic tests and how they may be used in planning for children who need assistance in developing good reading comprehension skills.

McGuire-Bumpus Diagnostic Comprehension Test (1971). This test accompanies the Croft reading series, a systems approach to the assessment and remediation of reading skills. The strengths of this approach to reading assessment are related to the manner in which reading comprehension is subdivided into specific skills. The Croft program specifies five levels of reading: literal, interpretative, analytic, critical, and creative. Each level involves specific objectives to be accomplished by children as they move through the five levels, each of which demands more sophisticated comprehension of material than the preceding one. Objectives associated with the first four levels of reading are shown in Table 9.1.

Tests of each level of reading comprehension are provided for primary (approximately grades 2.2 to 3.2) and intermediate (approximately grades 4.0 to 6.0) levels. Table 9.2 shows test items for the first four levels of comprehension at the primary grade level.

Wisconsin Design for Reading Skill Development (1975). This curriculum represents a management approach to the assessment and development of reading skills. It includes four major components: a description of the skills considered to be

Table 9.1 Objectives of Four Levels of Reading According to the Croft Reading Comprehension Curriculum

Literal Reading

1. Recognition of detail.
2. Translation of detail.
3. Recognition of pattern signal words.[a]
4. Recognition of the main idea.

Interpretative Reading

1. Understanding an implied detail.
2. Seeing the pattern of ideas.
3. Inferring the main idea.

Analytic Reading

1. Selecting the main question to be answered.
2. Selecting a suitable hypothesis.
3. Distinguishing between relevant and irrevelant details.

Critical Reading

1. Selecting a criterion as a basis for evaluation.
2. Selecting a judgment based on the chosen criterion.

[a] Pattern signal words refer to words whose functions designate patterns of classification (many, another, group), sequences (first, next, later, tomorrow), causation (why, because, as a result of), and comparison (different, compare, but, both).

Table 9.2 Examples of Test Items from the Primary Battery of the *McGuire-Bumpus Diagnostic Comprehension Test* (1971) for Four Levels of Reading

***Literal** Level*

Barry and Billy are brothers, but they look very different. Barry is tall and has straight black hair. His eyes are brown. Billy is short and has curly blond hair. His eyes are blue.

1. In this story, Billy
   (a) is tall
   (b) has blue eyes
   (c) has curly brown hair
   (d) has straight blond hair
2. Barry has
   (a) short legs
   (b) blue eyes
   (c) curly hair
   (d) dark hair
3. Some words that show this story compares things are
   (a) very different
   (b) black hair
   (c) blond hair
   (d) they look
4. This story is mostly about
   (a) how Billy and Barry look alike
   (b) why Barry has straight hair
   (c) what Billy looks like
   (d) how Barry and Billy look different

***Interpretative** Level*

First, heat some cooking oil in a big pan until it starts to smoke. Next, put in a half cup of popcorn and cover the pan. Keep shaking it until the popping stops. Then take it off the stove.

1. When the popping stops, the popcorn is
   (a) ready to shake
   (b) in a bag
   (c) burned
   (d) done
2. In this story, the ideas
   (a) show the reason for something
   (b) tell how things are different
   (c) are in a special order
   (d) tell the result of something
3. This story is mostly about
   (a) how to make popcorn
   (b) why the pan needs a cover
   (c) how much popcorn to use
   (d) when to stop shaking

(*continued*)

Table 9.2—*continued*

***Analytic** Level*

Jim went to Mr. Bart's store to buy some candy for his friend Russ. Russ liked every kind unless it was yellow. Mr. Bart had three big jars full of candy. One had lemon drops. Another was filled with chocolate squares. The third had jellybeans of all colors in it.

1. The main problem in this story is
   (a) How many jars of candy did Mr. Bart have?
   (b) Why didn't Russ buy his own candy?
   (c) Where did Mr. Bart keep the jellybeans?
   (d) What kind of candy should Jim buy?
2. Probably Jim should buy
   (a) some lemon drops
   (b) some jellybeans
   (c) some chocolate squares
   (d) some chewing gum
3. One thing that is not important to know in solving this problem is
   (a) lemon drops are usually yellow
   (b) the candy jars were big
   (c) chocolate is not yellow
   (d) some jellybeans are yellow

***Critical** Level*

The third-grade boys needed a baseball coach. "Let's ask Mr. Smith," said Pete. He'd be a good coach because he has a brand new motorcycle and he smiles a lot."

1. Before the boys choose a coach, one thing they should think about is
   (a) men with motorcycles are always good coaches
   (b) baseball coaches need to know something about baseball
   (c) Mr. Smith is Pete's uncle
   (d) third-grade boys don't need coaches
2. Therefore, the boys need to find out
   (a) where Mr. Smith bought his motorcycle
   (b) if Mr. Smith lets boys ride with him
   (c) if Mr. Smith knows anything about baseball
   (d) if Mr. Smith would play favorites

essential to success in reading, statements of behavioral objectives for developing the skills, tests of reading skills development, and resource files of teaching materials and procedures. Six reading skills are identified as follows:

1. Word attack.
2. Comprehension.
3. Study skills.
4. Self-directed reading.

5. Interpretative reading.
6. Creative reading.

The *Wisconsin Tests of Reading Skill Development (WTRSD)* (1975) are available in two forms, as a booklet for each developmental level or as single-skill tests that can be administered as needed. Separate tests of word attack, comprehension, and study skills are available for levels A through G (corresponding roughly to grades kindergarten through 6). Examples of level E (grade 4) test items representing some of these skills are shown in Table 9.3. The specific level of tests to be administered to a given child should be chosen on the basis of the child's approximate reading level and grade placement. Various question-and-response-type items are used in the tests, including true-false, multiple choice, fill-in-the-blank, and short definition.

The *WTRSD* may be administered individually or to groups. There are no time limits imposed and examiners may answer any questions children pose regarding directions or unfamiliar words or tasks. The purpose of the tests is to assess individual performance on specific behaviors related to reading skills; results are not compared to group norms, so reading "scores" are not obtained. Because the tests can be scored by hand, results are immediately available for use in planning activities to enhance further skills development. When a child has progressed through all levels of the Wisconsin curriculum, the following important objectives should have been accomplished:

1. The student will be able to analyze words phonically and structurally.
2. The student will be able to use maps, graphs, tables, figures, dictionaries, encyclopedias, and other reference sources to locate and obtain information.
3. The student will comprehend words, sentences, and passages through use of inference, context, and analysis of relationships.
4. Skills leading to self-directed, interpretative, and creative reading will be developed.

The degree to which a child meets the first three of these objectives can be measured precisely by the *WTRSD* and the results of the assessment used to plan for further skill development.

Math Achievement. At one time, hearing-impaired children excelled at mathematics in the early school years. Rote learning of the basic addition, subtraction, multiplication, and division facts was no more difficult for the hearing-impaired than for normally hearing children. Flashcards provided welcome visual clues, and math computation was the least of the hearing-impaired child's school problems. The advent of "new math" brought changes. Math computation was no longer based on the memorization of facts but on an understanding of certain

Table 9.3 Examples of Test Items for Each of the Seven Skills Evaluated by the *Wisconsin Tests of Reading Skill Development* (1977), Level E, Form P[a]

1. Word Parts—Prefixes

Select the prefix that will make the base word fit the definition given.

1. ______ + human = greater than the ability of a normal human being.
2. ______ + count = something must be counted again.
3. The whole family went to a *postgame* party. What does *postgame* mean in this sentence?

2. Context—Direct Clues: Application

Jerry is thinking about being a reporter someday. He is very good at writing *webly*, that is, clearly and understandably.

Because Mrs. Jones gave directions *webly*, they were

A. too long
B. hard to hear
C. very mixed up
D. easy to follow

3. Detail: Clauses

While Mrs. Stone went to buy groceries, Joan cared for Mrs. Stone's children. She had a terrible time. Little Bobby threw cookies on the carpet, and then his sister, Susie, stepped on them. Later the cat climbed over the fence, and Joan had to spend an hour looking for it. Ricky used lipstick to mark around the door frame. Then the new puppy dug a hole in the middle of the roses that Mrs. Stone had just planted. Joan knew that Mrs. Stone would be home by three o'clock. Joan couldn't wait.

1. Who had a terrible time?
   A. Joan
   B. Susie
   C. Bobby
2. What did Susie step on?
   A. flowers
   B. cookies
   C. lipstick
3. Ricky used lipstick to work around the
   A. door frame
   B. fence
   C. wall

4. Paraphrase: Complex Sentences

1. Since the afternoon had been very hot, Billy headed quickly for the lemonade pitcher when he got home.
2. Billy, who had been playing hard all day, stopped for a cool drink on his way home.
1. The heavy snowstorm wasn't anticipated by the weather service so the street crew was unprepared when the bad weather hit.
2. Because the blizzard hadn't been forecast, the plows and salt trucks were not ready when the snow started.

(*continued*)

Table 9.3—*continued*

---

5. *Central Thought: With Organizer*
   1. Do you think that bicycle riding is a form of transportation? What about walking? Can you name the many kinds of transportation? Many people own and operate cars. Some families have two or more cars. Others ride buses, trucks, or trains. Some people ride horses. Horses can also be hitched to carts and wagons. Boats transport people across bodies of water. Planes transport people very quickly. Pan Am Airlines flies many passengers to England.
      (a) Horses can be attached to wagons and carts.
      (b) There are many forms of transportation.
      (c) Walking is a form of transportation.
      (d) Many people own and operate cars.
6. *Conclusions: Direct Relationships*

   Eddie lives on a ranch. His father owns many horses and cattle. Eddie and his father use different saddles for different kinds of work. Eddie and his father are riding in a roundup tomorrow. When they ride in a roundup, they have to ride for a long time. When Eddie has to ride for a long time, he uses a large Western saddle. Eddie uses a light English saddle when he is racing. If he is just riding around the ranch for fun, Eddie rides without a saddle.
   1. Eddie will use a large Western saddle tomorrow.
   2. Eddie will use an English saddle tomorrow.
   3. Eddie will have to ride for a long time tomorrow.
   4. Eddie will ride without a saddle tomorrow.
7. *Sequence: Explicit Cues*

   When they finished putting everything on board, Carol and her father left the harbor. Carol headed the boat north toward Goat Island during the time that father checked the boat's equipment. Next he put up another sail so they would get to the island before dark. The boat began to go faster. Later Carol checked the compass because she couldn't see land. Then father repaired a worn rope while Carol looked for changes in the wind direction. Finally they both saw the island. It was about eight kilometers away. Soon father got out the rubber raft. They would use the raft to go ashore for the night.
   1. What happened just after father put up another sail?
      A. The boat began to go faster.
      B. Father repaired a worn rope.
      C. Father checked the boat's equipment.
      D. Both saw the island about eight kilometers away.
   2. What did Carol do at the *same time* father checked the boat's equipment?
      A. saw the island
      B. checked the compass
      C. looked for changes in wind direction
      D. headed the boat toward Goat Island

---

[a] The *Wisconsin Tests of Reading Skill Development*. Copyright 1977 by the Board of Regents of the University of Wisconsin System. Reproduced by permission of National Computer Systems, Inc.

concepts underlying them. "Number lines," "missing elements," and "sets" became the building blocks for mathematical skills, and their teaching was more verbally based than before. The consequence has been a reduction in the early advantage enjoyed by hearing-impaired children, along with poorer performance in math than previously noted.

Certain arithmetic concepts are verbally based. This is especially true for those math operations associated with upper elementary grades and beyond. Algebra, geometry, and other subsets of mathematics require a high level of thinking, based on verbal reasoning. Tests of mathematical skill consisting of computation problems only reveal operations that cannot be performed by the person being tested, but they provide no information concerning the reasons underlying the child's failure.

Several diagnostic tests of math skills are available on the market. Representative of these is *KeyMath* (Conally, Nachtman, and Pritchett, 1971), a comprehensive test of 14 skills associated with achievement in math. The authors of the test subdivide the skills into those representing content, operations, and applications of math concepts. The following subtests make up the *KeyMath* test (used here with permission):

	Subtest
Content	Numeration
	Fractions
	Geometry and Symbols
Operations	Addition
	Subtraction
	Multiplication
	Division
	Mental Computations
	Numerical Reasoning
Applications	Word Problems
	Missing Elements
	Money
	Measurement
	Time

KeyMath is appropriate for use with children in grades 1 through 9. Except for the first four subtests of operations, the test requires pointing, multiple-choice, or oral responses from the child being tested. *KeyMath* is an individual test and materials are colorful and interesting. Test items are arranged in order of difficulty and testing is terminated when the child answers two consecutive items incorrectly. Figure 9.1 contains examples of items from the test.

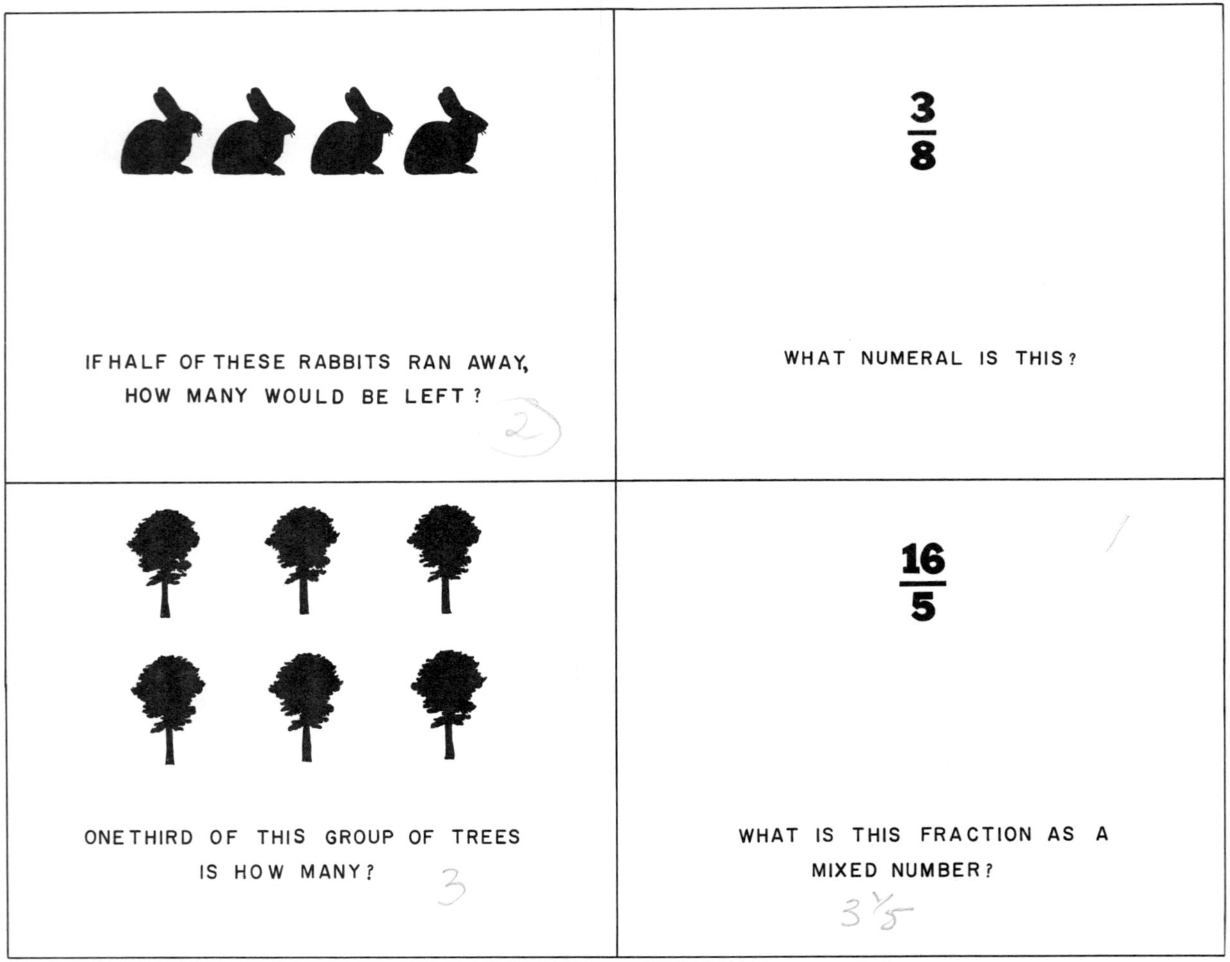
IF HALF OF THESE RABBITS RAN AWAY,
HOW MANY WOULD BE LEFT?
2
3/8
WHAT NUMERAL IS THIS?
ONE THIRD OF THIS GROUP OF TREES
IS HOW MANY?
3
16/5
WHAT IS THIS FRACTION AS A
MIXED NUMBER?
3 1/5

Figure 9.1. Examples of four items from the fractions subtest of the *KeyMath* achievement test. These items assess a range of knowledge from the third- to eighth-grade levels. (Reprinted by special persmission of American Guidance Service. *KeyMath Diagnostic Arithmetic Test* by Austin J. Connolly, Ed. D.; William Nachtman, Ed.D.; E. Milo Prickeet, Ed.D.)

The response sheet furnished with *KeyMath* allows the plotting of a profile of the child's responses. Raw scores can be converted into grade equivalent scores if a single measure of math achievement is desired. Of much more use to clinicians and teachers, however, is the profile, which indicates at a glance the areas of relative strength and weakness exhibited by the child. Furthermore, the nature of the test allows the examiner to determine the specific factors involved in a poor performance on a given subtest. Much of what is being tested consists of the vocabulary involved in math concepts and operations and the use of information in reasoning through problems. From the results of the test it is possible to determine which skills prerequisite to overall math achievement are lacking or poorly developed, and remedial programs can be planned.

Speech-language pathologists and audiologists do not teach math. It is an academic subject and, as such, the responsibility of the classroom teacher. However, they may reinforce verbal concepts involved in math reasoning by providing practice with new vocabulary and use of verbal information in problem solving. These are language tasks, and remediation of deficits in these areas often contributes significantly to achievement in the classroom. A child who cannot follow the directions to "round this number to the nearest 100" may require supplemental instruction in the multiple meanings of the word "round." The teaching of new vocabulary is a legitimate language remediation activity. As such it falls within the purview of speech-language pathologists and audiologists, who should be alert for ways to coordinate therapy with classroom instruction. Discovery of the language deficits directly associated with classroom tasks will save time and, perhaps, wasted effort. Therefore, administration of a test such as *KeyMath* provides information of value in planning by both teachers and clinicians.

Classroom teachers seldom have time to administer individual diagnostic tests. Unless other professionals (psychologists, resource teachers, or learning strategists) are available for early testing, speech-language pathologists and audiologists should collect diagnostic information on the children they serve as soon as possible. Legal requirements that school personnel develop an Individual Education Plan (IEP) for each child receiving special services lends emphasis to the need for early, thorough assessment for planning purposes. Speech-language pathologists and audiologists can contribute significantly to the IEP, as well as to remediation of language deficits that directly affect academic achievement.

REFERENCES

Balow, I. and Brill, R., An evaluation of reading and academic levels of sixteen graduating classes of the California School for the Deaf, *Volta Rev.*, 77, 255-266, 1975.

Baron, N., Linguistic consciousness: Prerequisites for learning to read and write. Address delivered to the Summer Institute on Applied Linguistics, Rhode Island School for the Deaf, 1975.

Carrow, E., *Test for Auditory Comprehension of Language*. Austin, TX: Learning Concepts, 1973.

Connolly, A., Nachtman, W., and Pritchett, E., *Keymath Diagnostic Arithmetic Test*. Circle Pines, MN: American Guidance Service, Inc., 1971.

Davis, J., Performance of young hearing impaired children on a test of basic concepts, *J. Speech Hearing Res.,* 17, 342–351, 1974.

Denton, D., A study in the educational achievement of deaf children. In *Report of the Proceedings of the 42nd Meeting of the Convention of American Instructors of the Deaf.* Washington, D. C.: U. S. Government Printing Office, 428–433, 1966.

Downs, M., The expanding imperatives of early identification. In F. Bess (Ed.), *Childhood Deafness*. New York: Grune and Stratton, 1977.

Dunn, L. and Markwardt, F., *Peabody Individual Achievement Test*. Circle Pines, MN: American Guidance Service, Inc., 1970.

Engelman, S., *The Basic Concept Inventory* (Field Research Ed.). Chicago: Follett Publishing Co., 1967.

Gentile, A., *Academic Achievement Test Results of a National Testing Program for Hearing Impaired Student: 1971*. Annual survey of hearing impaired children and youth. Gallaudet College Office of Demographic Studies, Ser. D., No. 9, 1972.

Goetzinger, C. and Rousey, E., Educational achievement of deaf children, *Amer. Ann. Deaf,* 105, 221–224, 1959.

Hester, M., Manual communication, *Proceedings of International Congress on Education of the Deaf.* Washington, D. C.: U. S. Government Printing Office, 211–222, 1963.

Holm, V. and Kunze, L., Effect of chronic otitis media on language and speech development, *Pediatrics,* 43, 833–839, 1969.

Jastak, J., Bijou, S., and Jastak, S., *The Wide Range Achievement Test Manual of Instructions*. Wilmington, DE: Guidance Associates, 1965.

Kaplan, G., Fleshman, J., Bender, T., Baum, C., and Clark, P., Long-term effects of otitis media: A ten-year cohort study of Alaskan Eskimo children, *Pediatrics,* 52, 577–585, 1973

Kessler, M., The effects of early middle ear disease on the auditory abilities of third grade children, Ph.D. Dissertation, University of Connecticut, 1978.

Kodman, F., Educational status of hard of hearing children in the classroom, *J. Speech Hearing Dis.,* 28, 297–299, 1963.

Ling, D., Rehabilitation of cases with deafness secondary to otitis media. In A. Glorig and K. Gerwin (Eds.), *Otitis Media*. Springfield, IL: Charles C Thomas, 1969.

McClure, W., Current problems and trends in the education of the deaf, *The Deaf American,* 18, 8–14, 1966.

McGuire, M. and Bumpus, M., *McGuire-Bumpus Diagnostic Comprehension Test*. New London, CT: Croft Educational Services, Inc., 1971.

Moores, D., An investigation of the psycholinguistic functioning of deaf adolescents, *Except. Chil.,* 36, 645–654, 1970.

Myklebust, H., *The Psychology of Deafness*. New York: Grune and Stratton, 1964.

Needleman, H., Effects of hearing loss from early recurrent otitis media on speech and language development. In B. Jaffe (Ed.), *Hearing Loss in Children*. Baltimore: University Park Press, 1977.

Paradise, J., Management of middle ear effusions in infants with cleft palate, *Ann. Otol. Rhinol. Laryngol.,* 85, 285-288, 1976.

Peterson, M., Achievement of hard of hearing students in regular public schools, Ph.D. Dissertation, Wayne State University, 1972.

Pugh, G., Summaries from the appraisal of silent reading abilities of acoustically handicapped children, *Amer. Ann. Deaf,* 91, 331-349, 1946.

Quigley, S. and Thomure, R., *Some Effects of a Hearing-Impairment on School Performance.* Champaign-Urbana: Institute of Research on Exceptional Children, University of Illinois, 1968.

Reynolds, L., The school adjustment of children with minimal hearing loss, *J. Speech Hearing Dis.,* 20, 380-384, 1955.

Ross, M., Definitions and descriptions. In J. Davis (Ed.), *Our Forgotten Children.* Minneapolis, MN: National Support Systems Project, Bureau of Education for the Handicapped, USOE, 1977.

Sprunt, J. and Finger, F., Auditory deficiency and academic achievement, *J. Speech Hearing Dis.,* 14, 26-32, 1949.

Trybus, R. and Karchmer, M., School achievement scores of hearing impaired children: National data on achievement status and growth patterns, *Amer. Ann. Deaf,* 122, 62-69, 1977.

Ventry, I., Effects of conductive hearing loss: Fact or fiction, *J. Speech Hearing Dis.,* 45, 143-156, 1980.

Vernon, M. and Brown, D., A Guide to psychological tests and testing procedures in the evaluation of the deaf and hard-of-hearing children, *J. Speech Hearing Dis.,* 29, 414-423, 1964.

Wisconsin Test of Reading Skills Development. Minneapolis, MN: Educational Systems, National Computer Systems, Inc., 1977.

Wrightstone, J., Aranow, M., and Moskowitz, S., Developing reading test norms for deaf children, *Amer. Ann. Deaf,* 108, 311-316, 1963.

Young, C. and McConnell, F., Retardation of vocabulary development in hard-of-hearing children, *Except. Chil.,* 23, 368-370, 1957.

CHAPTER 10

Educational Management

This chapter acquaints clinicians and teachers with some of the issues involved in the provision of educational services to hearing-impaired children. Although audiologists and speech-language pathologists are not responsible for the education of children in the sense that they teach them academic subjects, they are closely involved in certain aspects of their educational lives.

ROLES OF AUDIOLOGISTS AND SPEECH-LANGUAGE PATHOLOGISTS IN EDUCATIONAL MANAGEMENT

Audiologists are often the first professionals to confirm the diagnosis of hearing impairment. They advise parents as to the remedial steps necessary for the child, often making recommendations about school placement, advocating certain educational methodologies, or referring children and parents to specific educational programs. Audiologists also conduct parent-infant activities involving the use of amplification, auditory stimulation, and early language development. They frequently serve as members of a team of professionals within school settlings. To make intelligent recommendations, audiologists must be knowledgeable about the educational deficits associated with hearing impairment, methods of minimizing them, and the characteristics of educational programs as they relate to certain parameters of hearing impairment.

Except for the classroom teacher, speech-language pathologists are the school personnel who typically have the greatest amount of contact with hearing-impaired children. If audiologists or teachers of the deaf are not employed by the school system, speech-language pathologists constitute the only available professionals who have been trained even minimally in hearing and its impairment. They are viewed as experts in the subject and are expected to serve as a resource to other personnel. They often provide the only individual remedial help available to children with mild or moderate hearing impairments. Their knowledge of the relationship between language skills and educational demands can be instrumental in obtaining appropriate educational placement or ancillary services for the children they serve. Until school systems in general establish as a priority the adequate education of hearing-impaired children, much of the responsibility for these children will continue to rest with the speech-language pathologist. Fortunately, most of them can work effectively with hearing-impaired children with some additional training or orientation toward their language and educational problems.

MAJOR EDUCATIONAL ISSUES

There are three major issues concerning the education of hearing-impaired children about which speech-language pathologists and audiologists should be knowledgeable: (1) educational methodology to be employed, (2) residential versus day class placement, and (3) mainstreaming. Each of these topics is characterized by controversy, heated polemics, and few facts. It is easy for professionals just entering the field to become caught up in the issues as a result of the intense emotion associated with them. Clinicians "take sides," the identity of which often depends on the opinion and bias of those with whom they are associated, rather than on careful evaluation of the data available. Because they have few clinical experiences of their own to use as a basis for decision making, beginning speech-language pathologists and audiologists reflect the experiences of those who train them. This situation creates a problem of critical evaluation. Most professionals remember their successes more vividly and more readily than their failures. The clinical experiences reported by most of us tend to support our own points of view and illustrate the weaknesses of divergent views. The result is that the important anecdotal data (experiences) provided to young professionals are usually one sided and tend to prejudice them toward a given point of view.

If the issue was a theory of educational development in the abstract, involving much discussion but no practical application, the controversies surrounding the education of hearing-impaired children would constitute an interesting intellectual exercise, neither harmful nor helpful. This is not the case, however. When professionals argue vociferously over educational methodology, for example, they do not do so in a vacuum. Bewildered parents, confused administrators, a wondering public, and vulnerable children are caught in the turmoil. They have no way of evaluating the rhetoric that pours over them. In most cases, these people have no reasonable alternative but to go along with the view of the professionals associated with the first educational institutions they encounter. The results may be favorable or they may be a disaster, but they will too seldom be based on a rational evaluation of facts from which logical educational decisions can be made.

Hearing-impaired children are a heterogeneous group. Their hearing losses vary in degree from mild to profound, the onset of hearing loss may occur anytime in life, the ability to use residual hearing for the discrimination of speech is different for each child, the age of identification and intervention varies widely, the successful use of amplification depends on individual characteristics, the language status is variable, availability of remediation differs sharply, family support depends on factors too numerous to list, intelligence is as variable as it is in the normally hearing population, and many hearing-impaired children exhibit additional handicapping conditions ranging from orthopedic to visual. In view of these facts it would be absurd to assume that all hearing-impaired children can benefit from the same educational placement or the same educational methods. Flexibility in planning would appear to be essential. Careful evaluation of each child's status must be made before placement is decided on, and the latter should be reviewed periodically. The needs of the child must be related to the characteristics of the educational programs under consideration. To accomplish these logical steps, hearing professionals must set aside biases in favor of analysis and data, a move that would be considerably easier to make if more objective data were available. One of the most detrimental effects of the heated controversies that characterize the field of education of the hearing impaired is the fact that professional energies have been so dissipated and opinions so polarized that necessary research has not been accomplished. Although hearing-impaired children have been educated in the United States since the early 1800s, only a few carefully controlled studies of the efficacy of various educational procedures or placements have been reported.

Many factors contribute to the paucity of research into educational practices, including the heterogeneity of the population described above. Even so, more research would be possible if cooperation among programs and personnel were more common. It is not unusual for researchers to request permission from 25 to 30 different educational programs before finding one that will agree to cooperate in a research project. The level of distrust that has resulted from the polarity of views has been detrimental to the education of children, the collection of data, the development of improved teaching procedures, the establishment of placement guidelines, and the credibility of professionals. Audiologists and speech-language pathologists must try to avoid the mistakes of the past and approach the question of education of the hearing impaired with open minds and critical evaluation of existing data. Only under these circumstances will they be maximally helpful to parents, children, and educational institutions.

Educational Methodologies

The controversy surrounding the educational procedures to be used with hearing-impaired children has influenced all other aspects of their habilitation. It is difficult to describe the level of emotion that has been associated with the methods controversy. Personal confrontation with it is necessary in order to appreciate the level of near hysteria it often reaches. The roots of the controversy go back more than 200 years to Europe. When the first schools for the deaf were established in the United States they were influenced by European schools of thought, including different opinions regarding the educational methods to be employed. Moores (1978) devotes two chapters to a fascinating description of the history of education of the deaf in Europe and the United States. A less objective view of the controversy, often referred to as the "200 Years War," can be found in the impassioned pleas that have been published on every conceivable side of the issue. These may be found in hundreds of articles in the *Volta Review,* the publication of the Alexander Graham Bell Association for the Deaf (representing the *oral* point of view) and the *American Annals of the Deaf,* the publication of the Conference of American Instructors of the Deaf (CAID) (representing the *manual* point of view). In addition, books like those by Mindel and Vernon (1971), Pollack (1970), Ling (1976) and Schlesinger and Meadow (1972) present strong opinions in one direction or another.

At the time that the intense controversy developed, all hearing-impaired children were referred to as deaf. Diagnostic procedures were not developed, medical treatment of ear pathologies was not well developed nor available, and amplification was unheard of. Any noticeable degree of hearing loss was sufficient to require special educational procedures, if they were available. This fact helps to explain the nature of the controversy that centered around a single major question: Should hearing-impaired children be exposed to any form of manual communication? Early opinion on the subject was probably determined largely by the nature of the hearing losses encountered. If the population to be served consisted primarily of children with congenital, severe, sensorineural hearing losses, the observer was likely to support the use of manual communication. If a majority of the population consisted of children with acquired, moderate conductive or sensorineural hearing losses, the use of manual communication may have seemed unnecessary and inappropriate.

Unfortunately, there are no accurate descriptions of the early students in schools for the deaf, because there was no way of measuring the attributes of interest. We can only hypothesize that differences existed among children that influenced their teachers' choice of educational methodology. At any rate, the earliest schools for the deaf were enmeshed in the struggle, with proponents of each philosophy (oral or manual) seeking to prevail over the other. No effort was made to determine which of the methods might be efficacious with different types of children. The focal point of the controversy, the use of manual communication, became the rallying point for both sides, and sign language has been endowed with attributes of both heaven and hell.

Underlying the central question of whether or not sign language should be used with hearing-impaired children are several others. Would exposure to and use of sign language prevent the development of speech and speech-reading skills? Would use of sign language enhance or decrease linguistic and academic skills? Are social skills affected by the use of manual communication? Would use of sign relegate persons to life within a restricted community populated by other hearing-impaired people? What effect would the use of sign have on employment possibilities?

Professionals interested in the education of the hearing impaired have never hesitated to provide answers to each of these questions. Unfortunately, the nature of the answers can be predicted if the methodology advocated by the educator is known. Until the 1960s these questions were answered primarily on the basis of opinion, personal experiences with children, or wishful thinking. Meanwhile, the original educational methods (oral and manual) were being modified and expanded into a variety or procedures, most of which are still in use today.

Manual Method. The earliest schools for the deaf in the United States were based on the manual method (Moores, 1978). Two systems of sign language were used: (1) the methodical sign, which sought to represent the English language in word order and morphology; and (2) the natural sign, consisting of a visual language not based on English or any other spoken language. Reception and expression of language was through sign only. The belief that deaf persons could not be taught to speak persisted among manual educators for several years after the oral method was introduced. Altbough some manualists began to introduce speech work into the manual method in the late 1800s, many refused to do so until later. Soon, however, the manual method was largely extinct, having given way to the simultaneous method.

Oral Method. The oral method was brought to this country from Germany in the 1800s. The rationale for the method centers around the fact that hearing-impaired children grow up and live in a hearing world, in which humans communicate by the spoken word.

To be accepted in and by society, they must learn to express themselves through speech and to receive messages through lipreading. The method was initiated long before the advent of electronic hearing aids, so early oralism did not stress the use of hearing. Instead, lipreading was the receptive mode for the spoken word. Language development for young children was based on lipreading skills, and the method involved much drill on interpretation of lip movements. Because much of spoken language is not visible on the lips, the missing elements were taught in written form. Use of signs, fingerspelling and formal gestures were forbidden and often punished. The abhorrence of manual communication was based on the belief that its use would preclude the learning of speech and lipreading. Drill on speech was constant, and language was learned expressively at the same time it was learned receptively.

Considering the inefficiency of lipreading alone as a means of receptive communication, it seems miraculous that prelinguistically, deaf children were ever able to learn by this method. That some of them did is a tribute to the dedication of their teachers and parents and the perserverance of the individuals themselves. Many children failed to learn language by the oral method during the optimal years for efficient learning. Unfortunately, virtually no data were kept on the proportion of children who were able to benefit from oral teaching. Many educators now blame oralism for the poor achievement of hearing-impaired children because of its universal use with them during their best language learning years. This is probably an unfair assessment, because children exposed to other methods also exhibit severely reduced language and educational achievement. A more serious indictment of oralism is made by hearing-impaired adults who express deep resentment at having been deprived of a means of easy communication with peers and family during their childhood and youth.

With the introduction and widespread use of amplification the oral method began to be known as the *oral-aural* method. Children were encouraged to wear amplification and to use auditory input, however limited it might be, as an adjunct to lipreading.

Simultaneous Method. This approach to education of the deaf involved the use of some of the principles of oralism and some of manualism. Teachers spoke instructions to students, augmenting their speech with signs or fingerspelling for key words or concepts. The use of the two modes of communication was not systematic and varied from teacher to teacher in most schools. Until the early 1970s, schools using the simultaneous method rarely exposed children to sign in the classroom until approximately age 8 or 9. This practice was based on the premise that all children should be given a "chance to be oral." Children were exposed to sign by their peers in the dormitories or on the playground and no serious attempt was made to suppress its use. The simultaneous method is criticized by both proponents and opponents of sign language. The former claim that sign is used too seldom to be of benefit, and the latter claim that the use of any signs prevents the learning of speech. The lack of consistent use of either sign or speech can certainly be criticized on the basis of learning theory; indeed, the results obtained by simultaneous methods are not remarkable. Unlike other methods, its proponents rarely go on record describing the program or its successes. Its ambivalent attitude toward the usefulness of sign language probably resulted in the worst learning conditions possible for children. Children were instructed by the oral method until the optimal learning years had passed, but the use of speech was not endowed with high enough priority to be emphasized as a means of expression outside of class and beyond the age of 9.

Auditory Method. In the 1960s greater emphasis was placed on the use of residual hearing. Improved diagnostic techniques enabled professionals to identify hearing impairment at younger ages than was possible previously. The use of amplification, largely nonexistent until the 1950s, was stressed. The natural contribution of audition to language development was emphasized by educators, who insisted that all children could be taught to use their residual hearing as a tool for learning language. In their zeal these educators may have overestimated the number of children who could learn efficiently through the auditory system. Nevertheless, they served to focus attention on the usefulness of sound to hearing-impaired children. The auditory method involves intensive auditory stimulation in natural surroundings. Children learn to localize, imitate, identify and discriminate sound, and produce speech. Not only are signs and fingerspelling forbidden, but lipreading is also discouraged until the child has shown the ability to use audition effectively. The goal of the auditory approach is for the child to incorporate hearing into the personality (Pollack, 1970) and to become so adept in its use that special educational procedures are uneccessary. The auditory method, therefore, is designed for use with infants and toddlers. If successful, they will be educated in regular classrooms with normally hearing children. For this method to be maximally effective, children must be identified early in life and amplification (preferably binaural) introduced as soon as the hearing loss is identified. Parents must spend several hours a day in active stimulation of toddlers if they are to benefit optimally from this approach. The auditory method is also known as the acoustic or acoupedic method and is described in detail by Pollack (1970) and Whetnall and Fry (1964).

Rochester Method. Also known as *visible speech,* the Rochester method combines lipreading and fingerspelling. This method was initiated at the Rochester School for the Deaf in 1878 (Scouten, 1942). Based on the observation that many morphological and syntactic units of spoken language are not visible on the lips, this method seeks to augment lipreading and audition with a more visible form of language. Because, in theory, every letter of each word is provided to the hearing-impaired students through fingerspelling, they will learn the less visible components of the language more quickly. Signs are forbidden as inadequate representations of English. The combination of fingerspelling and lipreading has also been used extensively in Russia, where it is known as neo-oralism (Moores, 1972). Fingerspelling is easily learned as an expressive skill, although fingerspelling simultaneously with speech at normal speaking rates requires much practice. Reading rapid fingerspelling is a more difficult task, especially for persons who do not have to rely on it for communication.

Cued Speech. A relatively recent communication method, cued speech was developed at Gallaudet College by Cornett (1972). Recognizing that spoken language provides an incomplete representation of English when it must be lipread to be understood, Cornett developed a set of hand signals to accompany speech called cues. Utilizing eight hand shapes and four basic hand positions, a total of 32 cues are provided. Each hand shape represents three or four consonants from different viseme groups, easily distinguishable from each other on the lips (e.g., **t, m,** and **f**). Each hand position (placement at the body or face) represents two or three vowels from different viseme groups (**-a-, -i-,** and **oo**). By using the cues, homophenous words can be distinguished from each other on the basis of the hand shape and position employed. For example, the words *pop* and *mop* are identical on the lips, but the cues for **m** and **p** involve different hand shapes, thus allowing the lipreader to distinguish between the two words. Figure 10.1 shows the cues developed by Cornett.

Cued speech is an oral method in which the ambiguity associated with lipreading has been reduced to a minimum. Learning the cues themselves is not difficult, but combining them with speech in consonant-vowel clusters requires extensive practice. A knowledge of phonetics is necessary for accurate use of the system, because the phonetic components rather than the letters of the words spoken dictate the cues to be used. Once mastered, they provide additional information not available on the lips, thus enhancing lipreading ability significantly.

Total Communication. This method is also referred to as bimodal communication. It refers to the use of multisensory input systems and modalities for the reception and expression of language. Audition, lipreading, reading, sign, fingerspelling, and gestures are used to comprehend language, while speech, sign, gestures, fingerspelling, and writing are the modalities of expression. Any or all of these modes of communication may be used with individual children; none would be withheld when useful.

The rationale underlying total communication is based on two major premises. First, all hearing-impaired children are different and require different procedures, stimuli, and techniques if they are to learn as well as possible. For some children, auditory input can be used for the comprehension of language; for others, visual input will result in more efficient learning. Children who cannot lipread well will require other types of visual input. Some children will be able to learn to speak intelligibly, others will not. Therefore, hearing-impaired children should be exposed to as many forms of language as possible.

The second premise is that *communication* is the basis for most human endeavors. Its early development allows for meaningful interaction with others in the environment. This leads to the development of language skills and knowledge of

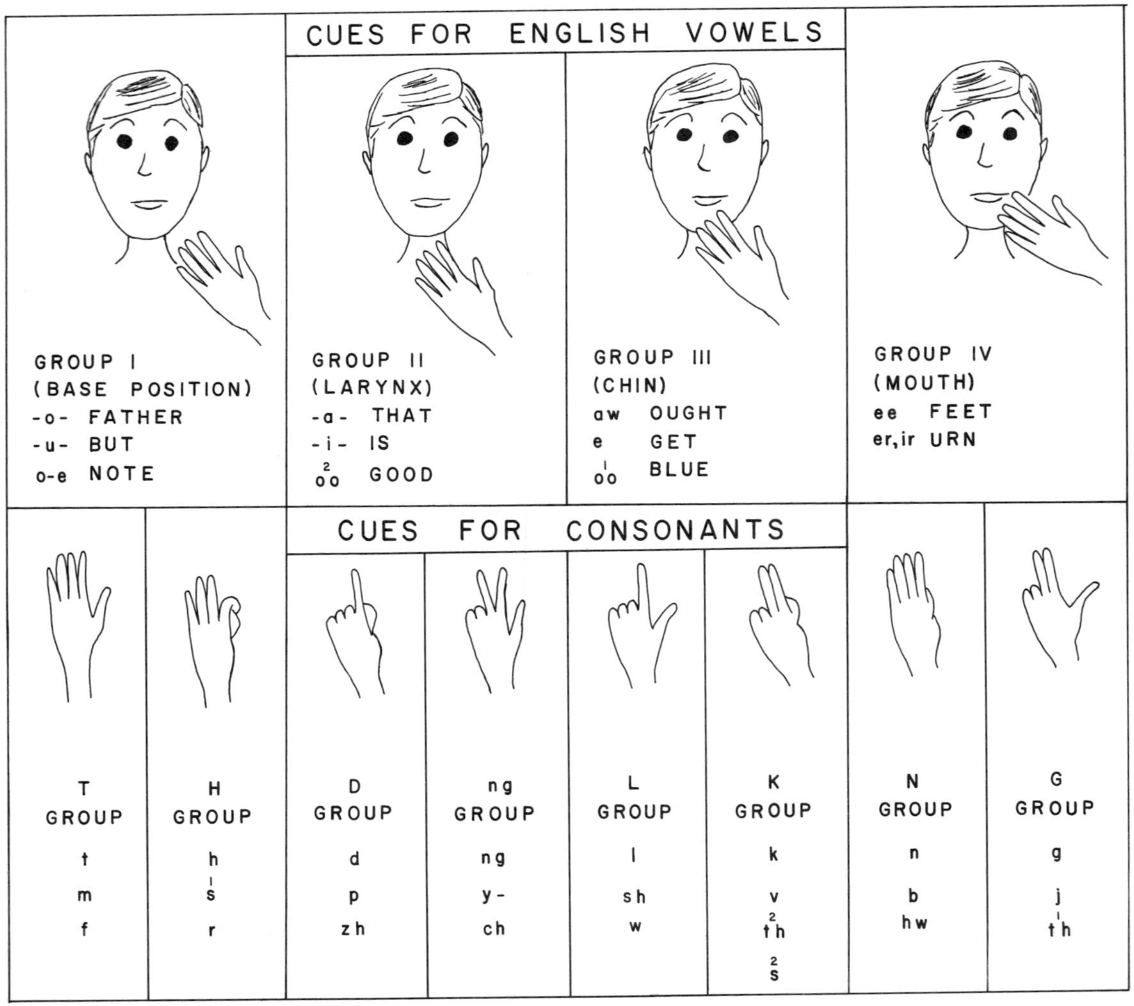

Figure 10.1. Cues devised by Cornett to represent various groups of phonemes.

self in relation to others through social interaction. Both reception and expression of language are necessary for communication and total communication provides a means for early development of both types of language skills. Pointing to the slow development of speech, lipreading, and auditory discrimination skills by many children, proponents of total communication advocate the use of sign with audition and speech as a means of developing rapid, two-way communication between young hearing-impaired children and others. Although early communication may depend on sign, other forms of language, such as speaking and lipreading, develop as children become proficient in the use of symbols and knowledgeable about the structures of the language to which they are exposed.

Total communication calls for the simultaneous presentation of speech and manual communication. This is not as easy to accomplish as it sounds, and it requires practice similar to that needed for facile use of cued speech and the Rochester method. Care must be taken to avoid "shortcuts," the most common of which is the omission of sign (Moores, 1978).

Critics of total communication assert that, in actuality, it is not "total," but simply the simultaneous method with a new name. The assumption is that persons using total communication often use sign alone. Other critics claim that every word is not signed, or that auditory input is not emphasized. In reality some programs designated as total communication do emphasize certain communication modes to the detriment of others. They are not total communication programs under those circumstances, but represent some other method or combination of methods. The most valid criticism of many total communication programs appears to be their failure to emphasize the use of residual hearing while concentrating on lipreading and sign as a means of comprehending speech.

Effectiveness of Educational Methodologies in Use

The two most prevalent methods in the United States today are oral-aural and total communication. As in the 1800s, the two major methods differ primarily in their attitude toward the use of sign in classrooms. The goals of both are similar: the development of communication skills for use in social, academic, and vocational endeavors. Only the means by which the goals are achieved distinguish the methods sharply. Rarely are either of the methods observed in pure form. According to recently reported research, teachers in oral-aural programs use many gestures for communication, and children use gestures and sign, especially when communicating with each other. Teachers in total communication programs often omit sign or fingerspelling, and children typically use one form of communication at a time, often speech alone (Weiss, Goodwin, and Moores, 1975). Table 10.1 shows the communication modes associated with the educational methods most widely used at present.

These authors also report a high degree of flexibility of hearing-impaired

Table 10.1 Communication Modes That Characterize Various Methods for Educating Hearing-Impaired Children

	Communication Modes Employed	
Method	*Receptive*	*Expressive*
Oral-Aural	Lipreading, hearing	Speaking
Auditory	Hearing	Speaking
Rochester	Lipreading, fingerspelling	Speaking, fingerspelling
Cued Speech	Lipreading (with cues)	Speaking
Total Communication	Hearing, lipreading, fingerspelling, sign	Speaking, fingerspelling, sign

children in various types of programs. They appear to be able to use three modes of communication with ease: oral-aural, oral-aural plus manual, and manual. Children appear to adapt the communicative mode to the situation, using more speech and speechreading with teachers or other normally hearing people and more manual communication with classmates, regardless of the type of program in which they are enrolled. If sign is not used, as in oral-aural programs, children develop a gestural system for use with each other (Weiss et al. 1975).

Trends in the popularity of educational methods used with the hearing impaired change from time to time. At present, there is a pronounced shift away from oral-aural programs toward total communication programs. While such shifts are to be expected, it would be unfortunate if either type of program existed to the exclusion of the other. Hearing-impaired children are a heterogeneous group; they require excellent teaching and a variety of approaches. The search for improved ways of teaching and stimulating children must continue if their educational status is to improve. This process is facilitated by healthy disagreement and dissatisfaction with the *status quo*. At the same time, the adversary relationship that has developed among advocates of the various methodologies is not conducive to productive research or improvement of teaching strategies. Proponents of each method feel compelled to defend practices of the past against all criticism. Guidelines are needed that can be used to determine objectively the optimal placement of children within methodologies. Their development will require recognition of the value of different approaches as well as careful investigation of the interaction between the characteristics of children and those of various educational programs. Every method has its successes; they are well documented in journals and books. Every method also has its failures, but they are documented only in national data pools that combine everybody's failures into statistics. What is needed is a careful, objective analysis of the proportion of successes to failures under all methodologies and an analysis of those factors contributing to each outcome.

Meanwhile, the decision regarding the educational method of choice for a given child must be made by someone based on some combination of factors. Because the major distinguishing characteristic of the two most commonly used methods revolves around the use of sign language, hearing professionals should be aware of the data that exist regarding the effects of the use of manual communication with hearing-impaired children.

Studies of the Effects of Using Manual Communication. Little or no investigation of the effects of the use or nonuse of sign language was reported until the 1960s. One reason for the lack of research was the prevailing philosophy among educators of the deaf and other professionals that all children should be given a chance to develop oral skills before sign was introduced as a last resort. That philosophy has at least two underlying assumptions: (1) it is "better" to be oral than to use sign, and (2) children will not be oral if exposed to sign. The first assumption cannot be investigated objectively, and the second proved difficult to study. Because children were not exposed to sign language until they had spent several years in school and, usually, had failed to progress satisfactorily, the effects of the use of sign could not be separated from other factors in the child's life. What was needed was a group of children who had been exposed to manual communication early in life, before failing under some other form of instruction. The only available group meeting that criterion consisted of deaf children of deaf parents who were exposed to sign language from infancy as the primary means of communication in the home. In the early 1960s studies were published comparing deaf children of deaf parents (called the *manual* group) and deaf children of normally hearing parents (called the *oral* group). As the data revealed, the designations of oral and manual were misnomers, but they served to distinguish the groups easily.

Early Studies of Deaf Children. Quigley and Frisina (1961) reported data for 16 nonresidential deaf children of deaf parents and 16 nonresidential deaf children of normally hearing parents. They measured vocabulary, lipreading ability, speech, and educational achievement. Only two differences were found between the groups. The manual group scored higher in vocabulary knowledge and the oral group scored higher in speech. There was no difference between the groups in lipreading and educational achievement.

Stevenson (1964) studied the records of 134 deaf children of deaf parents and a matched group of 134 deaf children of normally hearing parents. He reported that 38 percent of the manual group but only 9 percent of the oral group attended college. His results revealed that 90 percent of the manual children attained a higher educational level than their matched oral student.

Denton (1966) investigated the achievement test scores of the academic top 10% of deaf children in 26 schools for the deaf. The mean achievement level for the manual group was 8.2 grades and the mean for the oral group was 7.7 grades.

Stuckless and Birch (1966) investigated five areas of achievement in deaf children of deaf parents and deaf children of normally hearing parents. They found no differences between the groups in speech and psychosocial adjustment; the manual group was superior to the oral group in lipreading, reading, and writing skills.

In 1968 Meadow investigated matched pairs of deaf children of normally hearing and deaf parents. She reported that children with deaf parents ranked higher in self-image tests and in academic achievement than did children of normally hearing parents. The manual group scored 2.1 years higher in reading, 1.25 years higher in math, and 1.28 years higher in overall educational achievement than the oral group. The gap in overall achievement between the two groups increased with age. Teacher ratings of students revealed that the manual group was ranked higher in written language, willingness to communicate with strangers, absence of communicative frustration, use of fingerspelling and signs, maturity, independence, responsibility, sociability and popularity. There was no difference between the two groups on speaking or speechreading ability.

Quigley (1969) investigated the effects of the Rochester method (fingerspelling and speech) on certain academic and communicative skills of severely hearing-impaired preschool children aged 3 to 7. Comparing children educated by the Rochester method to children educated by the oral method, he found the former to be better in lipreading, three of five measures of written language, and five of seven measures of reading. The oral children were better on one measure of written language.

Criticisms of the Early Studies. These studies were criticized by educators of the deaf who opposed the use of manual communication. Objections to the studies centered on two major issues. First, the children of deaf parents were genetically deaf and thus were less likely to exhibit other learning problems associated with etiologies such as rubella or meningitis. In particular, brain damage was assumed to exist in at least some of the children of normally hearing parents. Second, the studies were criticized on the basis that, because of their ages at the time of the studies, the children probably did not have the benefit of a good preschool intervention program and were, therefore, not representative of properly trained oral children.

The first objection has little face validity when the characteristics of the children in the oral groups are considered. In each study, the IQ of the matched children was at least 104 and no evidence from psychologists, test results, or school performance existed to suggest that brain damage was present. Although one cannot argue with certainty that no differences existed in the central nervous systems of the two groups, the absence of any evidence of brain damage argues against the relevance of the objection.

In an effort to meet these criticisms, Vernon and Koh (1970) investigated the effects of genetic deafness. They controlled the variable of etiology and compared two groups of genetically deaf students. One group had deaf parents, while the other, whose parents were normally hearing, had deafness resulting from recessive genes. Educational achievement, reading, lipreading, speech intelligibility, and written language were assessed. The manual group achieved from 1.2 to 1.6 grades higher educationally than the oral group. Reading achievement was higher at all ages for the manual group and differences increased with age. There were no differences between the groups on speech or lipreading skills. The manual group was higher on written skills. Comparison of these students whose IQs were 110 or higher revealed that 82 percent of the manual group passed college entrance examinations while only 51 percent of the oral group did so.

Vernon and Koh (1971) also addressed the subject of the effects of preschool training on eventual achievement. They reported a follow-up study on three groups of 23 children, aged 15 years and older. Group 1 consisted of deaf children with normally hearing parents who had three years of preschool education at the John Tracy Clinic. Group 2 consisted of deaf children with normally hearing parents who had no preschool training. Group 3 consisted of deaf children with deaf parents who had no preschool training. The groups were matched under rigorous criteria (IQ differences of no more than five points, age differences within six months, and sex). The authors investigated academic and communicative achievement. Results indicated no difference between the two groups with normally hearing parents on academic achievement. The group with deaf parents scored at least one grade level above the other groups on achievement test scores. Sixty-eight percent of group 3, 47 percent of group 1, and 34 percent of group 2 passed college entrance exams. Teacher ratings of speech and lipreading ability revealed no differences among the three groups; group 3 scored higher in written language.

Balow and Brill (1975) also conducted a follow-up study comparing the academic levels of 15 graduating classes at the Riverside School for the Deaf in California. These authors reported significantly higher academic achievement levels in deaf children of normally hearing parents who were enrolled in the John Tracy Clinic nursery program as compared to those who had received no preschool training. However, their data also revealed higher academic achievement by deaf children of deaf parents (9.2 grade level) than by deaf children with normally hearing parents who attended the John Tracy nursery school (8.2 grade level).

Nix (1975) raised other objections to the studies showing superior academic performance of deaf children of deaf parents. He suggested that the studies are invalid because they are ex post facto rather than experimental studies. Nix particularly objected to the fact that many of the oral groups were no longer enrolled in oral programs at the time that the studies were conducted. He apparently overlooked those studies that included children attending oral programs at the time of the study. Phillips (1963) and McCroskey (1968) presented data for orally trained students who attended preschool and who did not. There were no differences between the groups in achievement in language arts, arithmetic, or in social skills.

Nix also questioned the ability of researchers to match groups precisely, the size of the subject pools, and the lack of random selection and assignment of subjects. The variables influencing the effects of deafness such as age of onset, training methodologies, etiologies, educational placement factors, and family status, to name but a few, are legion. Controlling all variables in studies of this nature is literally impossible. To insist on such a state of affairs is the same as advocating a complete absence of research in deafness and maintenance of the *status quo*. Rejection of findings obtained from small subject pools is especially invalid when the results of several studies conducted in a variety of geographical areas by various investigators reveal the same findings; that is, deaf children exposed to sign early in life reach higher achievement levels than those children who are not exposed to sign. In addition, there appear to be no detrimental effects of early exposure to sign on the learning of lipreading and speech skills. The consistency of these findings is remarkable in view of the variables involved, especially considering that deaf children of deaf parents live in relatively improverished surroundings. Family income is lower, there are fewer books and educational materials in the home, and children are exposed to fewer experiences outside the home (Schein, 1968). The consistent demonstration of superiority in language and academic skills by these children indicates that there must be something in the early experiences of the children that would account for their achievement. The most logical factor is early exposure to language in a form that is meaningful and nonambiguous.

Later Studies. Three further studies are of importance to this topic. Brasel and Quigley (1977) conducted a study designed to control many of the variables involved in comparison studies. They investigated the academic and linguistic skills of four groups of deaf persons. Two oral groups, designated as average oral (AO) and intensive oral (IO), were compared to manual groups, designated as average manual (AM) and manual English (ME). Group members were selected carefully. AO group members had attended oral schools, but without unusual participation by them or their parents. IO groups members attended oral schools and their parents were actively involved in all stages of their education. AM subjects had deaf parents who communicated with them via American Sign Language. They attended schools in which sign language was used by children and teachers. ME group members had deaf parents who communicated via manual English, in which English word order is preserved and some word endings are spelled or otherwise designated. Results of the study revealed no differences between the two oral groups in academic or linguistic functioning. A significant difference between the oral and the manual groups existed, in favor of the manual groups. Comparison of the two manual groups revealed a significant difference between the AM and the ME groups, with the latter being superior on all measures. Brasel and Quigley concluded that representation of the English language through signs and fingerspelling is the most effective means of fostering development of proficiency in English by deaf children.

Moores and his associates (Moores and McIntyre, 1971; Moores, McIntyre and

Weiss, 1972; Moores, Weiss, and Goodwin, 1973, 1974; Weiss, Goodwin, and Moores, 1975; and Moores, Weiss, and Goodwin, 1978) conducted a longitudinal evaluation of preschool programs for hearing-impaired children. Instead of seeking to determine which educational approach is the "best," they investigated several important components of a variety of early education programs representing various methodologies and educational settings. Measures of receptive and expressive communication abilities, academic achievement, cognitive development, communication patterns, and parental attitudes were obtained. Children were about 3 years old when the study began and were between 6 and 8 when the study was completed.

Results are described in detail in the original sources listed above. Major findings include the following:

1. Children from all programs scored well on prereading skills, more poorly on arithmetic skills. These data reflect the emphasis on prereading and reading skills in most preschool programs for hearing-impaired children. In academic skills the lowest scores were obtained by children in an auditory, parent-centered program. The highest scores were obtained by children in a Rochester method program with a cognitive-academic orientation.
2. Measures of use of residual hearing to understand speech revealed average auditory discrimination scores of 58 percent and 53 percent in two programs whose children were far superior to those in other programs. One of these was an auditory-oral program; the other was a program using total communication. The authors interpreted these results to mean that the use of manual communication *per se* has no effect on the use of residual hearing. Extensive training in auditory discrimination appears to result in better use of auditory information regardless of whether or not sign is also available.
3. Measures of the contribution of lipreading to receptive communication indicated the poorest use of this visual skill in children enrolled in oral-aural programs and the greatest use by children enrolled in total communication programs. The use of sign did not appear to detract from lipreading.
4. Intelligibility of speech production by children varied widely within programs, less widely among programs. Mean intelligibility ratings were highest for children enrolled in a total communication program (45.11 percent) and lowest for children enrolled in a program that was oral-aural until 1974, the final year of the project (29.90 percent). Use of sign language appears not to affect the intelligibility of speech adversely.
5. Regardless of the methodology advocated by the program, communication within the classroom was primarily gestural or sign. Teachers and children in oral programs relied heavily on gesture for communication. Con-

versely, teachers in total communication programs signed only a small proportion of the words spoken in class.

6. Parental attitudes differed among the programs. Those whose children were enrolled in oral-aural programs initially viewed the goals of the preschool program to be the development of speech and lipreading skills. Parents whose children were enrolled in total communication programs viewed the goals as the development of academic skills. By the end of the investigation, parental attitudes were the same, with emphasis given to the development of academic skills.

The authors of the several studies concluded that children may respond differentially to various educational procedures. None of the programs participating in the study appear to have the "answer" to the problems of educating deaf children. The children who achieved the highest were those with the most residual hearing who were exposed to total communication in a cognitive, academically oriented program. These investigators are pessimistic, however, about the overall communicative skills of the children studied. The speech of many children in each program was almost completely unintelligible. Attempts to communicate with strangers were rare and limited to gestures and a few words. The children processed sentences almost exclusively as S-V-O utterances, misinterpreting many messages as a result. Communication in English was best in written form. Even so, Moores et al. concluded,

> the programs studied appeared in general to be more successful than those studied in the past in the development of academic readiness and communication skills. The more successful programs had cognitive-academic and simultaneous oral-manual components from the beginning. The evidence suggests that it is harmful to delay either cognitive-academic training or the use of manual communication. Those children who do not receive such training and communication at early ages do not catch up by age eight. In fact, in some cases the gap widens. The least beneficial approach for the children studied included an aural-only methodology within a traditional socially-oriented nursery school framework. Although such an approach may be beneficial for an occasional child, there is no evidence to support its use from the beginning with profoundly hearing impaired children (Moores, Weiss, and Goodwin, 1978, p. 936).

Jensema and Trybus (1978) reported an attempt to correlate academic achievement with mode of communication. Although they do not represent an experimental study, the data are interesting and suggest caution in ascribing a cause-effect relationship between sign or speech and achievement. These authors reported the results of a national study of the relationship between academic achievement and the current communication patterns used by hearing-impaired children and their teachers and parents. Questionnaires were obtained that included descriptions of the current use of various means of communicating (including cued speech, speech alone, signs, fingerspelling, gestures, and writing). Communication patterns were also related to various characteristics of the children, such as age, onset and degree of hearing loss, family income, ethnic background, use of hearing aids, preschool attendance and hearing status of parents. Academic achievement was measured by the Stanford Achievement Test, Special Edition for Hearing Impaired Children (SAT-HI). The intercorrelations of the variables studied revealed complex relationships not easily described. Differences in a variety of characteristics influence the use of sign and speech. Therefore, the influence of communication mode on academic achievement is confounded with other important variables. The authors state, ''For example, hearing level, hearing aid use, and speech intelligibility form one cluster of variables which are related to communication patterns. Ethnic background and family income form another such cluster; both this cluster and the previous one are related to the educational placement of the hearing-impaired child, and this entire complex of variables is related to reported speech use and sign use'' (p. 16).

Jensema and Trybus suggest that definitive research into the effects of communication mode on academic achievement will be difficult to achieve, because it is unlikely that children exist who differ only on the variable of communication style. They concluded that, ''Taken all together, then, the available data suggest that while factors such as the child's hearing level and the family's income level have a large influence on the child's school achievement, variations in communication methods, specifically in the amount of speech used and the amount of signs used, have little relationship with achievement scores, given the existing national variations in the quantity and quality of use of those methods'' (p. 19).

There are few data regarding the use of sign or fingerspelling with moderately hearing-impaired children. Mills (1975) reported on the communicative and academic status of several children with moderate hearing losses who attended a total communication preschool program prior to full time enrollment in regular classes. All were achieving at grade level (third and fourth); one child had been held back for one grade. None of the children used sign to communicate, and videotaped interviews revealed that their speech was intelligible and natural sounding. Mills concluded that a total communication program that stressed the use of audition and speech as well as sign was not detrimental to the educational achievement or communication skills of children with moderate hearing losses.

A summary of the results of studies investigating the effects of manual communication on children's development is provided in Table 10.2. Although children respond differentially to various educational procedures and a case can be made for the use of each of them with some children at some time, critical evaluation of the research into the effects of the use of sign reveal one incontrovertible fact: there is no evidence that manual communication is detrimental to the development of hearing-impaired children.

Table 10.2 Summary of Results of Studies Investigating the Performance of Children Who Were Exposed to Manual Communication (Manual) and Those Who Were Not (Oral)

	Results				
Investigator	*Speech*	*Lipreading*	*Academic Achievement*	*Language*	*Social Adjustment*
Quigley and Frisina (1961)	Oral group superior	No difference	No difference	Manual group superior	—
Stevenson (1964)	—	—	Ninety percent of manual group scored higher than matched oral student	—	—
Denton (1966)	—	—	Manual group superior	—	—
Stuckless and Birch (1966)	No difference	Manual superior	Manual superior	Manual superior	No difference
Meadow (1968)	No difference	No difference	Manual superior	Manual superior	Manual superior
Quigley (1969)	—	Manual superior	Manual superior	Manual superior	—
Vernon and Koh (1970)	No difference	No difference	Manual superior	Manual superior	—
Vernon and Koh (1971)	No difference	No difference	Manual superior	Manual superior	—
Balow and Brill (1975)	—	—	Manual superior	—	—
Brasel and Quigley (1977)	—	—	Manual superior	Manual superior	—

Residential Versus Day Class Placement

The problem of choosing an educational environment for hearing-impaired children is a complex one, involving decisions on several levels. The most immediate one is whether a child should be placed within a local school system or at a residential facility for deaf children. This is a decision that may be faced several times within a child's educational life, regardless of the degree of hearing impairment involved. The nature of local programs changes, the needs of children differ from time to time, and distant programs may offer advantages and disadvantages that must be weighed as children develop. For example, the parents of a newly identified two-year-old deaf child are in need of immediate support services for themselves and for the child. Such services may not be available locally. The residential program designed to serve deaf children in that state may not accept 2-year-old children on a residential basis, and the school may be too far away to serve the child on a nonresidential basis. Under these circumstances parents face three choices: remain where they are without services, move to an area in which appropriate services are provided, or arrange for foster-home placement for the child in another area. The last two options require a decision as to whether to place the 2-year-old in the residential facility on a day-class basis or within a local school system elsewhere in the state. If services are available both locally and in the residential school, parents often receive conflicting opinions from professionals regarding which of these is most appropriate for a given child.

The residential versus local school decision also arises when children are already placed in either situation, but the placement does not appear optimal. This can occur when children are experiencing failure, and a change in the type or number of services seems advisable. Ideally, there should be open communication among programs serving hearing-impaired children within a state in order to facilitate optimal placement of all children. Unfortunately, this does not seem to be the case in most states. A brief historical note may help to explain the problem.

Development of Programs in Local Schools. The oldest programs for hearing-impaired children within a state are the state public residential schools for deaf children. For many years, these schools were the only organized educational facilities for children with any degree of hearing impairment. Children either attended regular classes within a local system, usually without support services, or they attended the residential school for the deaf. When speech-language pathologists and audiologists joined local school staffs, minimal support services became available and fewer moderately hearing-impaired children attended state schools for the deaf. By 1960 many local school systems had developed educational programs for severely hearing-impaired children, primarily at the preschool level (Moores, 1978). Most of these early programs were oral, staffed by speech and hearing personnel whose major interests lay in developing speech and language skills in the children they served. Educational needs of hearing-impaired children were not well understood by these personnel and were not established as a major priority. As these programs developed and as knowledge about language development and its relation to educational achievement grew, public school programs were instituted in which teachers of the deaf were employed, as well as speech-language pathologists. The development of self-contained classes for hearing-impaired children taught by teachers of the deaf grew out of early intervention programs, and gradually classes were established for older chlldren. Typically, local systems hired one special teacher for preschoolers, then expanded the programs into the elementary grades as the children aged. Many larger school systems developed junior and senior high school programs as well.

Personnel associated with residential schools reacted with alarm to the development of services for hearing-impaired children in the public schools. Much of their concern was legitimate, for many public school programs initially employed teachers without credentials in education of the deaf. The education of hearing-impaired children was often delegated to teachers and clinicians who were largely untrained to teach academic subjects to those children. Because severe hearing impairment constitutes a low-incidence condition, the establishment of a comprehensive program for hearing-impaired children requires a large population base. Brill (1975) estimated that a population of 60,000 *school children* is necessary if a school system intends to provide adequate educational services for elementary-aged, hearing-impaired children. More than three times that number is necessary for development of secondary school programs. Educators of the deaf feared that many local school systems would not have the resources necessary for the establishment of sound educational programs.

Nevertheless, the trend toward local education of hearing impaired children has continued. By 1974, census figures indicated that 70 percent of the children identified as deaf in the United States were being educated in day classes, and more than half of the total population were enrolled in public school classes (Moores, 1978). These data primarily reflect programming for hearing-impaired pupils in metropolitan areas in states that have pioneered services for this population. As late as 1966 a National Education Association study of programs for handicapped children revealed that fewer than 50 percent of the school systems enrolling more than 300 pupils made any special provisions for hearing impaired children (Lawrence and Kapfer, 1970).

Modern Relations Between Local and Residential Programs. Although many public school programs of today are staffed by well-qualified personnel and use a variety of teaching methodologies, animosities that developed in the early stages of the trend toward public school education of the hearing impaired have been slow to disappear. In many states there is an adversary relationship between local school programs and residential schools that seriously interferes with the provision of services. Parents are caught in the middle of an unhealthy competition for students by the two types of programs. It is a rare state in which there is genuine, nonhostile cooperation among all educational service agencies. There are hopeful signs, however, that some effort is being made to develop cooperative programs in which residential school students are integrated into public school classes to varying extents (Porter, 1975; Ross, 1976; Connor, 1976). A survey of 22 residential schools that encourage partial integration of selected students into regular classes was reported by Craig and Salem (1975). A total of 410 children were involved in the integration program reporting; all but 37 of them were judged to be benefiting from the regular school placement. The data indicate that most children were integrated at the high school level.

The Effects of Day or Residential Placement on Children. Few studies have been reported that investigate the effects of residential versus day class placement of hearing-impaired children. The data that do exist are inconsistent and difficult to interpret. Kaufman (1965) reported a follow-up study of academic achievement of pupils enrolled in a residential school for the deaf and pupils who had been transferred to public schools. Both groups demonstrated improvements in reading achievement scores four years after the initial testing. There was no significant difference between the two groups, both of which were small (42 residential and 11 day school students).

Craig (1965) investigated the self-concept development of 16 day school and 16 residential students, using a sociometric scale that required children to choose classmates with whom they would prefer to play, study, sit, and work. Subjects were also asked to estimate which children would choose them as desirable partners. Results indicated that the residential group rated themselves higher on the scale of self-acceptance than the nonresidential group and the deaf children attending day classes chose fewer partners than the residential students. Craig hypothesized that the higher self-acceptance and social expansiveness of the residential group resulted from the experience of close ties with school friends, a situation that is more probable when classmates are all deaf as opposed to when a majority of classmates are normally hearing.

A comparative study of children integrated into public schools and those enrolled in special schools for the hearing impaired was conducted by van den Horst (1971). Verbal achievement tests and social adjustment scales were administered to the two groups, which were matched for IQ, age, sex, degree of loss, type of loss, and hearing aid use. Results of the study indicated that the integrated group scored higher on the verbal achievement test but exhibited poorer social adjustment.

The variables involved in placement decisions make comparative research difficult to accomplish. The influence of degree of hearing loss and the presence of additional handicapping conditions on the decision to place in local or residential schools cannot be ignored. Although present placement can be controlled in studies, the characteristics of previous intervention strategies are often unknown for children in both placements.

There may be advantages and disadvantages to both residential and public school placement of hearing-impaired children. In deciding between them, several aspects of a child's development must be considered, including educational growth, social development, family relationships, and personality factors. Residential schools offer increased opportunities for social interaction with others. The fact that all students are hearing impaired eliminates the stigma of being different, at least within the school setting. Child-to-child communication is easier to establish and maintain, providing more opportunity for socialization. Although the proponents of integration stress the advantages of association with normally hearing children, many severely to profoundly hearing-impaired children do not actually interact socially with normally hearing children even though they are with them daily. Some advocates of residential school placement claim that association with other hearing-impaired children contributes to a healthier self-concept than is possible for children who are educated with normally hearing children. There simply are not enough empirical data to allow for objective evaluation of such claims.

Day class attendance allows a child to remain at home, living within the family circle, with all the advantages that implies. If communication patterns are well-established among family members, the hearing-impaired child learns much about the community, functioning within a family structure, and the relationship of family members to the outside world. This is important information for any child. A sense of place is developed through observing individual interactions within and external to the family. Children who grow up within a complete community also tend to develop greater independence than is possible in most residential schools for the deaf. The degree to which independence is fostered is somewhat dependent on parental attitudes and practices. It is possible for overprotective parents to discourage independent actions severely. Efforts toward fostering responsibility, self-discipline, and independent thought and action must be made by people in daily contact with the child in question, whether in a residential or family setting. There are no data that can be used to determine the relative success of families versus school personnel in this task.

Perhaps the most compelling argument for placement in either residential or local schools is the appropriateness of the educational experiences available in each. Children who require special classes in order to achieve academic success must attend programs that are staffed by qualified personnel and provide educational experiences commensurate with their needs. Children whose communicative skills allow for education among hearing students should have that opportunity. For some children, an academic track leading to postsecondary education is necessary. For others, vocational training, beginning early in life, will be essential. The availability of vocational training may be a compelling factor in the residential-public school choice. Finally, educational methodology may vary from one program to another, and should be matched to children's needs.

Mainstreaming

The most popular general trend in education at present is mainstreaming. The term refers to educational programming for children with physical and mental impairments in which students are educated primarily within regular classrooms with normal children. Support services of various types may be available but mainstreaming represents a move away from segregation of children who have handicapping conditions. Mainstreaming began with educable mentally retarded children (Dunn, 1968), and progressed rapidly to include other handicapped children. Court cases in which school districts were brought to trial for failure to provide an education to handicapped children provided additional impetus to the movement, which culminated in the passage of Public Law 94-142 (The Education of All Handicapped Children Act of 1975). Referred to as the "mainstreaming law" by some educators, P. L. 94-142 seeks to ensure educational services for heretofore unserved and underserved populations of children. The act requires that all handicapped children be educated in the "least restrictive environment" possible. Educators of the deaf have expressed concern over misinterpretation of that wording, citing the communicative problems associated with deafness that make placement within regular classrooms unsuitable for many hearing-impaired children (Brill, 1975; Garretson, 1977). These authors argue that the regular classroom may be the *most* restrictive environment for hearing-impaired children if their special communicative and educational needs are not understood and met.

Proponents of mainstreaming argue that association with normally hearing children in the learning environment will result in educational benefits, better social development, and improved communication abilities for hearing-impaired children (Craig, Salem and Craig, 1976). As is true of other areas of controversy surrounding the education of hearing-impaired children, this issue is difficult to study and quantify. Much of the literature consists of descriptions of local mainstreaming efforts (Northcott, 1973; Rister, 1975, Mills, 1975; De Salle and Ptasnik, 1976; Kopchick, 1977). Studies of the actual effects of mainstreaming on children are complicated by the number of programming options that are included under its rubric.

Continuum of Placement Options. Some educators have expanded the definition of mainstreaming to include any program for hearing-impaired children that exists within a public school setting (Brill, 1975; Moores, 1978). Although this is not an accurate interpretation of the term, it is applied often enough to warrant special mention. The variety of placement options found in public school settings is often referred to as a ''cascade of services'' (Ross, 1976), only a few of which actually constitute mainstreaming. The cascade includes the following placement options.

Self-Contained Classrooms. These classrooms are essentially day-class programs for hearing-impaired children. Class members may be integrated into physical education, art or shop classes, but their academic subject matter is taught by a teacher of the deaf within a classroom populated by other hearing-impaired children. There is infrequent contact between children enrolled in the class and normally hearing children who attend the school in which the classroom is located. Special effort must be made if the children in the self-contained class are to have meaningful contact with normally hearing children. Academic subject matter, language and speech are taught by the teacher of the deaf, with or without ancillary services from audiologists and speech-language pathologists.

Resource Room. A resource room for the hearing impaired is one to which children go for academic assistance for varying periods of time. The resource room is usually staffed by a teacher of the deaf, whose responsibilities include academic tutoring, pre- and postteaching of material covered in the regular classroom, and language and speech work (preferably with the assistance of a speech-language pathologist.) In some school systems the resource room is taught by other types of special education personnel, such as a learning disabilities specialist. The amount of time spent by a child in the resource room depends upon individual needs. A given child may spend two to three hours a day there; another may spend 30 minutes daily or an hour twice a week. Flexibility is a necessary attribute for the teacher and other school personnel. Children may be seen individually or in small groups by the resource room teacher. If resource room work is coordinated with classroom activities, frequent contact between regular and special teachers is necessary. The resource room teacher is not responsible for teaching all academic material; responsibility is usually limited to a few subjects in which a child is having difficulty. This placement option is frequently referred to as ''partial integration.''

Itinerant Teacher of the Deaf. If there are not enough hearing impaired children within or near a school building to warrant establishment of a resource room, their educational needs may be met by an itinerant teacher of the deaf. The itinerant teacher travels to more than one school, providing academic tutoring. Because of travel time, the itinerant teacher often spends less time with children than would be possible in a resource room setting. Children may be seen daily but are usually seen fewer times per week. Teachers of the deaf are not enthusiastic about this type of service provision. They cite the wasted time spent traveling and the reduced opportunities for contact with classroom teachers as the major disadvantages of this placement option. On the other hand, families tend to favor itinerant services, because children attend their local community schools with classmates who are also their neighborhood playmates. For children who require two to three hours a day of special support, itinerant placement may not be feasible unless other personnel, such as audiologists, speech-language pathologists, or reading specialists, are available to provide additional support.

Regular Classroom with Support Services. This placement differs from the ones described above in that children receive no services from teachers of the deaf. Support services are provided most often by speech-language pathologists, less often by audiologists, reading specialists, or educational strategists. Hearing-impaired children who require remedial academic work are not well served by this placement option, the most common one in most public schools. Small school systems cannot provide special personnel for a few children whose ages and hearing losses are heterogenous. For mildly hearing-impaired children who exhibit good academic skills, regular sessions with a speech clinician may constitute adequate support. For more severely hearing-impaired children, this placement option is usually not adequate to meet their needs.

Regular Classroom with No Support Services. Children enrolled in this placement may have their hearing tested periodically, but regularly scheduled support services are not provided. Thousands of hearing-impaired children receive no support services. Some children are able to succeed under these circumstances, if success is loosely defined. Occasionally services are available, but are not deemed necessary for many children who have been identified. More often, the need for service, is recognized, but they are simply not available.

Of these placement options, only the last three constitute mainstreaming, unless the time spent in a resource room is minimal.

Prevalence and Effects of Mainstreaming Programs. Craig, Salem, and Craig (1976) reported data from a questionnaire survey of programs serving hearing-impaired children. Estimates of the numbers of programs and students involved in mainstreaming or integration and the criteria for student selection were obtained. Results indicated that integration into regular classes was offered by 30 percent of the residential schools, 65 percent of the day schools, and 74 percent of the day classes that responded to the questionnaire. Not surprisingly, day classes located in public schools reported the largest percentage of deaf children who attend regular classes (53 percent of those enrolled), and residential schools reported the smallest (13 percent). Most of these students were enrolled in partial integration; mainstreaming in regular classrooms with and without support services was practiced in fewer than one-third of the programs surveyed.

These authors reported that students were selected for integration and mainstreaming on the basis of their communication skills, level of academic achievement, and degree of social development. It is interesting to note that improvements in these three areas were listed also as the *objectives* of integration. Also listed as objectives were "developing self-sufficiency" and "increasing interactions between deaf and hearing students.'' The evaluation of mainstreaming programs was accomplished largely by informal means. Programs reported using ''student report cards, informal evaluations, . . . special report forms and formal observation'' as evaluative data. No definitions of informal evaluations or formal observations were given.

Descriptions of national trends, local programs, and the achievement of individual students provide interesting data but do not indicate how well children succeed in the mainstream of education. Are the objectives sought by educators achieved and, if so, to what extent? What are the characteristics of children who are successfully educated in regular classrooms? In an effort to answer these questions, Reich, Hambleton, and Houldin (1977) compared the academic achievement, communication skills, and social adjustment of children enrolled in programs representing four levels of integration: regular classroom placement without services from a teacher of the hearing impaired (full integration), regular classroom placement with service from an itinerant teacher, placement in special classes with integration into nonacademic or academic courses (partial integration), and placement in special classes for all academic work (partial segregation). The authors reported that direct comparisons could not be made among the four programs because of important differences in the personal and social characteristics among student groups. Integrated students had significantly better hearing and communication skills than segregated ones. Although the data were seriously confounded by these differences, Reich et al. concluded that integration is beneficial to academic achievement, but detrimental to social adjustment. These conclusions were based on the fact that integrated students made better progress in academic development than segregated students, whose achievement fell further behind the norms the longer they remained in school. These findings could also be interpreted as the natural result of the language deficit imposed by more severe hearing impairment. Reich et al. reported that students who are successfully integrated have highly developed oral skills, at least average intelligence, and supportive parents. Children with more severe hearing losses require more specialized support services, but the degree of hearing loss is less important than the ability to comprehend speech. The authors concluded:

> However, even when oral skills are highly developed, children with severe and profound losses seem to require a great deal of special help in school, either from the school itself or from their parents. Children with moderate or marginal losses can usually be integrated if an itinerant teacher is available to provide periodic help. Most children who can be fully integrated without special help will only have losses in the mild or marginal category. But even these children should have periodic follow-up to make sure that they are continuing to progress in the setting.

Criteria for Mainstreaming. It appears important that school systems that purport to serve hearing-impaired children be able to provide most of the placement options described previously. If they cannot, they must establish soundly based guidelines concerning the types of hearing-impaired children the school system can and will serve. Criteria for selection of students for mainstreaming and integration have been suggested by several authors (Griffing, 1970; Northcott, 1973; Simmons-Martin, 1976; Hanners, 1976; Reich, Hambleton and Houldin, 1977) including the following:

1. Language skills within one year of those associated with chronological age or within the range exhibited by other members of the class into which the child will be placed.
2. Reading and writing skills within a year of other members of the class.
3. Evidence that the child can ''handle'' the regular curriculum.
4. Social maturity, including a strong self-concept, equal to or better than that of other class members.
5. Chronological age within two years of the average age of other children in the class.
6. Acceptance of hearing-impaired children by teachers and students.
7. Acoustic environment of the classroom that is conducive to learning by the hearing-impaired child or the use of special amplification to overcome a poor auditory environment.
8. Good oral communication skills.
9. Strong parental support.

Although the criteria are reasonable, the assumption that most mainstreamed hearing-impaired children meet them is not. Children who are most likely to meet these criteria fall into two major groups: (1) children with mild to moderate hearing losses, and (2) severely hearing-impaired children who have had the benefit of early intervention and who are excellent users of amplification. Unfortunately, many children who fall into the first category have been mainstreamed from their entrance into school without adequate assessment, placement or support services. Many are unidentified. They fall farther and farther behind in academic achievement while being passed through the school system with their peers (Peterson, 1972). Even when these children manage to achieve at some acceptable level, they do not realize their full potential. Thus, they are not convincing examples of the success of the mainstreaming philosophy. Most of the mildly and moderately hearing-impaired chlldren in the schools are widely scattered and have not received adequate support services. Studies that compare them with the minority who have received a variety of excellent support services, such as the ones described in the literature supporting the mainstreaming concept, have not been reported.

Children who fall within the second category may actually achieve better than the moderately hearing impaired, probably as a result of their greater visibility. Unlike those children with milder hearing impairments, they are better identified, wear amplification more often, and receive a greater variety of support services from hearing professionals and family members. If early intervention strategies were successful, these children have the language skills necessary for success in school plus the added benefit of continued services.

Although most proponents of mainstreaming stress the necessity of good oral skills for successful integration into regular classrooms, descriptions of some programs (Mills, 1975; deSalle and Ptasnik, 1976; Kopchick, 1977) indicate that children who use manual communication may also be successfully mainstreamed with the aid of interpreters or note takers.

Successful functioning in the regular classroom may also be dependent upon certain environmental factors. One of these is the acoustic nature of the classroom in which the child is placed. As discussed in Chapter 4, the average classroom has an ambient noise level that is higher than that acceptable for normally hearing listeners and far in excess of that acceptable for hearing-impaired listeners. It is not unusual for children whose speech discrimination scores in quiet are high (above 80 percent) to understand less than 30 percent of what is heard in noisy environments that simulate classroom conditions (Ross, 1972). Significant difficulty in discriminating speech in the classroom may be the most important factor affecting performance. Probability estimates of success in the regular classroom should be based on criteria that include measures of speech reception and discrimination in noise.

If classroom noise and reverberation patterns cannot be improved, amplification systems that minimize their effects should be used. The use of FM auditory training units, which require the teacher to wear a wireless microphone (radio transmitter) and the child to wear a radio receiver, may alleviate the effects of poor acoustic conditions to an acceptable extent. If neither of these options are possible, mainstreaming decisions must be made with great care, and frequent follow-up of children is mandatory. It is doubtful that 1 percent of the classrooms in the country could meet the acoustic standards optimal for hearing-impaired children. Furthermore, fewer than 20 percent of the identified hearing-impaired children in the schools wear adequate amplification (Ross, 1977). Obviously, mainstreaming is usually done under conditions that are less than ideal.

Although many educators have interpreted P. L. 94-142 to mean that local systems *must* serve all handicapped children within their districts, this does not appear to be either feasible or desirable in some cases. If population restrictions limit the types of services that can be offered by a single system, joint county, district, or area programs may be developed. When necessary, children should be referred to programs that are better designed to meet their needs. External referral is not popular with local administrators, because funding patterns are based on the number of children enrolled in a system. The "loss" of a child means loss of revenue, so placement decisions are sometimes made because of fiscal considerations.

Placement within or external to a school system should be based on a complete evaluation of the language, communication, academic and psychosocial status of each child. Infinite variations of these factors exist among children and must be considered carefully when placement decisions are made. Many children are appropriate candidates for partial integration or special class placement during portions of their educational lives, mainstreaming during others. Too often, children are assigned to classes on the basis of their physical size, geographic location, parental preference, a single test, informal observation, or the need for one more child in a class to justify hiring an additional teacher. Unfortunately, it is the exception rather than the rule for school systems to offer the complete cascade of services described above. Hearing professionals have a responsibility to educate other school personnel regarding the needs of hearing-impaired children. If they are successful, additional personnel and services may be added.

Team Approach. The current approach to serving hearing-impaired children in the public schools involves a team of professionals. P. L. 94-142 requires a joint effort between professionals and parents in the development of the IEP. The team of professionals necessary for adequate provision of support services has been described by Brown (1976) and Davis (1977a). Members include audiologists, speech-language pathologists, teachers of the deaf, psychologists, administrators, classroom teachers, and parents. The competencies required of the team as a whole are described by Brown as follows:

1. Ability to work as a team member on diagnostic and educational teams and with regular and special education school personnel.
2. Basic knowledge of learning theory and behavior modification.
3. Thorough understanding of normal child development, with emphasis on language acquisition and development.
4. Thorough understanding of informal and formal testing techniques, including intellect, language, achievement, speechreading, social skills, and so forth.
5. Ability to administer, interpret, and use formal and informal test data in planning appropriate instructional programs.
6. Knowledge of historical approaches in teaching hearing-impaired children (i.e., oral-aural, auditory, speech-reading, natural method, manual, total communication, and cued speech).
7. Knowledge and skills in providing parent education and counseling with parents of handicapped children, hearing-impaired pupils in particular. The ability to empathize with parents and children who are hearing impaired.
8. Knowledge of auditory processing, amplification, classroom acoustics, and so forth.
9. Knowledge of audiological testing procedures (i.e., air and bone conduction, speech audiometry, site of lesion, and the significance of varying degrees and types of hearing loss).

10. A personality and an understanding that enable acceptance of differences and what they mean. (Brown, 1976, pp. 82–83).

The team evaluates, devises and carries out remedial plans, provides resource information to each other and other school personnel, and monitors progress of the children being served. When school systems do not employ some team members, their services often can be contracted for on an individual or group basis. Personnel employed by other school systems, universities, community speech and hearing centers, or other agencies may be used as consultant team members.

Team Manager. The diversity of services offered by team members and the variety of evaluation and remedial needs exhibited by children necessitate the appointment of a team manager. Theoretically, any team member could serve as manager, or the role could be rotated among professionals. A more satisfactory approach would be to designate as manager the team member who is most knowledgeable about hearing impairment and the most conversant with the variety of services that may be needed. The identity of this person will vary from team to team but should be someone who is employed by the schools. The present authors strongly support the audiologist as the team member best suited to being manager. Because of their knowledge of hearing, hearing disorders and their evaluation and habilitation, amplification, and room acoustics, audiologists are best qualified to coordinate the efforts of the team. Audiologists seldom have case loads or classes that make consultation difficult to schedule. They may be able to arrange more time for making and following up on referrals, coordinating team efforts, and conducting evaluations, especially if team management is viewed as one of their primary responsibilities. They are especially well prepared to plan and execute monitoring systems for hearing aids and auditory training equipment, a vital ingredient in the successful education of hearing-impaired children.

Development of In-Service Training. Successful placement of hearing-impaired children in public school systems depends on adequate preparation of teachers and other school personnel. In the rush toward mainstreaming, the needs of the regular educators who are responsible for the day-to-day education of the children in their classrooms have received low priority. Children are often assigned to teachers who have recieved little or no information about hearing impairment. Literature describing the educational needs of hearing-impaired children may not be easily available to general educators. List of do's and don'ts may be provided (Gildston, 1973), but these refer primarily to communication with hearing-impaired children rather than to their educational characteristics and needs. A few brief discussions of hearing impairment in schoolchildren (Pollock and Pollock, 1971; Davis 1977b) are available that can be brought to the attention of teachers by special educators.

Teachers report a high level of frustration when asked to educate hearing-impaired children. Their schedules are often interrupted for special services, they may be asked to handle unfamiliar equipment, and they are expected to teach children with special needs about which they know little.

One of the major contributions to be made by speech-language pathologists, audiologists, and teachers of the deaf is the development and administration of in-service programs designed to acquaint school personnel with hearing impairment. Several in-service programs and sets of materials have been developed (Nober, 1975; Bitter and Johnson, 1975). They consist of information and materials considered to be important to those serving hearing-impaired pupils. Existing in-service programs are based on the experiences of those who developed them, because extensive empirical data on the status of hearing-impaired children within public schools or the perceived needs of personnel serving them are not available. A survey of public school personnel reported by Davis, Shepard, Stelmachowicz, and Gorga (in press) indicated that the in-service needs of various types of school personnel differ according to their preservice training and their past experiences with hearing-impaired children. The survey also showed that teachers of the deaf and speech-language pathologists differ significantly in their perceptions of the effects of moderate hearing impairment on children. In general, teachers of the deaf view moderately hearing-impaired children as having fewer academic and social problems than do speech-language pathologists. This may result from their comparing these children to deaf, rather than to normally hearing children. Because these two types of professionals are the most likely ones to be involved in in-service training at the local level, their disparate views may confuse school personnel unless in-service is carefully planned and coordinated.

Timing and Presentation Mode. Unless it is impossible to do so, in-service training should be presented to participants *before* the school year begins. Teachers and others will feel more comfortable about establishing an effective working relationship with special children if they know what to expect and whom to consult if problems arise. The uneasiness and resentment often experienced by teachers in the absence of adequate preparation are readily transmitted to children during their initial contacts. Support should be provided to teachers as a preventive measure. Information having to do with hearing aid monitoring, for example, should be known to teachers prior to their first contact with the child, so that a systematic procedure can be instituted from the beginning of the teacher-child relationship. A knowledgeable teacher provides children with feelings of security and sets the stage for positive working relationships.

If several teachers, administrators, or other professionals are in need of information about hearing impairment, some in-service training can be provided to all of them at the same time. If several *children* are involved, it is important that their individual characteristics (the results of hearing, language and academic evaluations) be discussed with the personnel serving each child. If assessment has not been completed, the information that is available can be shared along with a description of the need and plan for additional evaluation. It is essential to obtain the cooperation of administrators, teachers and other personnel early in the school year; the more information they possess, the more cooperative they will become. Professional jargon should be avoided, but examples and illustrations of principles will be helpful. Each topic should be discussed in general terms, then applied to the individual child or children to be served. Questions should be entertained before introduction of a new topic, so that areas of confusion can be cleared up and misunderstandings avoided.

In-Service Topics. The extent to which each of the following general areas of information can be discussed will depend on the time allotted for in-service training sessions and the nature of the children to be served. An attempt should be made to cover each topic. If several short sessions are to be held rather than one longer session, initial topics should stress the information most relevant to immediate classroom management of hearing-impaired children. Such items as hearing aid checks, classroom acoustics, and communication modes should have top priority.

In-service training should include discussion of the following:

1. *Characteristics of hearing loss(es) involved.* Each child's audiogram should be explained in terms of the probable effects of the hearing loss on the reception and discrimination of speech. The extent to which visual information will be necessary as an adjunct to hearing should be estimated. The effects of distance from the speaker to the child and the need to locate sound sources and emphasize visual materials should be explained.
2. *Communication modes.* The various receptive and expressive modes employed by hearing-impaired children in communication should be described. The importance of audition, supplemented by lipreading, to effective communication should be stressed. A major purpose of in-service training is to prepare personnel to help children achieve their potential. For moderately hearing-impaired children, the use of their hearing for learning is a primary goal. At the same time educators should be reminded of the need for facing the child and speaking clearly so that lipreading can also occur.

   If any of the children under discussion use manual communication, the nature of fingerspelling and sign language should be discussed. Care should be taken not to intimate that the manual forms of reception and expression are last-resort or undesirable modes of communication. Their practicality and contribution to effective communication should be made evident. If several children use manual communication, sign language instruction should be offered to teachers and children attending the school.
3. *Use of amplification.* General principles of amplification should be explained, without technical detail. The fact that hearing aids amplify *all* sounds but do not provide normal hearing should be stressed. The types of

hearing aids worn by the children involved should be shown and practice in manipulating controls and components provided. The need for daily hearing aid monitoring should be stressed. Instructions for conducting listening checks of hearing aid function can be given in oral *and* handout form and practice in completing the required steps provided. (See Chapter 4 for listening check instructions.) Hearing aid troubleshooting charts may also be distributed.

4. *Classroom acoustics.* The acoustic nature of classrooms should be described as they relate to the presence of hearing loss and the use of amplification. Suggestions can be given for reducing ambient noise and reverberation within classrooms (see Chapter 4). Optimal placement of children and teacher within a given classroom should be discussed. Alternate forms of amplification, such as FM transmitters and receivers, can be demonstrated, if appropriate.
5. *Language and educational characteristics.* The effects of hearing loss on language development should be presented briefly, then related to the specific deficits exhibited by the children to be served. The relationship between the language problem and the comprehension of instructions, curriculum materials, and communication with teachers and peers should be defined. Where possible, common classroom tasks should be divided into the subskills necessary for adequate performance. For example, a reading readiness activity that involves matching pictures to alphabet letters (dog to *d,* rake to *r*) requires certain basic skills and information. The names of the pictures must be known, the instructions must be audible, and the child must be familiar with the alphabet. Special vocabulary and phrases (*match, same as, draw a line between, connect,* and *begins with*) must also be comprehended. These subskills can then be related to the communicative and language status of the hearing-impaired children under discussion. Few pedagogic details and many brief examples will illustrate effectively the impact of language delay on educational achievement.
6. *Responsibility of team members.* If several professionals are available as members of a support team a brief explanation of the specific responsibilities of each should be made. If possible, each team member should be present and introduced. Questions addressed to these professionals are encouraged. Offers to serve as consultants should be accompanied by copies of scheduled visits to the school, office hours and telephone numbers, and requests to set a date for an initial visit to each teacher's classroom.

Follow-up of In-Service Training. The importance of rapid follow-up contact with participants in the in-service training cannot be overemphasized. At least one team member should visit teachers in their own classrooms as soon as possible. The visit should consist of observation, casual conversation, and an opportunity for the teacher to ask questions that have occurred. The first visit should be brief, informal and friendly. If problems are observed they should be mentioned casually, if at all. Only those problems that involve factors outside the immediate control of the teacher, such as noise sources or inoperative amplification units, should be brought up during the initial visit. Later, when a trust relationship has developed between the teacher and the team members, plans can be made jointly for working out any difficulties encountered. Specialists within school systems are sometimes resented by teachers, who may misinterpret the specialist's role or be threatened by their own feelings of insecurity in a unique situation. Some beginning clinicians react to their own insecure feelings by "coming on strong," thus adding to the tension that may exist between teacher and specialist. The first task of the hearing specialist within the school is to establish a friendly working relationship with school personnel, based on a mutual respect and understanding of the roles each has in the overall education of children. Children have received inadequate support services as a result of animosity among the personnel involved in their education, none of whom are willing to compromise on details, or admit that others are as important to the child's success as themselves. The development of personality conflicts and power struggles can be minimized when personnel understand the roles played by others who are involved in educational management. Time thus spent will reap important benefits and contribute to the successful management of hearing-impaired children in the schools.

REFERENCES

Balow, I. and Brill, R., An evaluation of reading and academic levels of sixteen graduating classes of the California School for the Deaf, *Volta Rev.,* 77, 255–266, 1975.

Bitter, G. and Johnson, J., *SYSTEMS O.N.E.* Salt Lake City: Educational Media Center, 207 Milton Bennion Hall, University of Utah, 1974.

Brasel, K. and Quigley, S., The influence of certain language and communication environments in early childhood on the development of language in deaf individuals, *J. Speech Hearing Res.,* 20, 95–107, 1977.

Brill, R., Mainstreaming: Format or quality? *Amer. Ann. Deaf,* 120, 377–381, 1975.

Brown, J., Contemporary programming for children with hearing impairments. In *Serving Hard-of-Hearing Pupils: Alternative Strategies for Personnel Preparation.* Report of a Summary Conference sponsored by BEH, USOE, Atlanta, 1976.

Connor, L., Deaf and hearing children at the Lexington School for the Deaf or Mainstreaming the special school. In G. Nix (Ed.), *Mainstreaming Education for Hearing Impaired Children and Youth.* New York: Grune and Stratton, 1976.

Cornett, R., *Cued Speech Parent Training and Follow-up Program.* Washington, D.C.: Bureau of Education for Handicapped DHEW, 96, 1972.

Craig, H., A sociometric investigation of the self concept of the deaf child, *Amer. Ann. Deaf,* 110, 456–478, 1965.

Craig, W. and Salem, J., Partial integration of deaf with hearing students: Residential school perspectives, *Amer. Ann. Deaf,* 120, 28-36, 1975.
Craig, W., Salem, J., and Craig, H., Mainstreaming and partial integration of deaf with hearing students, *Amer. Ann. Deaf,* 121, 63-68, 1976.
Davis, J., Personnel and services. In J. Davis (Ed.), *Our Forgotten Children.* Minneapolis, MN: National Support Systems Project, Bureau of Education for the Handicapped, USOE, 1977a.
Davis, J. (Ed.), *Our Forgotten Children: Hard of Hearing Pupils in the Schools.* Minneapolis: Audio Visual Library Service, University of Minnesota, 1977b.
Davis, J., Shepard, N., Stelmachowicz, P., and Gorga, M., Perceptions of hearing impairment held by school personnel: Suggestions for inservice training development, *Language, Speech and Hearing Services in the Schools,* in press.
deSalle, J. and Ptasnik, J., Some problems and solutions: High school mainstreaming of the hearing impaired, *Amer. Ann. Deaf,* 121, 533-536, 1976.
Denton, D., A study in the educational achievement of deaf children. In *Report of the Proceedings of the 42nd Meeting of the Convention of American Instructors of the Deaf.* Washington, D.C.: U.S. Government Printing Office, 428-433, 1966.
Dunn, L., Special education for the mildly retarded: Is much of it justified? *Except. Chil.,* 35, 13-20, 1968.
Garretson, M., The least restrictive environment, *The Deaf American,* 29, 25, 1977.
Gildston, P., Do's and don'ts for the classroom teacher. In W. Northcott (ed.), *The Hearing Impaired Child in a Regular Classroom.* Washington, D.C.: A. G. Bell Association, 1973.
Griffing, B., Planning educational programs and services for hard of hearing children. In F. Berg and S. Fletcher (Eds.), *The Hard of Hearing Child.* New York: Grune and Stratton, 1970.
Hanners, B., The audiologist as educator: The ultimate hearing aide. In G. Nix (ed.), *Mainstream Education for Hearing Impaired Children and Youth.* New York: Grune and Stratton, 1976.
van den Horst, A., Defective hearing, school achievements, and school choice, *Teach. Deaf,* 69, 398-414, 1971.
Jensema, C. and Trybus, R., Communication patterns and educational achievement of hearing impaired students, Series T, Number 2, Office of Demographic Studies, (August) 1978.
Kaufman, M., A follow-up study on reading test results of deaf children, *Amer. Ann. Deaf,* 110, 420-423, 1965.
Kopchick, E., Mainstreaming deaf students using team teaching, *Amer. Ann. Deaf,* 122, 522-524, 1977.
Lawrence, C. and Kapfer, M., The potential of current trends in public education for the hard of hearing child. In F. Berg and S. Fletcher (Eds.), *The Hard of Hearing Child.* New York: Grune and Stratton, 1970.
Ling, D., *Speech and the Hearing Impaired Child.* Washington, D.C.: A. G. Bell Association, 1976.
McCroskey, R., Final progress report of four-year home training program. Paper presented at A. G. Bell National Convention, San Francisco, 1968.

Meadow, K., Early manual communication in relation to the deaf child's intellectual, social and communicative functioning, *Amer. Ann. Deaf,* 113, 29-41, 1968.

Mills, M., Total communication in the public schools. Seminar presentation at the North Central Regional Conference, American Speech and Hearing Association, 1975.

Mindel, E. and Vernon, M., *They Grow in Silence: The Deaf Child and His Family.* Silver Springs, MD: National Association of the Deaf, 1971.

Moores, D., Neo-oralism and education of the deaf in the Soviet Union, *Except. Chil.,* 38, 377-384, 1972.

Moores, D., *Educating the Deaf: Psychology, Principles and Practices.* Boston: Houghton Mifflin, 1978.

Moores, D. and McIntyre, C., *Evaluation of Programs for Hearing Impaired Children, Report of 1970-1971.* Research Report No. 27, University of Minnesota Research, Development and Demonstration Center in Education of Handicapped Children, 1971.

Moores, D., McIntyre, C., and Weiss, K., *Evaluation of Programs for Hearing Impaired Children, Report of 1971-1972.* Research Report No. 39, University of Minnesota Research, Development and Demonstration Center in Education of Handicapped Children, 1972.

Moores, D., Weiss, K., and Goodwin, M., *Evaluation of Programs for Hearing Impaired Children, Report of 1972-1973.* Research Report No. 57, University of Minnesota Research, Development and Demonstration Center in Education of Handicapped Children, 1973.

Moores, D., Weiss, K., and Goodwin, M., *Evaluation of Programs for Hearing Impaired Children: Report of 1973-1974.* Research Report No. 81, University of Minnesota Research, Development and Demonstration Center in Education of Handicapped Children, 1974.

Moores, D., Weiss, K., and Goodwin, M., Early education programs for hearing impaired children: Major findings, *Amer. Ann. Deaf,* 123, 925-936, 1978.

Nix, G., Total communication: A review of the studies offered in its support, *Volta Rev.,* 77, 470-494, 1975.

Nober, L., *Hearing Impaired Formal Inservice Program.* Northeast Regional Media Center for the Deaf, 1975.

Northcott, W., *The Hearing Impaired Child in a Regular Classroom.* Washington, D.C.: A G. Bell Association, 1973.

Peterson, M., Achievement of hard of hearing students in regular public schools, Ph.D. Dissertation, Wayne State University, 1972.

Phillips, W., Influence of preschool training on language arts, arithmetic concepts and socialization of young deaf children, Ph.D. Dissertation, Columbia University, 1963.

Pollack, D., *Educational Audiology for the Limited Hearing Infant.* Springfield, IL: Charles C Thomas, 1970.

Pollock, M. and Pollock, K., Letter to the teacher of a hard-of-hearing child, *Childhood Educ.,* 206-209, (January) 1971.

Porter, G., The missing vital dimension in successful integration, *Volta Rev.,* 77, 416-422, 1975.

Public Law 94-142: The Education for All Handicapped Children Act, *Federal Register,* August 23, 1977, Part II.

Quigley, S., *The Influence of Fingerspelling on the Development of Language, Communica-*

tion, and Educational Achievement of Deaf Children. Champaign-Urbana: University of Illinois Press, 1969.

Quigley, S. and Frisina, D., *Institutionalization and Psycho-Educational Development of Deaf Children*. Washington, D.C.: CEC Research Monograph, 1961.

Reich, C., Hambleton, D., and Houldin, B., The integration of hearing impaired children in regular classrooms, *Amer. Ann. Deaf,* 122, 534–543, 1977.

Rister, A., Deaf children in mainstream education, *Volta Rev.,* 77, 279–290, 1975.

Ross, M., Classroom acoustics and speech intelligibility. In J. Katz (Ed.), *Handbook of Clinical Audiology*. Baltimore: Williams and Wilkins Co., 1972.

Ross, M., Model educational cascade for hearing impaired children. In G. Nix (ed.), *Mainstream Education for Hearing Impaired Children and Youth*. New York: Grune and Stratton, 1976.

Ross, M., Definitions and descriptions. In J. Davis (Ed.), *Our Forgotten Children*. Minneapolis, MN: National Support Systems Project, Bureau of Education for the Handicapped, USOE, 1977.

Schein, J., *The Deaf Community: Studies in the Social Psychology of Deafness*. Washington, D.C.: Gallaudet College Press, 1968.

Schlesinger, H. and Meadow, K., *Sound and Sign: Childhood Deafness and Mental Health*. Berkeley: University of California Press, 1972.

Scouten, E., *A Re-evaluation of the Rochester Method*. Rochester, N.Y.: Rochester School for the Deaf, 1942.

Simmons-Martin, A., The Central Institute for the Deaf demonstration home program. In G. Nix (Ed.), *Mainstream Education for Hearing Impaired Children and Youth*. New York: Grune and Stratton, 1976.

Stevenson, E., A study of the educational achievement of deaf children of deaf parents, *California News* (Berkeley: California School for the Deaf), 80, 143, 1964.

Stuckless, E. and Birch, J., The influence of early manual communication on the linguistic development of deaf children, *Amer. Ann. Deaf,* 111, 452–460, 499–504, 1966.

Vernon, M. and Koh, S., Effects of manual communication on deaf children's educational achievement, linguistic competence, oral skills, and psychological development, *Amer. Ann. Deaf,* 115, 527–536, 1970.

Vernon, M. and Koh, S., Effects of oral preschool compared to early manual communication on education and communication in deaf children, *Amer. Ann. Deaf,* 116, 569–574, 1971.

Weiss, K., Goodwin, M., and Moores, D., *Evaluation of Programs for Hearing Impaired Children: 1969–1974*. Research Report No. 91, University of Minnesota Research, Development and Demonstration Center in Education of Handicapped Children, 1975.

Whetnall, E. and Fry, D., *The Deaf Child*. Springfield, IL: Charles C Thomas, 1964.

CHAPTER 11

Assessment and Treatment of Psychosocial Problems

The psychosocial implications of hearing impairment have been of interest to investigators since the early 1800s. The fundamental question is the extent to which cognition depends on language development and vice versa. The manner in which the basic question is answered often determines the philosophy by which professionals operate in their contacts with hearing-impaired persons. Conflicting opinions and data exist to such an extent, however, that the suspicion arises that authors either are not talking about the same things or are defining them in different ways. A case in point is the word "language," which has not been defined precisely when used in conjunction with hearing impairment. Although authors do not say so, they appear to equate "language" with "English" or some other spoken linguistic code.

The extent to which cognition and language are interdependent has been argued vigorously by Ray (1847), James (1890), Binet and Simon (1910) and more recently by Myklebust (1953), Furth (1966), Shif (1969), and Tomlinson-Keasey and Kelly (1974). Moores (1978) reviewed the early literature and challenged the assumption that severely hearing-impaired people do not develop language. Moores suggested that investigations of dependence of thought on language or the reverse should not be centered on hearing-impaired subjects under the assumption that they have not developed language skills. Many of them have not developed adequate English skills; their language skills per se have not been measured. It may be unfortunate that the tools by which we measure language are usually measures of English, and measures of cognition are also English based.

PSYCHOSOCIAL CHARACTERISTICS ASSOCIATED WITH HEARING IMPAIRMENT

Difficulties in the comprehension and expression of the common code of their environment has influenced the assessment of various psychosocial skills in hearing-impaired persons. This is particularly true of investigations of intelligence and personality, but measures of social acceptance and self-concept are probably affected as well.

Intelligence

Studies of the effects of hearing impairment on intelligence have been limited to the deaf. Although the definition of deafness given by most investigators has been vague, it is clear that their subjects were severely hearing impaired. The view of the nature of intelligence associated with deafness has progressed through several stages since the early 1940s (Moores, 1978). Prior to 1950 the prevailing view held that deafness resulted in inferior intelligence compared to that of normally hearing persons (Pintner, Eisenson, and Stanton, 1941). Many studies contributed to this view, even though their results were inconsistent and difficult to interpret. Because performance-type activities were used as measures, investigators assumed that the verbal deficits associated with deafness had not influenced the subject's ability to perform on the tasks.

In 1953 Myklebust presented his *organismic shift theory,* concerning the intelligence of deaf persons. He disagreed with the early position that deafness resulted in inferior intelligence. Instead, Myklebust argued that deafness causes individuals to organize their perceptions of the world on a restricted basis. Personality, intellect, and behavior are qualitatively different from those of normally hearing persons. For lack of a better word, Myklebust described the result of the organismic shift as "concrete thinking." With little evidence to support this claim, he asserted that deaf children must function on a concrete level; because they cannot hear, their interactions with the environment leave them incapable of abstract thought and reasoning. Myklebust's statements have been used to support the need to emphasize the use of the auditory system in early infancy in order to prevent the development of concrete, rather than abstract, thinking skills.

Rosenstein (1961) disagreed with Myklebust's gloomy view of deafness and abstractions, citing the inconsistent and contradictory use of terms, assessment tasks, and interpretations of results by investigators. He postulated that when the linguistic nature of test items was beyond the experience of the children being tested, performance was poor. Rosenstein argued, therefore, for a *linguistic* deficit instead of a cognitive one. Furth (1964) reviewed literature on language and cognition and advanced an *experiential deficit* theory. He concluded that the performance of deaf persons on cognitive tasks was influenced by a lack of appropriate experience with similar tasks under favorable circumstances. Linguistic restrictions further limited understanding of the tasks.

Vernon (1968a) reviewed all available studies of intelligence in the deaf population from 1930 to 1966. Contrary to the popular view that deaf persons score below those with normal hearing on tests of intellectual functioning, Vernon's review revealed that deaf children were superior to normally hearing children in 13 of the 31 studies reported. He concluded that deaf children perform as well as normally hearing children on a variety of tasks designed to measure intellectual functioning. In a series of studies of children whose deafness was caused by various etiologies Vernon (1967a, 1967b, 1967c, 1968b) reported the incidence of multiple handicaps associated with different etiologies and their effects on IQ measures. These data illustrate the dangers of treating deaf persons as a homogeneous group, especially when discussing global characteristics such as intelligence.

By the 1960s most investigators had concluded that deafness does not result in intellectual deficit. In a way, this is surprising, in view of the relationship between the testers' knowledge of deafness and the results obtained. Vernon (1968a) showed that researchers who are experienced in the psychological evaluation of hearing-impaired children obtain fewer differences between deaf and normally hearing groups than inexperienced examiners. According to a survey reported by Levine (1974), 83 percent of the psychologists in the United States who were working with hearing-impaired children had no special preparation for the task, and 90 percent of them were unable to communicate in sign language. The Levine survey revealed that the most popular intelligence test in use with hearing-impaired children was the performance portion of the *Wechsler Intelligence Scale for Children (WISC)*. This test is described by Vernon and Brown (1964) as an appropriate test for use with this population. Unfortunately, however, the subtest directions involve verbal instructions that must be understood for optimal performance. The use of pantomime or visual aids for giving instructions, such as pictures or sequence cards, have been suggested by Murphy (1957), Neuhaus (1967), and Reed (1970). Sullivan (1978) investigated the performance of hearing-impaired children on the *WISC* when directions were (1) pantomimed, (2) given with visual clues, and (3) given in total communication, using speech, signs, and fingerspelling simultaneously. The children in her study all used total communication in their classrooms; they obtained significantly higher scores when instructions were given to them in the total communication mode. The overall difference in scores amounted to more than 20 IQ points.

Appropriate IQ Tests. In view of the influence of communication style on the results obtained, it is important to interpret intelligence test results with caution. Vernon and Brown (1964) discuss appropriate tests for use with hearing-impaired children; psychologists serving such children should be referred to their article as a guide to test selection. In general, tests should be administered that allow for separation of verbal and performance scores. Tests that yield a single score (*Stanford-Binet Intelligence Scale,* for example) are inappropriate for use with the hearing impaired because any existing language deficit will negatively influence the obtained IQ score. The *Stanford-Binet* test is widely used by school psychologists, however, and many hearing-impaired children have been labeled mentally retarded on the basis of its use. This is especially true of children whose hearing losses are not obvious. If hearing loss is not identified and reported to the psychologist prior to testing, misdiagnosis may occur. When the test protocol allows it, verbal, performance, and total scores should be reported separately so that a complete picture of intellectual functioning can be obtained. Hearing-impaired children typically show significant differences between verbal and performance scores on intelligence tests.

A few measures of intelligence have been standardized on populations of hearing-impaired children. The best known of these is the *Nebraska Test of Learning Aptitude,* norms for which are available for deaf and normally hearing children. Instructions are pantomimed for deaf, spoken for normally hearing children. The norms for deaf children can only be used if instructions are not spoken. Therefore, when the test is administered to children with any degree of hearing loss, the decision as to which norms will be used must be made prior to test administration and instructions given in the appropriate way.

As is the case with language and academic achievement, investigations of intelligence and hearing impairment have concentrated on deaf people. The studies reported have undoubtedly included subjects with moderate hearing losses, but their patterns of cognitive functioning have not been reported separately.

Personality and Emotional Adjustment

Another aspect of psychosocial development that has been studied is personality development. Unlike the area of intellectual assessment, this aspect of psychological evaluation does not use assessment tools that are recognized as being valid or reliable for a variety of populations. There are three major approaches to the assessment of personality structure: projective techniques, objective tests, and behavioral observations. The tests used will depend on the theoretical base adhered to by the individual psychologist. There are no personality tests designed specifically for use with hearing-impaired subjects. This is unfortunate due to the verbal nature of the available tests and the influence it may have on results obtained from hearing-impaired people.

Personality Traits of the Deaf. Most investigators have concluded that deaf persons exhibit atypical personality patterns. On the basis of projective and personality test data, they have been described as egocentric, impulsive, coercively dependent (Altshuler, 1962); neurotic and introverted (Pintner, Fusfeld and Brunswig, 1937); immature and submissive (Soloman, 1943); irritable, suggestible, and lacking impulse control (Levine, 1956); inadequate and inappropriate (Stewart, 1971); and aggressive (Heider and Heider, 1940).

Although Myklebust (1964) indicated that deaf persons' responses to the *Minnesota Multiphasic Personality Inventory (MMPI)* suggested psychosis, and Springer and Roslow (1938) reported a high incidence of neurosis in the deaf, studies of patients being treated for mental disorders revealed an incidence of psychosis and neurosis in the deaf population similar to that in the hearing population (Rainer and Altshuler, 1970). The major psychoneurotic reactions observed in hearing-impaired patients were anxiety based. Rainer and Altshuler concluded that deafness was not a significant cause of the anxiety, but may have contributed to early developmental factors that resulted in anxiety.

Descriptions of the personality traits associated with hearing impairment have also been made on the basis of surveys of teacher or counselor opinion. Meadow and Schlesinger (1971) administered a questionnaire to teachers and counselors at a residential school for the deaf. They found an incidence of emotional disturbance (12 percent) that was five times that associated with normally hearing children. Survey respondents also indicated almost three times as many behavioral problems in deaf students than would be expected on the basis of data for normally hearing children.

In a departure from the use of personality tests or teacher ratings of traits, Reivich and Rothrock (1972) gathered data from teachers of the deaf using a *Behavior Problem Checklist (BPC)*. The *BPC* consists of 65 descriptions of behavior that measure four dimensions: conduct disorders, personality disorders, inadequacy-immaturity, and socialized delinquency. Factor analysis of data for 327 deaf students revealed that the factors found for deaf children were more similar to than different from those of normally hearing children. Two factors that appeared to be unique to the deaf subjects were isolation and communication problems; they accounted for 10 percent of the variance. These results indicate that the behavior of deaf children is very similar to that of normally hearing hearing children, but is significantly influenced by two specific behavior clusters associated with deafness. Further research of this nature might yield more useful information than is currently available for understanding the behavior patterns of deaf persons.

People who have no contact with deaf adults may conclude from the available studies that deaf people are emotionally disabled. It is more difficult for persons familiar with this population to accept the descriptions of personality deviance that fill the literature. Far from exhibiting the antisocial behavior and poor coping mechanisms expected on the basis of research results, most hearing-impaired people are indistinguishable from normally hearing people with regard to their sociability, ability to function as integrated personalities, and approaches toward family and community life. The incidence of emotional disturbance appears to be similar to that in the normally hearing population. It is present, but it is not the norm. Under these circumstances, why are research results so negative?

Several factors may account for the results obtained. The test instruments used are not appropriate for the deaf population because they require advanced English language facility and oral communication skills. Projective tests, such as the *Rorshach* or *Thematic Apperception Test,* require subjects to describe ambiguous pictures or ink blots. The level of detail and imagination used in descriptions influences their scoring. In other words, subjects' personalities are judged by the content of their verbal output. Because the majority of the studies have been done with deaf people whose verbal output could be expected to be low, the tasks themselves were biased aginst the population with whom they were employed. Communication between examiners and subjects was limited by the oral skills of the subjects, which are not described. In only one study reporting Rorshach data were deaf students encouraged to use sign to express themselves (Levine, 1956). Unfortunately, the examiner did not sign and all students were enrolled in an oral school for the deaf where signing was actively discouraged (Moores, 1978).

Paper-and-pencil personality tests, such as the *California Test of Personality* and the *MMPI* require subjects to read and comprehend complex sentences, choose between pairs of sentences as a description of preferred behavior, or judge the degree to which activities or opinions expressed in sentence form are representative of their own behavior. Because the average reading achievement level of the deaf is below fifth grade, it is doubtful that many subjects understood the materials well enough to yield valid responses.

Another factor that contributes to the questionable validity of the reported research concerns the interpretation of responses on the basis of norms for normally hearing persons. Failure to identify with personality test statements such as "I am the life of the party" or "I can talk to strangers with ease," may result in high scores on introversion, withdrawal, or shyness scales, but they may also represent healthy adjustment to the inability to hear and understand conversation easily. Moores (1978) points out that the belief that persons are hostile toward you represents paranoia only if it isn't true. Many hearing-impaired people experience hostility or indifference from others, and their feelings of mistrust are well founded.

The inability of most researchers to communicate with hearing-impaired subjects also casts doubt on the results of personality studies. Donoghue (1968) reviewed the pertinent literature and suggested that the inability of examiners to communicate with hearing-impaired subjects contributed to judgments of emotional immaturity, rigidity, egocentricity, and paranoia.

Schlesinger and Meadow (1972) have questioned the validity of measuring personality traits in isolation and attributing personality differences that may be observed to deafness itself. Recognizing the influence of environment on personality development, they suggest an analysis of the entire life cycle of hearing-impaired persons if insight into their adaptive patterns is to occur. The model they propose is discussed later in this chapter.

Personality Traits Associated with Moderate Hearing Impairment. Several studies have compared the emotional adjustment patterns of moderately hearing-impaired people to other groups. One of the earliest studies was reported by Pintner (1942). He administered the *Aspects of Personality Test* to 1171 hearing impaired and 1208 normally hearing children in New York City. The hearing losses of the experimental group were not defined; some children were included in the group on the basis of teacher observation alone. Pintner found no differences between the two groups on measures of ascendance-submission or extroversion-introversion. He reported that children having "greater" hearing loss scored lower on overall measures of emotional stability.

Kahn (1957) attempted to measure the responses to frustration of three groups of 15 normally hearing, 15 moderately hearing-impaired, and 15 severely hearing-impaired children. Kahn did not define hearing loss in decibels, but in percentages based on the AMA method of determining degree of hearing loss. "Moderately" hearing-impaired children were described as having a 3 to 25 percent loss, and "severely" hearing-impaired children had losses greater than 25 percent.

Kahn administered a projective test of frustration in which children responded verbally to (1) pictures depicting events that might be frustrating to children and (2) an actual test of frustration, which required reproduction of complex block designs from examples providing too little information. Results of both tasks were interpreted by Kahn as favoring hearing-impaired children. They met frustration more constructively than their normally hearing peers, giving responses that emphasized solutions, alleviation of problems, and removal of frustration barriers. He concluded that hearing-impaired children respond more positively to frustration than normally hearing children do. Perhaps they have had more practice, although Kahn does not suggest this.

In 1966 Fisher reported the results of an investigation of the adjustment patterns of hearing-impaired and normal children. Hearing-impaired subjects consisted of 51 children with conductive hearing losses, 25 with ''perceptive'' losses, and seven with mixed losses. Results of the study indicated that hearing-impaired children were significantly less well-adjusted than their normally hearing peers. While 28 percent of the normally hearing children were classified as having ''unsatisfactory adjustment,'' 47 percent of the hearing-impaired children were so classified. Fisher reported that girls were more maladjusted than boys. Subjects exhibited the following adjustment patterns:

Hearing Impaired (%)		**Control (%)**
33	Demonstrative (aggressive)	65
26	Withdrawal	22
41	Mixed	13
100		100

These data indicate that hearing-impaired children are not more aggressive nor withdrawn than normally hearing children generally. Instead, hearing-impaired children seem to exhibit flexible patterns of adjustment, sometimes acting out when upset and withdrawing at other times. If anything, they appear to be less likely to engage in aggressive behavior as a means of resolving conflict than normally hearing children, who use this avenue of release more frequently than any other. It can be hypothesized that the different patterns of adjustment are related to self-concept and self-assurance, but data do not exist at present to support that contention.

As part of a larger study, Goetzinger, Harrison, and Baer (1964) investigated the emotional adjustment of 20 children with hearing losses between 20 and 35 dB (no reference given). Estimates of adjustment came from teachers, who rated few of the hearing-impaired children as good or excellent in attitudes, manners, or general emotional behavior compared to normally hearing children matched for age and sex. Teachers also judged the hearing-impaired children to exhibit a higher incidence of introversion, poor work habits, shyness, need for encouragement, and emotional variability. The last item seems to corroborate Fisher's findings regarding the employment of a mixture of aggression and withdrawal in the emotional adjustment patterns of hearing-impaired children.

Myklebust (1964) administered a personality test to adults whose hearing losses were congenital or adventitious. He identified the latter group as hard of hearing. Myklebust found differences between males and females within groups and between groups. He concluded that all hearing-impaired subjects exhibited poorer emotional adjustment than the normally hearing controls. Emotional maladjustment was greatest for deaf males, least for hard-of-hearing females. Within both groups, males indicated poorer adjustment than females. The hard-of-hearing groups appeared more depressed than the deaf. Myklebust concluded that hard-of-hearing adults are more aware of hearing loss as a handicap than are the deaf. Unfortunately, the effects of degree of hearing impairment are confounded with age of onset in the study.

The studies reviewed above illustrate the difficulties inherent in making definitive statements about the personality traits or emotional adjustment of hearing-impaired persons. Moderately hearing-impaired subjects do not appear to differ significantly from normally hearing persons in emotional adjustment. By contrast, deaf persons are described as being seriously maladjusted. In view of the problems inherent in the research reported above, it is unlikely that either of these extremes is an accurate representation of the psychosocial status of persons with hearing impairment.

Social Acceptance and Self-Concept

There is increasing concern among professionals regarding the social status of hearing-impaired children and adolescents. Hearing loss is often described as an isolation disorder, contributing to feelings of loneliness and rejection. The concept of self that develops when interaction with others is restricted influences overall social functioning. Whether they attend special educational programs or are being educated with normally hearing peers, the degree to which children are able to interact and the ease with which they establish meaningful relationships with others are important to their maturation. The move away from residential school placement and toward public school education has emphasized the importance of adequate social skills in hearing-impaired children. Unfortunately, there are no guidelines for use in fostering development of these skills. Indeed, little is known about the status of the existing social skills of the hearing-impaired population.

Measures of Social Adjustment. The nature of social problems is such that they do not lend themselves easily to investigation. The measurement of feelings of isolation and insecurity in social situations is a chancy thing. How can a numerical value be placed on the degree of acceptance experienced by children or the degree to which they are included in social activities by others? What measure can be made of the quality of social interactions? Because of the methodological difficulties involved, more opinions than data are available on the subject. Some proponents of mainstreaming minimize or ignore social problems. They cite testimonial evidence of hearing-impaired children's popularity among normally hearing classmates. The latter are described as interested, helpful, concerned, friendly, and supportive. By contrast, hearing-impaired children and their teachers report a more negative view of the social realities involved. Children report having few friends, being teased or ignored, and feeling inadequate in social situations. Teachers report a high incidence of social maladjustment among hearing-impaired children regardless of the degree of hearing loss involved.

Interview Data. The most direct evidence of the social status of hearing-impaired children was reported by Peterson (1972). She conducted interviews with hearing-impaired children from two types of educational placements to elicit self-appraisal regarding their academic and social status. Ten children who were enrolled in regular classes were compared to eight children from special classes; a group of normally hearing children was also interviewed. The mainstreamed group received minimal support services from a speech-language pathologist; students in the special program were enrolled in resource or self-contained classrooms with some integration. Each child was asked to describe problems being experienced. Peterson identified three problems common to all three groups: occasional difficulty with a particular teacher or course, limited communication with parents, and sibling rivalry. Hearing-impaired children reported a high incidence of social problems. The most striking difference between the two groups of hearing-impaired children was their adjustment to having hearing losses and defective speech. The students who attended regular classes were resentful of their hearing aids and speech problems, and they seemed at a loss as to how to cope with the social problems encountered. By contrast, students from special placements showed good adjustment to their hearing aids; they seemed to have more friends and to be capable of coping with the everyday problems they faced.

The following excerpts from Peterson's interviews are typical of the comments made by the mainstreamed children:

> The student was then asked if she were experiencing any other difficulties. She began to tear and said that she did not have any friends. She then related an occurrence of the previous day. She had written a note to a classmate asking that she eat lunch with her. The classmate agreed but did not meet her at the appointed place; later the classmate was found in the cafeteria sitting with a group of girls. The classmate claimed to have forgotten the date but did not invite the student to join the group, rather she terminated the conversation by saying that perhaps they could eat together another time.
>
> She also reported that on many occasions she had approached groups of girls in the halls or cafeteria, but, "I don't know what they are talking about and I don't know what to say, and when I ask they say they will tell me later, but they don't. The girls laugh a lot especially when the boys are around, but I can't hear what they are laughing at. Sometimes I think they are laughing at me but I can't think of any funny things to say to them. My older sister always says funny things at home and every night I try to remember all the funny things she has said so that I can say them at school the next day, but I just can't remember them." The girl also said, "I even bought a book about how to make friends but that didn't help either. I just don't know how to do it."
>
> When asked about other problems, the student began to cry. She said that she had one friend who was also in the teacher-counselor program, but they were only friends at school. She explained that, "The kids don't like me. They can't understand what I say, but they don't ask me to repeat things anymore. They don't want me around." The student was equally distressed at the fact that she would be entering high school soon and if there was no teacher-counselor program in the high school, she would have no friends

> at all. She then said that her mother had told her to tell her classmates that some children wear glasses, braces, etc. The subject commented, "Even if you wear glasses you talk right and people don't think you're 'different' or 'weird'." She then appealed for any suggestions regarding how she might proceed to acquire a few friends. . .

Sociometric Measures of Social Status. Two other types of investigations provide data relevant to the social status of hearing-impaired children: measures of self-concept and social acceptance. Measures of the social status of hearing-impaired children have come primarily from sociometric procedures employed within classrooms. Elser (1959) conducted a study designed to compare the social position of hearing-impaired children with that of normally hearing children in the same classrooms. He measured general social status, friendship, reputation, and accuracy of perception by children as to who would choose them as friends. The friendship measure required children to name three children in the class whom they would and would not choose as friends, playmates, or lunchroom associates. The reputation measure involved guessing who was best and worst at playing games, who was most and least popular, who was smartest and least smart, and so on. The perception measure required children to name classmates they thought had or had not selected them for a friend or playmate. Status was determined by combining the results of the measures.

Results of the sociometric testing revealed that hearing-impaired children were not as accepted as the average by their classmates. There were few differences in the friendship measure, although the children least accepted as friends were those whose losses fell between 39 and 49 dB and those not wearing hearing aids. Elser hypothesized that children are more accepting of handicapped children who are clearly identified as such, possibly because attempts to "hide" a hearing loss result in behavior that is unacceptable to peers without some obvious reason. Hearing-impaired children did not enjoy as favorable a reputation as the average member of their classes. Estimates of their ability to play games, popularity, rating as a good sport, and ability to get their lessons easily fell below the average. There were no differences on ratings of personality. The accuracy of perception of who would choose them as friends was no different for the hearing impaired than the normally hearing children. According to Elser's data children with hearing impairments fall into the bottom third of their classes in status among their peers. Elser concluded that sociometric measures were not good bases for placement decisions but might offer supplementary information to educators concerning the social status of hearing-impaired children.

Kennedy and Bruininks (1974) investigated the peer status and self-perceived peer status of first- and second-grade hearing-impaired and normally hearing children in regular classrooms. Children with hearing loss were divided into two groups whose losses ranged from 45 to 74 dB and from 75 to 110 dB (no reference given). Three sociometric tests were used to measure social acceptance and perceived social acceptance. Results of the sociometric measures indicated that hearing-impaired and normally hearing children do not differ in their ability to perceive their own social status accurately. Generally, hearing-impaired children achieved social acceptance equal to their normally hearing peers, but ratings were more variable for this group than for normally hearing children. Degree of popularity varied widely among hearing-impaired children, with some being very popular and others being very unpopular. Children with more severe hearing losses were accepted better than those with less severe losses. These data corroborate those of Elser (1959) regarding the effects of degree of hearing loss on acceptance by hearing peers.

Bowyer and Gillies (1972) reported data on the social and emotional adjustment of deaf and "partially deaf" children enrolled in residential and public schools in England. Unfortunately, the authors do not define the designated categories of hearing impairment, other than to state that hearing for speech ranged from a "mild" loss to "no hearing for speech." Two teacher rating scales and two nonverbal tests of emotional adjustment were administered. Bowyer and Gillies concluded that children in the regular schools "cope satisfactorily" and that the ability to speak and understand speech are related to children's ability to "get on well" with adults and children.

Reich, Hambleton, and Houldin (1977) investigated socioemotional development of hearing-impaired children who were integrated into regular classes. Although their integrated subjects' academic achievement improved over time, social adjustment deteriorated. Comparisons of hearing-impaired children who were integrated at least partially and those who attended only segregated classes revealed no differences between the two groups in self-concept.

Measures of Self-Concept. The perception that individuals have of themselves influences many aspects of their behavior, including relations with others (Rogers, 1961). These social interactions in turn influence the further development of self-concept; we see ourselves as others see us (Raimy, 1971). There is some disagreement about the extent to which linguistic functioning influences self-concept development. However, if interaction with others is an important ingredient in perception of self, it is reasonable to assume that reduced communication skills might lead to altered perceptions of one's relation to the environment.

Many different instruments have been devised for the measurement of self-concept. Wylie (1961) describes various tests and their uses, concluding that most procedures fail in their attempt to evaluate the self as a whole. Most of the tests and procedures available have been used in only a few studies, yielding too few data on which validity and reliability measures can be obtained. Aspects of self-concept that are often measured are self-acceptance, self-esteem, and congruence between the real self and the ideal self. Attempts have been made to correlate the total self-concept with other factors, such as respect for others, effective daily functioning, goal setting, ability to influence others, goal-reaching behavior, and school achievement, to name a few (Wylie, 1961; Coopersmith, 1967; Fitts, 1972).

Several studies investigating the development of self-concept in hearing-impaired children have been reported. Craig (1965) compared children's responses on a perceptual sociometric test. Children were asked to identify the names of other children with whom they would like to perform some activity (going to the beach, sitting next to) and to estimate which of the other children in their classes would choose them for the same activities. Craig's major findings were that hearing-impaired children were significantly less accurate than normally hearing children in their perception of self as rated by their peers, and exhibited lower self-expansiveness by choosing fewer companions for the various activities than normally hearing children did. Craig's subjects included both residential and nonresidential hearing-impaired children. The latter named the fewest number of preferred companions, indicating greater isolation from peers.

Titus (1965) investigated the relationship between self-concept and emotional adjustment by requiring children to write 20 statements about themselves. Titus found that children who had high adjustment scores were also those who interacted most often with others.

Meadow (1969) investigated self-concept as it relates to hearing status of parents and family climate. Hypothesizing that deaf children whose parents are also deaf would develop healthier self-concepts than those whose parents are normally hearing, Meadow presented an adjective check list to students in a residential school for the deaf. Children checked one of six adjectives (lazy, pretty or handsome, smart, nice, mean, silly) based on their own evaluation of self and on the perceived evaluation of mothers, fathers, teachers, counselors, girls at school, boys at school, and normally hearing people. Results of this measure were correlated with teacher and counselor ratings of self-esteem, self-confidence, and adjustment to deafness and with family climate ratings obtained by family interviews.

Meadow found that deaf children of deaf parents exhibited significantly better self-concepts and were judged as having better emotional adjustment than deaf children of normally hearing parents. High self-esteem was also associated with a favorable family climate, good school achievement, and communication skills. Family characteristics that influenced self-concept differed for normally hearing versus deaf families. Children whose parents were deaf scored high on self-image if the parents were actively involved with other deaf families. Children whose parents were normally hearing scored higher on self-esteem if they were firstborn or only children and if their mothers were not employed outside the home.

Valone (1971) investigated the effects of early hearing impairments on the self-concept of 43 students from a residential program and 30 students from day programs for the deaf. He found that strong self-concept was related to sex (males exhibiting poorer self-esteem than females), communication skills, and school setting (day school students showing better self-esteem than residential school students).

The results of these studies must be considered in light of the limitations inherent in measures of self-concept. In the absence of validity and reliability estimates for the measures used, the test instruments themselves should be viewed with caution. Whether they measure self-concept or not is largely undetermined. Therefore, the practical implications of the data obtained are difficult, if not impossible, to judge. It is possible that the inconsistencies reported in the preceding studies result from the gross nature of the measurement tools and the difficulty of explaining the tasks to children with communicative problems. The results of these and similar studies call attention to the complexities involved in attempts to estimate perceptions held by hearing-impaired persons and to establish associations between these perceptions and other aspects of their personal lives. At least the authors whose studies are reported here have attempted to investigate aspects of personal development that relate to interaction with peers, teachers, and family, rather than concentrating on identifying traits whose labels are of limited value in understanding and planning for hearing-impaired children.

Attitudes of Others Toward the Hearing Impaired. Attitudes of others significantly affect the development of self-concept and the ability to interact with others. Rejection, either real or imagined, is usually met with withdrawal, at least temporarily. Rejection also causes reevaluation of self and frequent judgments of failure, whether such feelings are justified or not. Any consideration of social adjustment in hearing-impaired persons must take into account the level of hospitality that exists in the various environments in which they seek to function. Much of the existing data describing attitudes toward handicapping conditions have not concentrated on hearing impairment specifically. A few studies have, however, or their results can be interpreted to apply to hearing loss as well as other disabilities.

Assuming that teacher attitude would significantly affect a child's ability to function within a regular classroom, Harasymiw and Horne (1976) administered a questionnaire to teachers designed to elicit attitudes toward serving disabled children. Teachers who had served handicapped children and those who had not were exposed to in-service training and compared to a control group of teachers. Results indicated that, although basic attitudes toward disabilities remained unchanged, in-service training resulted in liberalized opinions regarding the manageability of disabled students. Teachers reported being less anxious after training, but no data are available concerning actual changes in teacher behavior resulting from the training.

Shears and Jensema (1969) investigated the relationships between normal and handicapped persons that bear on social isolation. They hypothesized that expressed attitudes toward various handicapping conditions would depend on the closeness of the relationship experienced with the person exhibiting the handicap. Ten categories of disabilities were established and persons were asked to indicate the situations under which they would accept people representing each. Situations ranged from living in the same country to marrying. Deaf persons were more acceptable than mentally ill and retarded persons, but less acceptable than amputees, wheelchair patients, and blind persons. The most visible disabilities were most acceptable and disabilities that carry a social stigma were least acceptable. The percentage of persons who would accept a deaf person under the varying social conditions are shown in Table 11.1.

Table 11.1 The Percentage of Respondents Who Would Accept a Deaf Person Under Each of Six Conditions (Shears and Jensema, 1969)

Conditions	*Percent*
Would live in same country	100
Would speak to	95
Would live in same neighborhood	80
Would work with	67
Would have as friend	53
Would marry	10

Shears and Jensema identified six dimensions that contributed to the stereotypes associated with the various disabilities: (1) visibility of the affliction, (2) interference with the communication process, (3) the social stigma associated with the disability, (4) the reversability of the disability, (5) the extent of incapacity, and (6) the difficulties involved in everyday living routines. The last three factors were more important as relationships became closer and more intimate.

An investigation of actual and perceived attitudes of normally hearing people toward deafness was reported by Schroedel and Schiff (1972). Response of deaf and normally hearing college students to attitude scales revealed more negative attitudes toward deafness on the part of the deaf than the normally hearing. Furthermore, deaf subjects perceived the attitudes of normally hearing persons to be more negative toward deafness than they actually were. Schroedel and Schiff concluded that normally hearing persons exhibit a "mildly positive" attitude toward deafness. The authors suggest caution in interpreting these results, stating, ". . . the possibility exists that attitude scores of deaf persons reflect actual experiences, while hearing persons have not thought much about their feelings toward deafness, and give spuriously positive scores. . ."

Emerton and Rothman (1978) investigated the attitudes of normally hearing college students toward deafness before and after exposure to deaf students at the Rochester Institute of Technology (RIT). Attitudes toward deafness were mildly positive initially, but became slightly negative by the time of the second survey. The change was not statistically significant. Attitudes seemed to fall into two groupings, with positive ratings occurring primarily on one-to-one interpersonal characteristics and negative ratings occurring on social expectation items. Deaf students were seen as friendly, patient, warm, and helpful. They were also judged to be immature and overemotional, to exhibit inappropriate classroom behavior and poor social manners. Emerton and Rothman suggest that the slight negative trend in attitudes may be related to conflict between the ideal and the real norms held by normally hearing persons. They recommend that future research concentrate on social norms and interactions rather than on psychological characteristics.

Neuhaus (1969) studied the attitudes of parents toward children and toward deafness. The parents and teachers of 84 deaf children were administered attitude and behavior rating scales, respectively. The congruency of maternal and paternal attitudes was measured also. Neuhaus' major findings were that parental attitudes toward children were more influential on children's behavior than their attitudes toward deafness. Maternal attitudes affected the emotional adjustment of their children more than paternal attitudes, which affected emotional adjustment only after the age of 8. When parents' attitudes were congruent, the result was better adjustment for the child. When parents' attitudes did not agree, the child's emotional adjustment was more influenced by the mother's attitude than by the father's. Parental attitudes in general became more negative as their children grew older. Implications of these findings and the role of parents in the emotional development of hearing-impaired children are discussed in a later section of this chapter.

Obviously, many factors are involved in the psychosocial development of hearing-impaired children. The inconsistencies of the reported research and the difficulties involved in measuring the factors involved have discouraged professionals from devoting the necessary attention to this important topic. It may be that social and emotional adjustment are too individualized and multifaceted to measure with an acceptable degree of accuracy.

ASSESSMENT OF SOCIAL-EMOTIONAL DEVELOPMENT

The formal assessment of intelligence, personality, and emotional adjustment is the responsibility of the psychologist. Psychological evaluations of hearing-impaired children should only be made by persons well-trained in assessment and knowledgeable about hearing impairment. The role of the speech-language pathologist, audiologist, and teacher of the deaf is to recognize symptoms of possible intellectual or adjustment problems and refer children exhibiting them to psychologists. Referrals should be accompanied by descriptions of the factors leading to concern about the child's development. Accurate referrals are enhanced if clinicians or teachers do not confuse social problems with emotional disorders or behaivor differences with personality defects. Labels must be avoided in this sensitive area. Once a child has been described as "emotionally disturbed," the label may never be eliminated. People reading the description establish predetermined expectations that may influence their interactions with the child in question. The result is often a self-fulfilling prophecy that is avoidable.

To maximize the effectiveness of preventive measures and psychological referrals, school and clinical personnel should become adept at observing and describing behavior objectively. There are two approaches toward the description of social behavior that are appropriate for use by clinicians and teachers: observation of behavior and sociometric data.

Observation of Behavior

The natural environment of the child serves as the setting for behavior observation. Interactions occurring during play, in the classroom, in therapy sessions and at home are important sources of information about a child's ability to interact with others. No special arrangements are necessary for observing in these situations, although the observer must make an effort to see the child in the various settings. Psychologists, teachers, speech and hearing personnel, and other specialists may serve as observers.

There are no norms for interpreting the significance of the behavior noted, but this does not constitute a disadvantage. The range of behaviors considered normal is quite wide. Environmental circumstances affect behavior at any given moment and must be considered when evaluating its significance. The purpose of documenting behavior is to increase understanding of the child's relationship to the environment and others within it. Behavior that is observed should be described objectively. If the behavior appears to be contributing to poor social relations or appears indicative of more serious problems, the child can be referred to a psychologist for evaluation and/or therapy. The following are guidelines for behavior observation.

1. Opportunities should be planned in which the observer can watch the child on several occasions. If classroom behavior is of major interest, several classroom observations at different times should be made. If general social behavior is the most important to be noted, the child should be observed during several different activities in different settings. Careful documentation is made of the situation in which the recorded behavior occurs.
2. Activity considered to be problem behavior should be described in writing. Definitions of any terms used by the observer should be clear. For example, a child should not be described as "withdrawing." Instead, the behavior eliciting that label should be defined in detail. "Susan suddenly turned and walked to the far corner of the room, where she sat with her back to the other children, staring at the floor. She remained there until class was dismissed." Observers should refrain especially from use of terms such as uncooperative, hyperactive, impulsive, domineering, violent, cruel and the like without complete descriptions of the behavior observed.
3. Conditions or events preceding the problem behavior should be described. Example: "Immediately before Susan walked away from the group, Tom

held her painting up and said, laughing, 'This is the funniest looking car I've ever seen.' " To do this, careful attention is necessary, so that precipitating behavior can be identified as well as possible. Obvious factors leading to important behavior are easily noted; subtle factors involving actions seemingly unrelated to the child under observation are more difficult to note and describe but may be important.

4. Reinforcement contingencies affecting the behavior should be noted. The behavior of others in the situation that feeds into, modifies, or eliminates the problem behavior should be delineated. A list of precipitative factors can be generated for a given child as well as a list of reinforcers that appear to be effective in modifying behavior.
5. Attempts on the part of the child to control self-behavior should be noted and described accurately.
6. General observations regarding the child's social relationships should be made. Inclusion in group activities, acceptance on teams or by individuals as a work or play partner, degree of social interaction during daily activities, observations of preferences for younger or older playmates, and other evidence regarding social interaction should be noted over a period of time.
7. Behavioral observations should be compared to those of other professionals or parents. Isolated problem behaviors should not be heavily weighted. Use of labels such as "emotionally disturbed" or "social isolate" should be avoided. These terms are best left to psychologists, who should themselves use them sparingly.

Sociometric Scales

The social position occupied by a child relative to peers may be obtained by use of several sociometric scales. The validity and reliability of the various scales and tests are not well established. This does not preclude their use as long as the data obtained are interpreted as general estimates only. Sociometric activities require children to identify classmates or peers who meet certain criteria. Often children are asked to estimate how they are perceived by others using the same criteria. A typical sociometric scale consists of asking children to list three classmates with whom they would like to go to the beach, study, or be friends. Another requires that classmates be identified as most and least friendly, smart, cooperative, and so on. The data obtained from children are used to establish a sociogram, a graphing of the relationships among the children participating in the task. Lines are drawn between individual children and those for whom they express favorable feelings. The pattern of classroom acceptance becomes visible at a glance.

Sociometric devices yield a large amount of data per class. If only certain children are of interest, data not pertaining to them may be ignored. Of particular interest is whether the hearing-impaired child is viewed as capable or incapable and as a desirable companion or not. Data from the children named by the hearing-impaired child as desirable are important, because they can indicate whether or not the warm feelings expressed are reciprocated. The social isolate may not be named by anyone for anything, either positive or negative. These are the children who are in the greatest difficulty socially. They are ignored and irrelevant as far as classmates are concerned.

A number of sociometric devices exist, depending on the purpose for which they are to be administered. A discussion of sociometric scales and their use is provided by Fox, Luszki, and Schmuck (1966). Classroom teachers should be consulted before plans are made for use of sociometric tests. They can assist in determining whether or not sociometric testing is feasible and help choose a test that will meet the purpose of its administration.

PREVENTION AND REMEDIATION OF PSYCHOSOCIAL PROBLEMS

Efforts to establish goals for post hoc improvement of social or emotional development have been sporadic and largely unsuccessful. Professionals do not agree on the extent of the problem or even whether or not it actually exists. Suggestions for improving social interactions and acceptance of special children are limited to classroom explanations of the disability (a plea for understanding and empathy based on increased knowledge); demonstrations of hearing aids or sign language; or establishment of a buddy system, in which the hearing-impaired child is paired with a classmate who can explain procedures or otherwise interpret situations.

The more complex mental health needs of hearing-impaired persons were largely ignored until the 1950s, except for research studies that sought to identify personality deviances in the population. Mental health services still are rare. Although mental illness and emotional problems appear to occur among the hearing impaired in the same proportion as in the normally hearing population, treatment programs that meet the needs of persons with hearing loss have been slow in developing. Based on 15 years of experience, Rainer and Altshuler (1970) made a series of recommendations for improving mental health services for the deaf. Among their suggestions was the observation that many problems of the hearing impaired could be prevented if adequate counseling services were provided to parents and child care workers when children are very young.

Factors Influencing Mental Health

For prevention measures to be successful they must be based on a thorough understanding of the factors that may contribute to poor mental health in hearing-impaired persons.

Parental Reactions. Parents of handicapped children face a crisis in their lives when confronted with diagnosis of the disability. Their reactions consist of a series of strong emotions similar to those involved in the grief reaction described by Kubler-Ross (1969). Several authors have described the emotional stages through which the parents of hearing-impaired children progress as they struggle to accept the child and the impairment (Mindel and Vernon, 1971; Schlesinger and Meadow, 1972; Moses, 1974; and Moores, 1978). These include shock, denial, anger, guilt, and frustration.

Tracing a typical family's experiences with a severely hearing-impaired child will illustrate the process. The parents anticipate the birth of the child with excitement, speculating on its sex and other characteristics. The baby is born and appears healthy in every respect. Sometime during infancy the parents begin to suspect that the baby does not hear normally. Rather than upset the other, each parent worries silently, hoping their fears are unfounded. Eventually, they seek professional help, usually from a pediatrician or family doctor. All too often, their fears are met with indifference or hostility on the part of the physician. The parents are advised not to compare children's development and to wait until the child is "old enough" to be tested. The diagnosis of deafness is usually made by a specialist several months to a year after the parents initially seek a professional opinion. During this time anxiety increases as the parents become convinced that something is wrong but are unable to obtain concerned assistance from knowledgeable professionals. They cannot ignore the symptoms of hearing loss, but cling to the hope that they represent a minor problem that can be easily solved. When the diagnosis is made and verbalized to them, parents react with shock, denial of the reality and seriousness of the loss, and anger at the delay involved in obtaining diagnosis and help.

Denial Reactions. Denial is a powerful defense mechanism, and it is fueled by the conflicting opinions of the physician who discounts the parents' fears and the specialist who confirms the hearing loss. During the denial stage, parents frequently visit many specialists hoping to find someone who will allay their fears by presenting an alternative diagnosis or the promise of effective treatment. They welcome statements from family members about how late cousin Joe talked or how stubborn Aunt Alice was, refusing to pay attention to anyone until she was 3. During this stage, some parents grasp at any promise of "cure," embracing acupuncture, spinal manipulation, and faith healing. The denial stage may be a lengthy one, and a few parents never work through it satisfactorily.

For most parents, however, there eventually comes a time when they can no longer deny the reality of the hearing loss. At this point other emotions occur, the expression of which are considered somewhat unacceptable by our society. One of these is anger, which contributes to the "why me?" reaction.

Anger. At first parents are angry because it seems unfair that such an event has happened to them. They ask themselves, "What have we done to deserve this?" Later their anger may result from the dawning realization that this is a permanent problem they face; it will not go away and it will affect their lives forever. Because they have been conditioned by societal pressures from childhood not to express anger overtly, parents rarely share their feelings of rage openly with anyone, including each other. Strong emotions usually emerge in some form, however, so the anger may be displaced in a variety of directions. For example, it may be directed toward the child. In extreme cases child abuse may occur; more commonly, parents will adopt a "hands off" policy, in which the child is not disciplined at all for fear that anger cannot be controlled. Frequently, parents will adopt passive attitudes, delaying the purchase of a hearing aid, neglecting to bring the child to therapy, and not following through on activities at home.

Anger may also be directed at the professionals who are serving the family. Recommendations and opinions may be challenged, attempts to serve the family may be thwarted, and, in rare cases, lawsuits may be filed on the basis of real or imagined grievances. When anger is directed at other family members, tensions may develop in the family that eventually destroy the marriage. Blame may be assigned for the hearing loss, one or the other parent may be accused of being uninvolved in the problem, or activities and attitudes unrelated to the hearing impairment may emerge as points of conflict.

A very common focus for anger is to turn it inward. Parents may be angry at their perceived inadequacies to deal with the entire problem. They may also be angry with themselves for being angry, as well as for unrelated shortcomings they attribute to themselves. When anger is turned inward it manifests itself as depression. In extreme cases, depressed persons become immobilized, unable to make decisions or to carry through with recommendations. Anger can be a very destructive emotion if it is not dissipated in harmless ways.

Guilt Reactions. Virtually all parents, especially mothers, eventually answer the question, "Why did this happen to me?" with what they consider to be a reasonable response: they blame themselves. Parents appear to have an incredible capacity for guilt. With no basis in fact they establish cause-and-effect relationships between an infinite variety of their own actions or thoughts and the presence of hearing impairment in the child. Such diverse items as cutting the child's hair before age 2 (an old wives' tale), failing to take vitamins throughout pregnancy, engaging in sexual intercourse during pregnancy, experimenting with drugs, becoming pregnant at the wrong astrological moment, and speaking harshly to a mother-in-law have all been reported as causative factors by guilt-ridden parents. In the case of hereditary deafness, guilt for being the carrier of a genetic trait for deafness *and* for being selfish enough to have a baby under such circumstances is common. Interestingly enough, deaf parents of deaf children appear to experience less guilt and to adjust more quickly to the diagnosis of deafness in their children than hearing parents (Meadow, 1967). Parents are likely to express feelings of guilt to family members and others, but the feelings seldom dissipate as a result. One of the most difficult guilt feelings to handle from the professional's point of view, is that rooted in the belief that the hearing impairment is a result of "God's will," as punishment for previous sins.

Anxiety reactions. The emotions of anger and guilt are accompanied by anxiety, especially as the parents begin to realize the extent of the impact that the child's hearing impairment may have on the family. Financial problems arise from the need to purchase amplification devices, enroll the child in remediation programs and preschools, and, perhaps, change employment settings in order to obtain adequate services for the child. Anxiety often results from inadequate professional services provided to parents, whose questions are not answered and for whom appropriate courses of action are not laid out. Many audiologists and physicians provide excellent diagnostic services, but virtually no remedial ones. Parents report a dismal failure on the part of these professionals in helping them understand the nature of the problems associated with hearing impairment or in referring them to resources that can. They feel impotent, confused, angry, and frustrated.

Parental Acceptance. If they receive the proper guidance and support, most parents will eventually reach a stage of acceptance of the child and the reality of the hearing loss. Acceptance may take several forms. Healthy acceptance involves an understanding of hearing impairment and its probable effect on the child's development. Parents use support services, enter into remedial efforts cooperatively, and provide a warm, accepting atmosphere in which the child may grow and develop. At the same time, the needs and desires of other family members are also important, and decisions that affect the entire family are made on the basis of what is best for the unit as a whole.

A less desirable acceptance pattern involves an unhealthy identification with the hearing-impaired child (Mindel and Vernon, 1971). This adjustment pattern is most common to mothers, whose lives tend to revolve around the child with the impairment. A symbiotic relationship may develop in which the child is overly dependent on the mother, who serves as a buffer between the child and the rest of the world. If the communication problem is severe, the child's knowledge of the world is filtered through the mother and her values and ideas are adopted. Because no differing opinions and a limited number of facts are available, the child may develop a remarkably narrow view of the world and its events and people. This type of acceptance reflects a failure to satisfactorily work through all the emotions described above. Devoting one's life to a single child's welfare is usually the result of unresolved guilt feelings.

Societal Expectations. Many of the emotional reactions experienced by parents can be attributed in part to society's attitude toward handicapping conditions in general. This country was founded on the Puritan work ethic, and Americans tend to evaluate individual worth in terms of productivity. In their essay, "The Handicapped Society," Lukens and Panter (1969) point out that Americans are identified to others by what they *do,* rather than by what they think or who they are. Such a value system places little worth on those individuals who cannot be expected to produce normally. This attitude is unspoken but pervasive and parents react to it subconsciously. The knowledge that they have produced a child who may not live up to society's expectations increases their feelings of guilt and anxiety.

Reactions of Professionals. The value systems inherent to our society affect professionals as well as parents. As teachers, clinicians, or healers they interpret their responsibilities to families to consist of making hearing-impaired children *normal.* The standard of normality adopted usually centers around modes of communication because they are the primary focus of remediation. As a result, the seriousness of the impairment and its probable effects are deemphasized. Instead, normal communication is established as both a goal and a procedure by which to obtain the goal. Parents are often discouraged from communicating with children by any means other than speech, regardless of the individual child's ability to process spoken language adequately. For some children, this advice is appropriate; for others, it is not.

Professionals are in a position of power relative to the parents and the child, whose attitudes they influence significantly. Most normally hearing parents of hearing-impaired children have never known a deaf individual, and previous experiences with hearing impairment are likely to be limited to hearing loss in elderly family members. Parents need advice and counsel; they do not know how to help their child nor what steps to take for remediation. Any opinion or advice offered by the professional under these circumstances is likely to be considered a "truth" and therefore more infallible than is warranted. In their zeal to serve the child, some professionals make pronouncements about communication ("He will not learn to speak if allowed to sign," or "She will not use her hearing if allowed to lipread") that are unproven oversimplifications of the communication process. Parents do not have the knowledge and experience necessary to evaluate these statements objectively.

In addition, professionals stress the necessity of extensive effort by the parents if the child is to progress. They are instructed to work with the child more or less constantly. Because the recommended procedures are presented as the best possible alternative, failure of the child to make adequate progress becomes a parental failure, never a professional one. The poster displayed in a famous school for deaf children that proclaims, "There are no failures. There are only parents who do not try hard enough," illustrates the point. When children fail in this atmosphere their parents experience guilt feelings that are instilled by professionals. The impact of overly optimistic or seriously biased professional advice is described by Moores (1978):

> . . . the major obstacle facing deaf people is well-meaning but misinformed hearing individuals. This includes hearing parents who, no matter what their intentions, reject or

> overprotect their deaf children and fail to provide them the security of knowing love with no strings attached. . .
>
> The problem lies in the misuse of power exerted by so many professionals over the lives of deaf individuals from the time of diagnosis through adulthood. There are guilty practitioners in all fields—pediatricians, audiologists, otologists, psychologists, educators, social workers, counselors, and myriad others. There is little chance for improvement until the insensitivity of hearing professionals is reduced and the paternalistic and maternalistic attitudes of such people, with their assumptions of superiority, are obliterated (p. 152).

Professionals and parents embark, therefore, on an emotion-laden task, frequently experiencing shared misgivings, anxieties, and hope.

Children's Reactions. It would be miraculous if children exposed to such an emotional atmosphere were not affected by it. The exact nature of the effects has not been established, but can be hypothesized on the basis of knowledge about child development and the influence of environmental factors on its stages. Schlesinger and Meadow (1972) have suggested using Erikson's model of development of man as a framework for discussion. Erikson (1968) hypothesized that individuals must progress through a series of eight sequential stages, each of which involves a developmental task that must be successfully completed. Schlesinger and Meadow (1972) have described the impact of deafness on the task of each stage. Of greatest importance to this discussion are the first three stages:

1. Basic trust versus mistrust: infancy.
2. Autonomy versus shame and doubt: early childhood.
3. Initiative versus guilt: childhood.

In the first stage, *basic trust versus mistrust,* infants must develop a sense of trust in their environment accompanied by warm feelings toward other persons. This is established primarily by loving interactions between mother and child. Infants learn to associate a variety of stimuli with caretaking activities in which basic needs are met. Parents who are anxious, angry, fearful, or depressed may be unable to respond normally to the infant. Reduced hearing deprives the infant of soothing sounds or sounds associated with need fulfillment. Included in the latter would be the sound of footsteps approaching, doors opening, and kitchen activities. Reduction in either parental response or auditory input alone might not affect the child adversely; if neither are available the effects are likely to be more serious.

The second stage, *autonomy versus shame and doubt,* is adversely affected by deafness largely because of the struggle to make the child normal. During this stage the young child develops a sense of individuality, of being able to control events. This is the stage in which children discover their ability to say "no" and to make some decisions on their own. Power struggles often occur between parents and children during this stage over the degree of independence to be allowed. Bodily functions are increasingly under the control of the child and provide a battleground between parent and child. For hearing-impaired children speech may become the major battleground (Schlesinger and Meadow, 1972). If it does, resentment may undermine efforts at communication. If the child is unsuccessful at attempts at speech, feelings of failure may develop at a time when the child should be developing a sense of self as an independent, well-functioning individual. Parents who are plagued by anger and guilt during this stage may become overprotective or punitive, thus reducing the child's feelings of autonomy and power.

During the third stage the child's task is to develop feelings of *initiative rather than guilt*. Children begin to move into the world, to observe events and people and test themselves against them. Children learn that some behaviors are permissible and others are not. They ask many questions and exhibit "motor exuberance." Schlesinger and Meadow (1972) suggest that much of the aggressive acting out seen in hearing-impaired children may result from their reduced ability to engage in "verbal exuberance."

During this stage children develop awareness of various role models as representative of future activities they may pursue or accomplishments they may reach. If deaf children are not exposed to deaf adults during this period, they may fail to identify realistic role models or to successfully develop the initiative necessary for achievement during succeeding stages.

One of the tasks involved in the third stage is the development of self-discipline based on knowledge of society's expectations; therefore the parents' consistency of and underlying attitude toward discipline is important. Parents who have not worked through their own feelings of guilt, anger, or depression may provide inconsistent discipline or engage in authoritative practices that teach children little about their own role in behavior management. In extreme cases of inconsistent management, children may not establish cause-effect relationships that might govern their behavior. Such children seek boundaries to their behavior constantly, "trying" adults repeatedly until some limits are established. Behavior such as this can be detrimental to remedial efforts unless it is modified. Punitive measures may simply contribute further to a child's failure to develop initiative during this stage.

Because development of self-concept and successful passage through the stages described above are largely dependent on parental reactions and behavior, the importance of helping parents achieve a healthy level of acceptance of reality is apparent.

Classroom Factors. As children grow older, increasing influence is exerted over them by factors external to the family. In particular, school personnel such as teachers and clinicians assume authoritative roles. The attitudes and expectations with which these personnel approach hearing-impaired children may influence their acceptance by other children. The teacher sets the tone for classroom behavior.

Insecurity on the teacher's part regarding classroom management of a specific child may result in ambivalent or negative feelings that are transmitted to class members. Children may observe accurately attitudes toward others that have never been expressed openly. In turn, the child in question detects unspoken attitudes and internalizes them. The underlying attitudes and emotions are usually subconscious and nondeliberate on the part of all involved, a fact that contributes to the frustration and attitude of helplessness that surrounds the problem of classroom tolerance of exceptional children.

Several suggestions have been offered by parents and professionals to minimize social problems within the classroom. The first step is to increase the teacher's self-confidence by providing adequate in-service training in hearing impairment. Chapter 10 contains a description of in-service topics and procedures. Once the teacher is able to understand and cope with the effects of hearing loss, it is less likely that attitudes toward the hearing-impaired child will differ from those toward other class members. Increased confidence will allow the teacher to view the child as simply someone to be educated. Class members will be more likely to view the hearing-impaired child as just another peer.

The second step is to make class members aware of hearing impairment and its probable communicative effects. The present authors have mixed feelings about this approach toward classroom management unless it is well managed and incorporates consultant expertise. Existing data suggest that children who are observably hearing impaired are accepted best by normally hearing children, suggesting that all hearing-impaired children might be accepted if their hearing losses were known (Elser, 1959; Kennedy and Bruininks, 1974). It makes sense, then, to inform children that a fellow class member is hearing impaired. They are more likely to attribute any unusual behavior to the hearing impairment rather than to less acceptable causes and to be more tolerant as a result.

However, these assumed benefits must be balanced against the embarrassment and associated resentment that may be experienced by the hearing-impaired child when the impairment is made public knowledge and becomes a topic of conversation. Many hearing-impaired children consider themselves damaged and inferior. They refuse to wear hearing aids or seek to conceal them. They long to be "like everybody else," and resent efforts and events that affirm their differences. These include therapy sessions, preferential seating, and other activities that call attention to the hearing loss. The damage to a child's ego caused by an announcement or discussion of the hearing loss, no matter how well intentioned, could be severe. The decision to discuss in class a particular child's hearing loss should be made only after consultation with a psychologist or others who are familiar with the child in question. Certainly the child's feelings about the matter should be explored and considered prior to a decision. Individual privacy should not be violated without consent by authority figures unless absolutely essential.

Exploring the child's feelings might also serve a useful purpose in personal adjustment. Acceptance of self as a hearing-impaired person is important to a child's mental health. Conversations or counseling with the child and the parents could result in positive attitude changes that may have significant consequences for classroom management and future development. Making peers aware of the effects of hearing impairment is probably desirable, but should be done as a part of a coordinated effort to help the child adjust to the social environment. General discussions of hearing impairment in all classrooms in the school might increase tolerance for hearing-impaired children, but the benefits have not been established and the time required might be better spent in other activities.

A third suggestion for increasing social acceptance is the establishment of a *buddy* system. The hearing-impaired child is assigned a classmate, who provides information about homework, class activities, and social events. This system can work well if the individuals involved are friends or if all class members are divided into pairs for purposes of reminding each other of important things. If the hearing-impaired child is the only one with a buddy, the stigma of being identified as different arises again. If the buddy resents the role, less rather than more social acceptance may result. The establishment of a buddy system should depend on careful assessment of the classroom situation and the hearing-impaired child's status within it. If the system is established in Kindergarten and continued throughout school, it may be accepted by all children as a part of classroom life. If initiated suddenly in an upper grade, it may simply serve to set the hearing-impaired child even farther apart than before.

Peer Factors. Peer pressure is a lifelong human experience that is particularly acute during adolescence. Most people prefer not to be considered different from their peers except in minor ways. When differences do occur, their nature is not as important as their perception. Communities of people dress alike, use the same slang language (oh wow, neat, like you know), engage in similar social customs, and style their hair the same. Any noticeable deviation from the accepted group norm may be considered weird or a sign of snobbery, especially among adolescents. Peer acceptance is of consequence to everyone, but some people are more affected by it than others. Because all individuals are, indeed, different in many respects, most children and young people perceive themselves as aberrant in some way, at some time. Skinny legs, protruding ears, cowlicks, and flat chests are deplored. Although physical differences such as these cause consternation, they are not particularly unique. Careful observation of schoolmates will reveal dozens of skinny legs and protruding ears. While not considered desirable attributes, these traits do not constitute a stigma.

Hearing loss, on the other hand, is rare enough to be considered a serious abnormality. It is also an invisible condition that can be successfully hidden under certain circumstances. Refusal to wear hearing aids or auditory training equipment represents an effort to avoid the stigma of hearing impairment. If speech is normal and communication on a one-to-one basis is not seriously affected, the hearing loss may be undetected by others. Behavior is likely to be affected in some respect, however, catching the attention of peers. Failure to respond to a distant greeting or a casual remark may be interpreted by others as snobbish behavior. Volunteering the same incorrect answer given by another child in class because the preceding exchange between teacher and child wasn't heard is embarrassing and interpreted as "strange" by classmates. If academic achievement is poor, the hearing-impaired child may be considered "dumb." Misunderstanding of casual conversations or frequent requests to repeat messages make a child seem "weird." Children who are intolerant of their own minor differences are not likely to be accepting of social mistakes as serious as these.

Children and adolescents strive to conform to peer standards because they fear peer rejection. They do not comprehend the fact that their friends may be as panicked about peer opinion as they are. It would be unreasonable, therefore, to expect hearing-impaired children to accept their differences as unimportant or barely noticeable to others. Once they have been laughed at or teased for failing to hear correctly, any social slight or interpersonal problem that occurs is probably interpreted as resulting from the presence of hearing loss. The effort that must be expended to appear normal and to keep up with peers can only be imagined.

Communication is the key to peer contact and acceptance. When one of the communicators is hearing imparied, the process requires more effort and time. Statements must be repeated, messages are misinterpreted or lost altogether, misunderstandings cause frustration or resentment, and certain communication situations cannot be managed satisfactorily. Telephone conversations may be difficult; whispering is impossible; conversations cannot be held in the dark. For some normally hearing children, even minor restrictions such as these are too discouraging to allow friendships to develop. The impact of reduced ability to communicate normally increases as children grow older. Social contacts shift from play activities involving building blocks, hammers, and pegs to games involving complex rules or role play. In adolescence social behavior consists primarily of long conversations about peers, music, TV, movies, extracurricular activities, and the opposite sex. Everybody uses the same slang, knows the same jokes, communicates in the same code. Hearing-impaired children are at an obvious disadvantage unless they have developed excellent communication skills. Even so, the environments in which most social contact takes place (in crowded rooms, in the presence of loud music, in gymnasia) reduces the probability that communication can be carried on with ease. The result is increased social isolation with age. By the time dating begins, the usual adolescent anxieties associated with it have been magnified. If dating partners are teased for going out with a hearing-impaired person, the problem is exacerbated. A lack of dates is seen as rejection because of the hearing loss. The fear of being left out may cause the young person to become too eager for acceptance, to try too hard, thus alienating others further.

The problems described above are common to many teenagers. If they are experiencing success in other aspects of their lives or have strong self-concepts, most young people pass through adolescence with few permanent scars. For children who must struggle for success in every aspect of their lives, peer rejection during adolescence may be of significant importance to their mental health.

Acceptance of hearing-impaired children by their peers may be enhanced by open communication concerning the impairment. Much of the indifference and many of the personal slights on the part of normally hearing children are not deliberate. They occur because children lack knowledge of the realities of hearing impairment and the feelings of those who experience it. Frank discussions among children about their feelings and intentions may alleviate resentment and misunderstandings. The consciousness of both normally hearing and hearing-impaired children may be raised by so-called "rap sessions." Discussions must be led by someone who can prevent emotional damage from occurring should they take an accusatory turn. Children must want to discuss the matter; they often exhibit reticence and an unwillingness to be honest that are detrimental to group discussions. The results of group discussion among peers have not been reported, so the success of the procedure is not documented.

If reaction to real or imagined peer rejection seems severe, it may be advisable to refer the affected child to a psychologist or the family for mental health counseling services.

Parent Counseling

Speech-language pathologists, audiologists, and teachers of the deaf can contribute significantly to the prevention of psychosocial problems in hearing-impaired children through parent counseling. Unfortunately, most contacts between these professionals and parents consist primarily of information giving rather than counseling in the truest sense. The hearing loss is explained, remedial or educational plans are described, hearing aid care is demonstrated. Many professionals, such as audiologists or physicians, meet with parents infrequently, often under serious time constraints.

Speech-language pathologists and audiologists are well trained in evaluation and remediation techniques to be employed with the client. They feel most comfortable explaining these procedures, their purposes and results. The emotions that accompany exchanges between parents and clinicians are more difficult for the average clinician to handle. As a result, emotions are usually ignored, suppressed, or unrecognized. According to parents, their emotional state often makes it impossible for them to comprehend fully the facts and opinions presented during so-called counseling sessions. Once the diagnosis of hearing impairment is verbalized, they may be overwhelmed by shock and anxiety and find it difficult, if not impossible, to listen attentively to complex explanations. Parents leave the session flooded with unidentified feelings, unspoken questions, and a general feeling of uncertainty and helplessness. Although they may have been encouraged to ask questions, they were unprepared to do so. When they recall the counseling session their overall impression is that the clinician presented information hurriedly, most of which they cannot recall. Many parents report bitterly that the professionals consulted seemed to have no interest in the emotional turmoil they felt and to feel little responsibility for referring them to other professionals who might be of help. Parents recall not knowing what to do and being too emotionally labile to organize themselves effectively. With few exceptions they value highly the first professional who shows interest in their feelings or spends unhurried time discussing their fears or needs. Much of the trauma associated with the diagnosis of hearing loss could be alleviated by effective parent counseling that includes both information giving and an opportunity for parents to express their feelings and emotional needs.

Unless an effort is made to provide it, a situation in which parents feel comfortable in expressing their feelings and voicing their concerns about their own role in the child's development will not occur. In spite of the fact that they are experiencing painful emotions, parents will not express them (and often will not confront them) in the absence of an environment that encourages emotional release. A basic requirement of such an environment is the establishment of a trust relationship between parents and the professional involved.

There are two essential characteristics associated with clinicians who are successful parent counselors: (1) they are accepting of a wide variety of behaviors and emotions and (2) they have highly developed listening skills.

Acceptance. A trust relationship will develop only if the clinician is accepting and nonjudgmental. Understanding and acceptance of one's own emotions is an important attribute for a clinician to have; the ability to listen and accept emotions expressed by others is another. Respect for the parents is essential. They must be viewed as capable individuals who have the major responsibility of facilitating their children's development. As such they are full partners in the habilitation to be planned and carried out. Their opinions are valid; their feelings are important; their cooperation is essential. The establishment of this cooperative effort is founded in mutual trust and respect. The professional cannot be viewed as an authority figure who judges actions or utterances and finds some of them unacceptable. Parents cannot be viewed as necessary evils to be tolerated or manipulated. Feelings as well as procedures must be explored together so that all involved share a complete understanding of the expectations, desires and limitations that affect the habilitation process.

It takes time for a trust relationship to develop, but the professional's actions and attitudes may speed up or retard the process. The following behaviors will contribute to the rapid development of a working trust relationship between clinician and parents.

1. Verbal and nonverbal messages must be congruent. It is not enough for the clinician to verbalize acceptance of or interest in the parents' feelings. Words and actions must reflect the same message. The statement, "I'm interested in how you feel about this," will be more believable if the clinician is sitting back in a chair, relaxed, and looking directly at the parent than if sitting on the edge of the chair, stacking papers, and looking at the clock. Clinicians should consciously observe their own nonverbal behavior and work toward eliminating distracting or contradictory mannerisms.
2. The clinician should be relaxed and unhurried. It is important that parents feel that they are not imposing unduly on the time of the clinician. The quickest way to end a counseling session prematurely is to hurry into the room, sit poised on the edge of the chair, speak rapidly, ask questions, nod energetically while the parent speaks, and change the subject often. The obviously hurried atmosphere is transmitted to the parents regardless of *what* is being said. It is not always possible for beginning clinicians to be relaxed, especially when counseling emotional parents. However, if they consciously relax and concentrate on the parents' needs, nervousness soon disappears and counseling skills improve.
3. Clinicians must be honest with parents and with themselves. It is difficult to respect someone who pretends knowledge or feelings that are not real. Parents often ask questions that are difficult to answer, and clinicians must be able to say, "I don't know." Some questions may be referred to physicians, psychologists, or others. Questions concerning the outcome of therapy should be answered as honestly as possible without undue pessimism or unwarranted optimism. Clinicians who are thoroughly familiar with the research literature regarding remediation of hearing impairment will be able to share this knowledge with parents in tactful, helpful ways.

    If the clinician is affected emotionally by the counseling session it may not be necessary to say so, but it is unwise to try to hide the fact. Sometimes clinicians are temporarily overwhelmed by unusual problems facing families, such as the accidental blinding of a deaf child, the diagnosis of multiple handicaps in several children in the family, or the sudden death of a parent. Attempts to disguise feelings of sadness or depression will probably result in behaviors that may be misinterpreted by parents as coldness, lack of concern, pity, or even anger. Obviously, the purpose of counseling is not to provide an emotional outlet for the clinician. The focus must always be on the parent and the clinician's emotional status is secondary. It should never intrude on the session, but may be mutually recognizable by parent and clinician in passing. On the other hand, no matter how concerned the clinician is, it is doubtful that strong emotions will be experienced as sharply as they are by parents. Statements such as, "I know how you feel," are met with scepticism and, sometimes, with anger and resentment by parents, especially if they are made by young clinicians who are not parents themselves.

4. The clinician should not become defensive. When parents are struggling with strong emotions they may displace anger, resentment, and frustration in the direction of the clinician. Sometimes these emotions are expressed openly in the form of accusations or complaints. At other times they are expressed through passive noncooperation. Clinicians must not take these parental actions personally. One purpose of counseling is to help parents release negative feelings and understand their relation to effective management of the child. They need to understand that their feelings are based on a natural emotional reaction to the specific problems involved in having a hearing-impaired child. This goal will not be accomplished if clinicians react with anger, resentment, and frustration of their own.

Active Listening. The most important attribute of the counseling clinician is the ability to listen carefully to both the *content* and the *emotion* conveyed in parental statements. Active listening occurs when clinicians are able to elicit meaningful comments from parents and to interpret the emotional content underlying what is actually said. Until it is safe to do so, parents will express verbally only what they believe to be acceptable to the listener. Active listening involves attending carefully to these "acceptable" statements and responding to them in a way that results in further disclosure of the emotion underlying them. For example, the statement, "I'm not worried about her future; I know she will be just fine," can be interpreted as evidence of calm acceptance and confidence in the future if content alone is observed. However, if the words are spoken while a handkerchief is twisted in both hands and in a voice cracked with emotion and strain, it is naive to assume that the content of the statement represents everything the parent is communicating. An alert clinician would suspect that the statement represented what the parent would *like* to believe. The combined verbal and nonverbal messages express anxiety about the child's future. Nonverbal messages are not always obvious. Careful observation of both verbal and nonverbal message components is essential to accurate listening and to the development of an effective counseling atmosphere.

Active listening skills can be developed with special instruction and practice and include the ability to identify emotional content, to elicit emotions congruent with actions, and to reflect emotion accurately. It is beyond the scope of this book to provide instruction in these counseling techniques. They are so important to adequate service to parents, however, that all speech-language pathologists, audiologists, and teachers of the deaf should receive training in them. When clinicians can listen empathetically, they can provide an atmosphere in which parents may openly express the "unacceptable" emotions they experience as a result of having a hearing-impaired child. Once these emotions are expressed and accepted as normal, parents are relieved of the burden of denying their own feelings.

The clinician has no solution for the emotional pain the parent feels and does not bear responsibility for it. Parents must work through the anger, guilt, and anxiety themselves. For many this is accomplished with dispatch once they feel free to talk about their feelings openly. For others counseling by professionals trained in psychotherapy may be necessary. Speech-language pathologists and audiologists will be better prepared to make the necessary referrals if they have listened carefully to parents and allowed them to reveal their emotional status freely.

Parent Support Groups

Parents frequently obtain their greatest emotional support and assistance from other parents. There are two ways in which professionals can foster interchanges among parents. One method is to establish a network of parents who volunteer to contact those of newly identified hearing-impaired children. Because of privacy considerations, the new parents must agree that their names can be given to others. The professional (usually the audiologist) then calls a volunteer parent and arranges for the personal contact. Some audiologists simply furnish the name of the volunteer to the new parents, who place the call themselves. For many parents this is a difficult call to make, and it is easier to accept a call than to initiate it. In either event, the volunteer parent offers to serve as a resource regarding community programs, activities, and services. Invitations to parent meetings or other activities are made. In general, the new parents are given a sense of belonging and of having someone to turn to who has experienced the same problems they now face.

Another source of support to the family is the parent group. Many parent groups rely on professionals for direction and guidance; others are more independent. The potential of the parent group as an emotional support has not been fully realized. Too many parent groups meet for business purposes, plan a fundraising event, hear an "expert" speak on some aspect of deafness, and go home. Groups designed for the parents of moderately hearing-impaired children are almost nonexistent. Group meetings that include an exchange of experiences, solutions to problems, or emotional reactions are rare. As a result, each parent must struggle with the emotions, questions, and everyday problems individually; the wheel is reinvented again and again.

Fostering Parent-Child Communication. The uncertainty and resentment experienced by most parents directly affects their ability to communicate openly with their children. At a conference sponsored by the Northeast Regional Media Center for the Deaf in 1971, deaf adolescents reported their major concern to be a lack of communication with their parents. These deaf children felt that their parents' failure to accept their deafness and its ramifications contributed significantly to the breakdown in communication between parent and child. An outcome of this conference was the development of special materials to be used by parent groups to enhance their knowledge and acceptance of themselves and their hearing-impaired children. Entitled *Parent-Child Communication,* the materials consist of 45 transparencies depicting typical experiences of the parents of hearing-impaired children and a manual with suggestions for their use. These materials may be obtained from the Northeast Regional Media Center for the Deaf.

The transparencies are drawings that represent events in the lives of parents and children, beginning during pregnancy and ending in adolescence. Parents are shown ''testing'' a child's hearing with a spoon and a pan, reading conflicting opinions regarding educational methodology, observing normally hearing children at play together, and engaged in other activities and observations directly related to the hearing-impaired child. Each transparency is accompanied by suggested questions and topics for discussion by the parents. The manual is for use by the group facilitator, who introduces the transparency and leads the discussion of it. Figure 11.1 shows a typical transparency. Some of the questions suggested for discussion

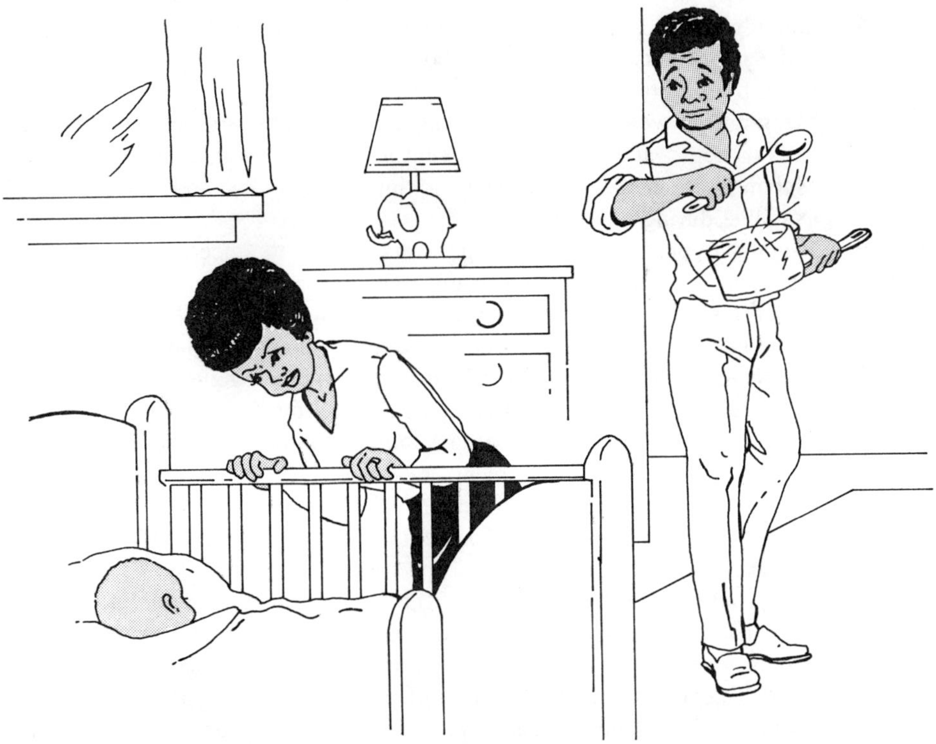

Figure 11.1. Example of *Parent-Child Communication* series transparencies for use with parent groups. (Produced under a grant from U.S. Office of Education, Bureau of Education of the Handicapped, OEG-0-73-0534.)

are: What have the parents said to each other? Who initiated this testing? Who suggested the possibility that your child might be deaf? What was the other parent's reaction? Who initiated the home tests which you performed? How did your child respond? How did you respond to your child's response or nonresponse? The questions are designed to elicit a discussion of the feelings that parents experienced at the time this event occurred in their lives.

Successful initiation of parent education or parent counseling programs requires considerable effort on the part of the professional involved. Parents may have been involved previously with typical parent groups and may have preconceived ideas about their worth. The most effective incentive to attend meetings occurs as a result of satisfaction among parents, so word-of-mouth support from other parents is helpful. This is more likely to happen if the professional has established a trust relationship with parents during individual contacts.

The most successful parent counseling groups share the following characteristics:

1. The group facilitator is open, nonthreatening, accepting of parents, and nonjudgmental. An atmosphere of cooperative effort between professional and parents exists, in which authoritative answers or opinions are not given by the group leader.
2. Meetings are well advertised. Parents are invited by newsletters, personal calls or notes, and reminders are sent just before the meeting is held.
3. Meetings are held at a convenient time for parents, and child care is available during meetings.
4. Parents are encouraged to help plan and execute the meetings. Topics for discussion and materials to be used are chosen by parents with input from the professional about the availability of resources.
5. Meetings are regularly scheduled and have planned agendas. Sufficient time is allowed for parents to become comfortable together. Once discussion begins, it is not hurried and participation by all is encouraged.
6. Parents are encouraged to continue thinking about topics between meetings. If appropriate, assignments may be given for interim activities. Parents should decide on the nature of these assignments, which may include checklists of parental behavior or attempts to practice the communicative skills discussed at the meetings.
7. The groups are relatively small. A group of 10 to 14 parents allows for diversity of opinion and experience without being so large that it threatens parents who are shy or must be encouraged to share their thoughts with the group. Ideally, both parents will attend, so a nucleus of five to eight couples is a reasonable basis for establishment of a group. Where possible parents of children of varying ages should be included. Parents of older children have experienced most of the problems faced by parents of young children and can share their solutions or frustrations.

Audiologists, speech-language pathologists, psychologists, or teachers may serve as group facilitators. Some training in counseling and group dynamics is beneficial, but extensive experience in group counseling is not necessary. Materials should focus on parental feelings associated with common events in their lives and provide a means of encouraging the sharing of emotions with other parents for support purposes. Many husbands and wives have never discussed their feelings openly with each other and express surprise at the similarities of their emotions. Lines of communication can be established between husband and wife, other parents, and parent and child as a result of carefully planned parent meetings.

Effective parent support through counseling or group discussions is essential to the mental health of the child. Unresolved emotions cause many parents to become overprotective, less demanding, critical, or generally nonsupportive or noninvolved in the child's life. Children who live in an anxious atmosphere are likely to develop their own anxieties about functioning in the family and in the larger community. Their attempts at socialization with peers, their concept of themselves as capable persons, and their willingness to move out into the world to develop their abilities with confidence are affected by the emotional and communicative climate of the home. Assistance to parents in resolving the intense feelings associated with having a hearing-impaired child should be a priority for persons concerned with the habilitation of these children.

Behavior Management of Children

The behavior of children of the most immediate concern to clinicians is that which occurs during clinician-child contacts. There are many behaviors that detract from the purpose of the interaction between clinician and child. Delaying tactics, refusal to perform tasks, disruptions of activities, objection to going or staying with the clinician, and inattention to tasks all constitute negative behaviors that interfere with remediation efforts. It comes as quite a shock to beginning clinicians when a well-planned therapy session disintegrates into a battle of wills between adult and child.

Successful behavior control occurs as a result of pleasant, but firm consistency. Children exhibit the behaviors listed above for a variety of reasons. Some are directly related to the immediate situation and others reflect general behavior patterns. Anxiety in a new situation, uncertainty as to what is expected, fear of failure, and a search for authoritative limits may all contribute to a given set of behaviors. The clinician's task is to minimize anxiety and uncertainty as much as possible and maximize motivation to participate in the treatment tasks. Several steps are involved in achieving these goals.

Establishing Objectives. The clinician should have the objectives of every treatment session firmly in mind. For an initial visit they may include the basic ones of separating child from parent, involving the child in planned activities, or keeping the child in the therapy room. Both behavioral and treatment objectives should be established that have two characteristics: they must be within the child's capabilities, and they must be relevant to the eventual goals of treatment. For each early encounter a minimum acceptable level of performance by the child should be predetermined. For example, if the major goal is to conduct a language evaluation, the basic objective may consist of establishing a cooperative point-to-the-picture response. If the child exhibits negative behavior that is difficult to control, completion of an entire test or procedure may not be possible. For purposes of future participation, however, the essential point response on request must be established sooner or later. If this is the basic objective, within the child's ability and relevant to the overall treatment goals, it should be accomplished before terminating the session. If this is not accomplished, the struggle to control the child's behavior will begin again at the next session. It will be more difficult then, however, because the precedent of victorious noncooperation has been set, and the child's behavioral limits are still in doubt. To avoid power struggles that end in a frustrated deadlock, step-by-step objectives should be set that will lead eventually to the desired goal.

Setting Behavior Limits. Behavior limits must be established and apparent from the outset of treatment. Many clinicians find behavior lists helpful. A written or pictured checklist of desired behaviors is prepared in poster form and kept visible throughout the treatment session. Table 11.2 depicts a typical behavior list. Spot checks of the listed behaviors are made throughout the session. Praise or points, stars, or other tangible reinforcers may be given when actual behavior matches expectation. Reinforcement of positive behavior is more effective for increasing incidence of the desired behaviors than punishment of negative actions. When children have difficulty attending and abiding by the established rules, the clinician must be alert for any relevant behavior that can be reinforced positively. Once the child experiences the pleasure resulting from receiving praise or some sort of token, there will be an increase in acceptable behavior and a decrease in actions that do not result in favorable responses. The process may be slow at first, but it is effective for all but a few children. The behavior list provides a nonverbal reminder of acceptable behavior for the child.

Table 11.2 Examples of Rules Used to Establish Behavioral Limits During Remedial Sessions

Behavior Checklist
1. Are you sitting in your chair, ready to work?
2. Are you paying attention (looking and listening)?
3. Are you waiting for instructions?
4. Are you keeping materials on the table?
5. Are you finishing tasks promptly?

If behavior limits are established from the beginning, time that would be wasted in power struggles can be used in beneficial treatment activities. Therapy cannot occur when behavior is uncontrolled. If adults are consistent in their reactions to each type of behavior exhibited by the child, behavioral limits are soon recognized and accepted.

Reacting Consistently and Calmly to Unacceptable Behavior. For most children a simple reminder of the behavior rules that have been established is sufficient to prevent serious behavioral problems. Occasionally, however, children will refuse to cooperate to the extent that a session breaks down. *If refusal influences a basic objective of the session,* the clinician may have to insist on appropriate performance. There are three common approaches to uncooperative behavior control, depending on the nature of the child's refusal.

If the child adopts a passive form of refusal, the clinician simply waits. After assuring the child that the desired behavior must occur before the session is terminated, the clinician should relax and wait patiently for the child to perform. An occasional reminder that the task remains to be completed is acceptable, but constant urging is not a good idea. No other activities or materials should be available to the child during the interim. A reassuring smile can remind the child that the clinician is comfortable with the situation and confident of eventual success. Some adults prefer to maintain a solemn face, but anger and punitive actions are inappropriate behaviors for the clinician. *The eventual goal of all behavior management procedures is to help the child establish self-discipline that will carry over into other settings.* Events leading to self-control should be as pleasant as possible under the circumstances.

At times children exhibit negative behavior that is or could be destructive to themselves or others. Violent actions occur when the child loses control for whatever reason. The clinician may have to use physical restraint to prevent damage to persons or things. The child should be held firmly. Talking in a soothing tone of voice will help reduce tension, even if the child cannot hear or understand what is said. At least the clinician will feel calmer, a state that will be transmitted to the child by nonverbal means. Statements such as "I know, I know, it will be all right. You're OK now," can convey sympathy and concern without making demands or giving unwelcome advice. As the child begins to calm down the clinician can gradually relax, releasing the child slowly as control is regained. The role of the adult is supportive, but expectations are obvious to the child.

Occasionally children are unable to control their behavior in spite of the measures listed above. Periods of "time-out" may be necessary, in which the child is taken to a designated spot in the room and required to remain there for a set period of time. It is essential that the spot be barren, uninteresting, and removed from any activity that may be going on nearby. After the specified period, the child is brought back to the ongoing activity. The clinician behaves normally, showing calm expectation that the child is now ready to cooperate. Most children detest the boredom of time-out periods. They receive no attention and no stimulation, the desire for which often precipitates unruly behavior.

Control of special instances of unacceptable behavior may require the assistance of parents or other professionals. For example, the separation of children from parents is usually a problem only for very young children. It must be frightening for a 2-year-old to come into a strange building full of strange people and then be separated from the parents and taken into an unknown situation. Some toddlers react with fright and, given a choice, elect to remain with family members. Others exhibit only momentary anxiety, which subsides quickly once the parents are out of sight and interest in therapy activities develops. If the child is genuinely frightened, the parents may accompany child and clinician to the therapy room. After the child explores the room, the parent should leave. In extreme cases, the parent may need to leave for a short time, return, leave for a longer time, return, and so on, until the child feels comfortable with the room and the clinician. When in the therapy room, parents should remain in the background, deferring to the clinician as the decision maker. Most young children quickly lose their dependence on the parent if the clinician and activities are interesting and success can be achieved.

One of the most difficult behavior problems to manage is a lack of motivation toward therapy. Although temper tantrums and refusal to sit and be quiet represent immediate, overt, disruptive behaviors, they are more easily controlled than a passive attitude of bored tolerance. Children who exhibit this attitude may eventually complete a task after deliberate delays and avoidances. They express failure to understand instructions, even though they are not new and have been understood previously. What appear to be deliberate mistakes are made, evaluated without interest, and eventually corrected. Requests for decisions or expression of ideas are met with bored shrugs and "I don't know." Any activity involving the use of materials or tools (such as pencil or scissors) is performed with agonizingly slow movements. These efforts at sabotage may occur during every therapy session, with different clinicians, and in the face of a variety of activities and procedures.

Children exhibit this type of behavior as an expression of hostility. It is seldom limited to the therapy room. Investigation reveals that the behavior exists at home, at school, and, to a lesser extent, with playmates. Many passive children have a history of temper tantrums and overtly uncooperative behavior in the past. Clinicians and teachers should establish desired behavior lists (which may include items such as "Finishes tasks quickly") and reinforce active, nondawdling behavior consistently. A program of behavior modification should be devised, preferably by a psychologist, that can be carried out in each environment in which the child functions. Parents should be enlisted as active participants in the behavior control program. Children such as these should be monitored closely by psychologists or other mental health professionals. In addition to effects on personality and social development, well-established patterns of hostile passivity are detrimental to achievement in a variety of areas due to successful resistance to learning.

Establishing a Favorable Emotional Atmosphere in Therapy. The emotional climate within the treatment session will contribute to a child's behavior. An atmosphere of open, friendly respect for the child by the adult is conducive to cooperation. It should be obvious that the clinician is in charge of the session, and that activities will be completed through a cooperative effort by clinician and child. The child should be encouraged, but not cajoled. The clinician is interested in the child's point of view, but is not deterred from completion of the planned task. The clinician's quiet confidence in the child will set the stage for mutual respect and effort.

Arranging Tasks So That the Child Achieves Immediate Success. Success increases motivation, contributes to feelings of competence, and allows pride in accomplishments. Most adults do not continue to attempt activities at which they fail consistently; certainly, they would not enjoy them. Many of the tasks presented to hearing-impaired children in therapy are difficult for them. To ensure cooperation, treatment sessions should begin with activities that allow some degree of success. This does not mean that the tasks should be so simple that they are boring, but that they can be achieved with reasonable effort. As confidence increases, tasks are made more complex or the level of expected performance is increased.

Much uncooperative and negative behavior is related to the nature of the tasks to be performed. If they are boring, irrelevant, or too difficult or confusing, children may refuse to complete them as a protest against inappropriate demands. It is essential, therefore, that therapy or classroom activities be founded on the baseline data obtained for the child by assessment procedures. Once appropriate activities are chosen, what is expected from the child should be explained carefully. To avoid uncertainty, oral instructions should be accompanied by visual clues. For example, if the task involved the identification of word classes, cards bearing the designations of "noun," "verb," "adjective," and so on should be provided as visual reminders of the task to be performed. The use of visual aids is essential to most hearing-impaired children, especially when new tasks or concepts are introduced. Creating them will also help the clinician focus on the essential information necessary to understanding the task at hand.

Children who are loved and accepted by others have a good chance of developing self-confidence and well-adjusted personalities. Audiologists and speech-language pathologists cannot ensure that the children they serve will be loved and accepted, but they can contribute to the development of an accepting environment by being aware of the factors that affect children and their own roles in influencing them. The clinicians who are most effective in this regard are those who understand the basis of human emotions and are comfortable with their own and the emotions of others.

REFERENCES

Altshuler, K., Psychiatric considerations in the adult deaf, *Amer. Ann. Deaf,* 107, 560-561, 1962.

Binet, A. and Simon, T., An investigation concerning the value of the oral method, *Amer. Ann. Deaf,* 55, 4–33, 1910.

Bowyer, L. and Gillies, J., The social and emotional adjustment of deaf and partially deaf children, *British J. Educ. Psych.,* 42, 305–308, 1972.

Coopersmith, S., *The Antecedents of Self Esteem.* San Francisco: W. H. Freeman and Company, 1967.

Craig, H., A sociometric investigation of the self concept of the deaf child, *Amer. Ann. Deaf,* 110, 456–478, 1965.

Donoghue, R., The deaf personality: A study in contrasts, *J. Rehab. Deaf,* 2, 35–51, 1968.

Elser, R., The social position of hearing handicapped children in the regular grades, *Except. Chil.,* 25, 305–309, 1959.

Emerton, R. and Rothman, G., Attitudes toward deafness: Hearing students at a hearing and deaf college, *Amer. Ann. Deaf,* 123, 588–593, 1978.

Erikson, E., *Identity, Youth and Crisis.* New York: Norton, 1968.

Fisher, B., The social and emotional adjustment of children with impaired hearing attending ordinary classes, *British J. Educ. Psych.,* 36, 319–321, 1966.

Fitts, W., *The Self Concept and Performance.* Research Monograph No. 5. Published under a grant from Social and Rehabilitation Service, 1972.

Fox, R., Luszki, M., and Schmuck, R., *Diagnosing Classroom Learning Environments.* Chicago: Science Research Association, Inc., 1966.

Furth, H., Research with the deaf: Implications for language and cognition, *Psychol. Bull.,* 62, 145–162, 1964.

Furth, H., *Thinking Without Language: Psychological Implications of Deafness.* New York: The Free Press, 1966.

Goetzinger, C., Harrison, C., and Baer, C., Small perceptive hearing loss: Its effect on school-age children, *Volta Rev.,* 66, 124–131, 1964.

Harasymiw, S. and Horne, M., Teacher attitudes toward handicapped children and regular class integration, *J. Spec. Educ.,* 10, 393–400, 1976.

Heider, F. and Heider, G., An experimental investigation of lipreading, *Psychol. Monogr.,* 52, 124–133, 1940.

James, W., Thought before language: A deaf-mute's recollections, *Amer. Ann. Deaf,* 35, 135–145, 1890.

Kahn, A., Responses of hard of hearing and normal children to frustration, *Except. Chil.,* 24, 155–159, 1957.

Kennedy, P. and Bruininks, R., Social status of hearing impaired children in regular classrooms, *Except. Chil.,* 40, 336–342, 1974.

Kübler-Ross, E., *On Death and Dying.* London: Collier-MacMillian, 1969.

Levine, E., *Youth in a Soundless World: A Search for Personality.* New York: New York University Press, 1956.

Levine, E., Psychological tests and practices with the deaf: A survey of the state of the art, *Volta Rev.,* 76, 298–319, 1974.

Lukens, K. and Panter, C., The handicapped society. In *Thursday's Child Has Far To Go.* Englewood Cliffs, NJ: Prentice-Hall, Inc., 1969.

Meadow, K., The effect of early manual communication and family climate on the deaf child's development, Ph.D. Dissertation, University of California, 1967.

Meadow, K., Self-image, family climate, and deafness, *Social Forces,* 47, 428–438, 1969.

Meadow, K. and Schlesinger, H., The prevalence of behavioral problems in a population of deaf school children, *Amer. Ann. Deaf,* 116, 346–348, 1971.

Mindel, E. and Vernon, M., *They Grow in Silence: The Deaf Child and His Family.* Silver Springs, MD: National Association of the Deaf, 1971.

Moores, D., *Educating the Deaf: Psychology, Principles, and Practices.* Boston: Houghton Mifflin, 1978.

Moses, K., Issues in parent counseling: An introduction to mourning theory. Miniseminar presentation at the American Speech and Hearing Association, Las Vegas, Nevada, (November) 1974.

Murphy, K., Tests of abilities and attainments. In A. Ewing (Ed.), *Educational Guidance and the Deaf Child.* Manchester, England: Manchester University Press, 1957.

Myklebust, H., Towards a new understanding of the deaf child, *Amer. Ann. Deaf,* 98, 345–357, 1953.

Myklebust, H., *The Psychology of Deafness.* New York: Grune and Stratton, 1964.

Neuhaus, M., Modifications in the administration of the WISC performance subtests for children with profound hearing losses, *Except. Chil.,* 33, 573–574, 1967.

Neuhaus, M., Parental attitudes and emotional adjustment of deaf children, *Except. Chil.,* 35, 721–727, 1969.

Peterson, H., Achievement of hard of hearing students in regular public schools, Ph.D. Dissertation, Wayne State University, 1972.

Pintner, R., Some personality traits of hard of hearing children, *J. Gen. Psych.,* 60, 143–151, 1942.

Pintner, R., Eisenson, J., and Stanton, M., *The Psychology of the Physically Handicapped.* New York: Crofts and Co., 1941.

Pintner, R., Fusfeld, I., and Brunschwig, L., Personality tests of deaf adults, *J. Gen. Psych.,* 51, 305–317, 1937.

Raimy, V., *The Self Concept as a Factor in Counseling and Personality Organization.* Office of Educational Services, Ohio State University Libraries, 1971.

Rainer, J. and Altshuler, K., *Expanded Mental Health Care for the Deaf: Rehabilitation and Prevention.* New York: New York State Psychiatric Institute, 1970.

Ray, L., Thoughts of the deaf and dumb before instruction, *Amer. Ann. Deaf,* 1, 149–157, 1847.

Reed, M., Deaf and partially hearing children. In P. Mittler (Ed.), *The Psychological Assessment of Mental and Physical Handicaps.* London: Methuen, 1970.

Reich, C., Hambleton, D., and Houldin, B., The integration of hearing impaired children in regular classrooms, *Amer. Ann. Deaf,* 122, 534–543, 1977.

Reivich, R. and Rothrock, I., Behavior problems of deaf children and adolescents: A factor-analytic study, *J. Speech Hearing Res.,* 15, 93–104, 1972.

Rogers, C., *On Becoming a Person: A Therapist's View of Psychotherapy.* Boston: Houghton Mifflin, 1961.

Rosenstein, J., Perception, cognition and language in deaf children, *Except. Chil.,* 27, 276–284, 1961.

Schlesinger, H. and Meadow, K., *Sound and Sign: Childhood Deafness and Mental Health.* Berkeley: University of California Press, 1972.

Schroedel, J. and Schiff, W., Attitudes toward deafness among several deaf and hearing populations, *Rehab. Psych.,* 19, 59–70, 1972.

Shears, L. and Jensema, C., Social acceptability of anomalous persons, *Except. Chil.*, 36, 91-96, 1969.

Shif, Z., *Language Learning and Deaf Children's Thought Development*. Moscow: Institute of Defectology, 1969.

Soloman, J., Psychiatric implications of deafness, *Mental Hygiene*, 17, 37-52, 1943.

Springer, N. and Roslow, R., A further study of the psychoneurotic responses of the deaf and hearing child, *J. Educ. Psych.*, 29, 590-615, 1938.

Stewart, L., Problems of severely handicapped deaf: Implications for educational programs, *Amer. Ann. Deaf*, 116, 362-368, 1971.

Sullivan, P., A comparison of administration modifications on the WISC-R Performance Scale with different categories of deaf children, Ph.D. Dissertation, University of Iowa, 1978.

Titus, E., A study of self-concept and adjustment of deaf teenagers, Ph.D. Dissertation, University of Missouri, 1965.

Tomlinson-Keasey, C. and Kelly, R., The development of thought processes in deaf children, *Amer. Ann. Deaf*, 119, 693-700, 1974.

Valone, F., The study of self concept and anxiety as it relates to marginal status in the moderately hearing impaired population, *Dissertation Abstracts*, 31, 5646, 1971.

Vernon, M., Rh factor and deafness: The problem, its psychological, physical and educational manifestations, *Except. Chil.*, 34, 5-12, 1967a.

Vernon, M., Meningitis and deafness, *Laryngoscope*, 10, 1856-1874, 1967b.

Vernon, M., Prematurity and deafness: The magnitude and nature of the problem among deaf children, *Except. Chil.*, 34, 289-298, 1967c.

Vernon, M., Fifty years of research on the intelligence of the deaf and hard of hearing, *J. Rehab. Deaf*, 1, 1-12, 1968a.

Vernon, M., Current etiological factors in deafness, *Amer. Ann. Deaf*, 113, 106-115, 1968b.

Vernon, M. and Brown, D., A guide to psychological tests and testing procedures in the evaluation of the deaf and hard of hearing children, *J. Speech Hearing Dis.*, 29, 414-423, 1964.

Wylie, R., *The Self Concept: A Critical Survey of Pertinent Research Literature*. Lincoln: University of Nebraska Press, 1961.

PART Three

ADULTS

CHAPTER 12

Communication Problems of Adults

The onset of hearing loss can occur at any age and from a variety of causes. Typically, acquired hearing loss occurs after the age of 40; the majority of the hearing-impaired population are adults whose hearing was normal until adulthood, who have completed average educational programs, who have had productive work experiences, and who have well-established family and social relationships. As a result the effects of hearing impairment on these clients is quite different from those experienced by hearing-impaired children, and the habilitation planned for them differs in many respects.

The fundamental effect of acquired hearing loss on adults is a reduction in the ease with which they communicate with others. Unlike children, hearing-impaired adults have no difficulty expressing themselves through speech or writing; it is the reception of speech that creates problems for them. The once clear, complete acoustic information constituting spoken language is now less intense and distorted, making listening a difficult task involving concentration and effort. As a result of this basic effect, social and vocational activities are affected also, leading to the need to modify interaction patterns in order to communicate effectively. Because most adults do not welcome changes in basic life-style, emotional adjustment to hearing impairment is necessary. This is often a difficult accomplishment and one that can interfere with successful rehabilitation.

Even though hearing loss is disruptive to easy communication, it usually occurs gradually and may not be recognized by the hearing-impaired person as easily as by others in the environment. Consequently, some hearing-impaired adults consult audiologists, not because they consider themselves handicapped, but because someone else does. This distinction is an important one for purposes of assessment and rehabilitation.

Before planning the rehabilitation program to be used with an adult, the audiologist should be aware of the general characteristics of hearing impaired adults and the nature of the communicative, psychological and social effects of the hearing loss. Some of this information can be obtained during routine audiological assessment, which will not be discussed here. Other information is collected through case histories, interviews, observations, and special procedures, such as the administration of lipreading tests or self-assessment scales. Collection of the baseline data necessary for planning rehabilitation is the focus of the following discussion.

CHARACTERISTICS OF HEARING-IMPAIRED ADULTS

There are three important factors to consider when describing the characteristics of people who acquire a hearing loss in adulthood. These include the incidence of hearing loss among adults, the major characteristics of the hearing loss, and the psychosocial aspects of impairments in general and hearing loss in particular. Each of these factors significantly influences the need for rehabilitation programs, the elements of those programs, and the prognosis for successful rehabilitation.

Incidence of Hearing Impairment in Adults

Precise statistical incidence data are not available or are incomplete in important ways. The Subcommittee on Human Communication and Its Disorders (1969) reviewed four large, well-publicized studies conducted since 1936. Based on a population of 200,000,000 Americans, the subcommittee concluded that there were approximately 236,000 (1.18 per 1000) deaf individuals of all ages and sexes; that approximately 6 million (30 per 1000) additional Americans have bilateral hearing impairments of a significant degree; that an additional 2.5 million (12.5 per 1000) have significant unilateral hearing impairment; that about 700,000 Americans with hearing impairments also have some degree of handicapping visual problem; and that there are no reliable data on the prevalence of hearing loss by cause, pattern of loss, or the prevalence of *dysacusis* (defined as the "garbling of audible speech").

The subcommittee reported that approximately 55 percent of the hearing-impaired population are men and that of the 6 million individuals with bilateral hearing impairments, 13 percent are between 17 and 44 years of age, 27 percent between 45 and 64 years, and 54 percent are 65 or older. They also reported that 36 percent have hearing losses (ISO 1964 reference level) of less than 36 dB through the frequency range 500 to 2000 Hz in the better ear, 43 percent have losses between 37 and 56 dB, 13 percent between 57 and 76 dB, 5 percent 77 and 86 dB, and 3 percent have hearing losses greater than 87 dB. The conclusions are that 81 percent of the population with significant bilateral hearing loss is 45 years of age or older and that 92 percent have losses less than 77 dB.

The National Center for Health Statistics (1967) estimated that 13 percent (133 per 1000) of individuals over the age of 65 have significant bilateral hearing loss, while the American Speech and Hearing Association (Spahr, 1971) conservatively estimated the incidence to be between 13 to 25 percent. The Metropolitan Insurance Company predicted an incidence rate of 129 per 1000 (12.9 percent) for the age group 65 to 74 and 256 per 1000 (25.6 percent) for those over 75 years of age (Willeford, 1971). Precise figures are unknown but it appears that at least 4.4 percent of the population is afflicted with significant hearing impairments. Whether the incidence is as high as the 15,400,000 (approximately 6.5 percent of the population) estimated by the hearing aid industry (Anonymous, 1977) remains to be determined.

These figures suggest that over 90 percent of the hearing-impaired individuals in the United States are in the age groups to which this chapter is addressed. Furthermore, 92 percent of the adult group have average hearing losses less than 77 dB, which means they have substantial residual hearing for rehabilitation with amplification, all other factors being equal. An estimated 80 percent of all hearing-impaired individuals have auditory cues available to them even in the unaided situation (average hearing losses less than 56 dB). The fact that incidence of hearing loss increases noticeably with age (81 percent of the hearing impaired are over the age of 45) poses a problem in rehabilitation because of the nature of the impairment associated with aging. In addition, the situation is compounded by other factors: for example, the National Council on Aging (Tiven, 1971) reported that of the 20,000,000 Americans over age 65, 25 percent live in poverty, many suffer from social isolation, about 25 percent live alone or with nonrelatives, about 25 percent live without telephones, 5 percent live in institutions and about 10 percent are unable to leave their residence because of infirmity.

Audiologic rehabilitation of the aging is complicated by complex problems related to economic and sociological factors, general states of health and well-being, and a poorly understood service delivery system. Many elderly adults do not secure needed services because of limited financial resources and lack of third-party payment mechanisms for hearing rehabilitation. For many, adequate transportation is lacking and limitations of physical stamina preclude use of inexpensive public transportation. Many are concerned about physical safety on the streets and in unfamiliar neighborhoods. Others simply do not know what to do about their hearing problem or whose services to seek. Because hearing loss is not considered a threat to general health and does not produce physical discomfort, the problems cited above become significant barriers to obtaining needed rehabilitative services.

If all hearing-impaired people are to have access to audiologic rehabilitation, the challenge to the service delivery system is apparent. It is conservatively estimated that a minimum of 64 percent (excluding for the moment the 36 percent with better ear losses of less than 36 dB) or close to 4 million people with bilateral hearing loss and an unknown proportion of people with unilateral hearing loss are potential candidates for amplification, but only 2 million people presently possess hearing aids (Anonymous, 1977). In addition, there is evidence that these hearing aid users need improved quality and quantity of pre- and post-fitting service. The findings relative to the poor condition of hearing aids worn by children and the inadequacy of repair services (see Chapter 4) suggest that a similar situation may exist for adults. Much remains to be done to provide for the initial and continuing needs of the unserved and underserved hearing-impaired population. Public awareness of the importance of periodic hearing screening must be increased so that medical attention, behavioral modification, and rehabilitation procedures can be instituted at the earliest possible time.

Hearing Loss Characteristics

Adventitiously hearing-impaired adults display diverse hearing loss characteristics. Numerous etiologies, varying amounts of hearing loss, a variety of audiometric patterns, variations in type and amount of loss in the two ears, a wide range of auditory discrimination scores, and differences in age of onset and duration are apparent. Because our concern is nonmedical rehabilitation, it is assumed that the client has had appropriate medical management including a differential audiologic workup (Olsen and Matkin, 1978). The aspects of hearing loss to be discussed here should provide necessary background information and orientation to the receptive problems of the adult population and factors that limit, complicate, or compromise improvement of auditory function.

General Considerations. Adults may present hearing losses of a conductive, sensory, mixed, neural, or central origin. However, because approximately 81 percent of potential clients are over 45 years of age, the great majority seen in an audiology clinic will have sensorineural hearing losses related to presbycusis and noise-induced hearing loss. This does not necessarily mean, however, that 81 percent of a clinic population will be over the age of 45, because the odds are against older people seeking otologic or audiologic services for reasons cited earlier. A census count maintained by one of the authors over a two-year period in a medical school audiology clinic located in a metropolitan community revealed that 58 percent of the clients evaluated were over the age of 19, but only 16 percent were over 66 years of age. The clinic provided audiological services for over 2800 clients during the two-year period and offered a wide range of evaluative and rehabilitative services to people of all ages on a self-referral basis. Because national incidence figures suggest that 54 percent of the hearing impaired are over age 65 it is unfortunate that this age group accounts for such a small percentage of cases seen in a hearing clinic, but it reinforces earlier statements and suggests some unmet needs.

In addition to presbycusis and noise exposure, other primary or contributory causes of hearing losses in adults may be ototoxic reactions to drugs, head trauma, Meniere's syndrome, labrynthine otospongeosis, or space-occupying lesions along the neural pathways. In terms of degree of hearing loss, incidence data suggest that no more than 8 percent have pure-tone average losses in excess of 77 dB and that 79 percent have average hearing losses no worse than 56 dB. A variety of pure-tone audiometric threshold patterns are seen; however, since presbycusis and noise-induced hearing loss are the two most common causes in adults, audiometric curves displaying sloping, high-frequency sensorineural loss are characteristic. Unilateral hearing losses occur and some clients will have bilateral unequal and asymmetrical losses, but most adults will have bilateral equal and symmetrical pure-tone configurations. The auditory discrimination characteristics of this population will vary considerably due to etiological factors and may not necessarily be equal bilaterally. Many adults will also complain of tinnitus and, to a lesser extent, vertigo and dizziness.

Noise-Induced Hearing Loss. Maas (1972) reported that as much as 50 percent of the work force is exposed to sufficiently high levels of noise to warrant concern about eventual hearing impairment. Daily exposure to noise of 90 dBA or higher is known to be injurious; however, there is evidence that noise levels exceeding 80 dBA are harmful to some people. At present the U. S. Department of Labor requires employers to maintain a hearing conservation program for workers in areas exceeding the 90 dBA level. Until all individuals are adequately protected, noise-induced hearing loss will continue to be a significant etiological factor. More detailed information about environmental noise, its effects and management, is available in Brandy and Studebaker (1978), Henderson, Hamernik, Dosanjih, and Mills (1976), and Lipscomb (1978).

Glorig (1958) classified hearing losses caused by environmental noise into two types: *occupational hearing loss,* caused by noise exposure in the work place; and *sociocusis,* changes in hearing caused by long-term exposure to the ambient noise of modern society. Hearing loss caused by noise can also be classified on the basis of severity or duration of exposure. *Acoustic trauma* occurs as a result of a one-time exposure to an extremely high-intensity sound having a sudden onset. It may be of short duration, but not necessarily. An explosion, for example, could produce instantaneous permanent damage to the middle-ear mechanism and the cochlea. Firearms, while not as dangerous, can also produce acoustic trauma. The more common type of exposure, *noise-induced hearing loss,* denotes the insidious hearing loss that accumlates over months and years due to exposure for several minutes or hours per day to moderately high-intensity noise. It occurs as a consequence of daily exposure to nosie levels sufficiently high to produce auditory fatigue resulting in measurable temporary threshold shift (TTS). Although the ear can recover from fatigue after noise stimulation has stopped, repeated daily assaults of occupational noise eventually produce a permanent threshold shift (PTS). This degenerative process can be accelerated by additional exposure to high levels of noise around the home and from participation in noisy leisure and recreational pursuits.

Noise-induced hearing loss is of cochlear origin and is characterized by a high-frequency hearing loss first noticeable as a downward notch in the region of 4000 Hz on the audiogram. As the loss progresses the notch becomes deeper and wider, although hearing may remain near normal at 2000 Hz and below. Somewhat better hearing at 8000 Hz than at 4000 and 6000 Hz is observed (Ward, Fleer, and Glorig, 1961). Because tolerance thresholds do not tend to increase correspondingly, loudness recruitment, defined as an abnormal increase in loudness, is almost always present as a manifestation of this cochlear damage.

It is tempting to regard these high frequency cochlear losses as filters, producing reductions in word scores that are predictable by viewing the pure-tone audiogram as a bandpass filter (Ward, Fleer, and Glorig, 1961). However, as discussed in Chapter 2, this view is not consistent with the difficulty encountered in attempts to rehabilitate people with such losses. Recent studies indicate abnormal findings at adjacent frequencies showing thresholds in the normal range (Humes, Schwartz, and Bess, 1979). Although individuals with mild-to-moderate noise-induced hearing loss may achieve high auditory discrimination scores in quiet that suggest normal speech reception, a better indication of the handicapping effects of the loss are obtained by evaluating performance under more life-like conditions such as testing against a noise or competing background message. Such testing combined with the client's assessment of communication difficulties is a more relevant index of rehabilitative need.

Presbycusis. Presbycusics represent the largest etiological subgroup in the adult hearing-impaired population. Presbycusis encompasses all changes in auditory performance associated with the aging process. For many years this degenerative condition was thought to be accurately described by changes in auditory sensitivity, but sufficient information (Willeford, 1978) is available to reveal it as a complicated condition that challenges the evaluative and rehabilitative skills of the audiologist. It is characterized by physical and physiological changes from the pinna through every state of auditory processing to the cortical level. Antonelli (1978) has described aged individuals as showing evidence of reduced ability in acquiring new information, weakened memory (especially short term), lengthened reaction time, reduced concentration and attention powers, reduced hearing and vision sensitivity, and emotional and psychological problems. Structural changes occur in the external, middle and inner ear, including neuroepithelial degeneration, ateriosclerosis of cochlear vessels and calcification of the basilar membrane in the basal turn, cochlear nerve degeneration, and cellular degeneration of the brain (Hinchcliffe, 1962). Willeford (1978) added cellular degeneration at the brain stem level to update Hinchcliffe's observations.

On the basis of study of human temporal bones, Schuknecht (1964) identified four types of presbycusis. *Sensory presbycusis* is characterized by atrophy of the organ of Corti and the auditory nerve fibers at the basal end of the cochlea, which probably produces an abrupt high-frequency hearing loss. *Neural presbycusis* results from loss of neurons in the auditory pathways, causing further reduction in auditory discrimination beyond that associated with the simple filtering effects of high frequency loss. *Metabolic presbycusis* involves atrophy of the stria vascularis. The stria vascularis functions to sustain biochemical and bioelectric function of endolymph. Atrophy, according to Schuknecht, results in a flat loss of sensitivity across frequencies. *Mechanical presbycusis* occurs as a result of changes in stiffness of the basilar membrane or other structures of the cochlea and manifests itself in a descending threshold curve.

It is unlikely that an individual would exhibit only one form of presbycusis, because it appears to be a degenerative process involving the entire auditory system with any combination of types and degrees of involvement possible. The singular effects of aging alone have not been isolated, because the observable manifestations of presbycusis are probably contaminated by factors not directly related to aging. Important factors might be diet, anxiety, sociocusis, health history, use of drugs and alcohol, and inhaled pollutants.

A reduction in hearing sensitivity occurs with increasing age (Glorig and Roberts, 1965; Corso, 1963 a and b; Hardick, 1979). Changes associated with presbycusis become evident in the third decade of life and worsen with each additional decade. The hearing loss is characterized by more loss in sensitivity for high tones than low tones with males tending to have more impairment at all ages. The loss of sensitivity is bilateral and symmetrical.

In addition, the individual with presbycusis demonstrates reduced ability to understand speech, as measured by word or sentence materials, which may range from mild to severe and often is inconsistent with predictions based on the degree of loss of sensitivity. Gaeth (1948) was the first to describe reductions in discrimination that seemed inconsistent with the loss in sensitivity. He named the phenomenon "phonemic regression" and observed that it occurred most frequently in adults over the age of 50. Pestalozza and Shore (1955) provided additional evidence by comparing discrimination performance of young and aging subjects with similar amounts of sensitivity loss. These authors confirmed Gaeth's observation and further showed that there was no significant relationship between the loss in discrimination and audiometric slope. Other studies (Melrose, Welch, and Luterman, 1963; Goetzinger and Rousey, 1959; Goetzinger, Proud, Dirks, and Embrey, 1961; Olsen, 1965) have documented the existence of abnormal speech discrimination among the aging. Konig (1957) reported that older people tend to have larger than normal difference limens for frequency. The altered resolving power of the ear may produce distortion that precludes normal discrimination.

The differentiation of peripheral and nonperipheral factors affecting discrimination of speech has served as the basis for further study. Because central auditory problems are associated with poor performance on difficult listening tasks, researchers have examined the performance of aging individuals with distorted, compressed, or complex speech listening tasks. Bocca and Calearo (1963), Harbert, Young, and Menduke (1966), Bergman (1971), Smith and Prather (1971), Marston and Goetzinger (1972), Jerger (1973), Garstecki and Mulac (1974), Konkle, Beasley, and Bess (1977), and Antonelli (1978) have shown that aging individuals perform poorer than younger people and that those with presbycusis perform most poorly. Findings are suggestive of central auditory pathway degeneration as the basis for the poorer discrimination of aging subjects. Furthermore, reduction in performance may be independent of the amount and configuration of peripheral hearing impairment. There is some evidence (Olsen, 1965; Blumenfeld, Bergman and Millner, 1969) that reduced performance is additionally influenced by changes in attention span, increased irritation, and tension resulting from listening in a competing noise situation.

Areas of auditory function other than speech discrimination have not been studied as extensively; for example, findings relative to loudness recruitment are inconclusive. Pestalozza and Shore (1955) found no loudness recruitment in 50 percent of their presbycusic sample. Goetzinger, Proud, Dirks, and Embrey (1961) found no loudness recruitment in 22 percent of their aged subjects. Harbert, Young, and Menduke (1966) found no loudness recruitment in 70 percent of their aged subjects; and Jerger, Shedd, and Harford (1959) found loudness recruitment, as measured by the Short Increment Sensitivity Index (SISI), to be quite unpredictable with presbycusic subjects. Jerger (1973) investigated the relationship between recruitment, as defined by the level of the acoustic reflex, and discrimination loss in elderly subjects and concluded that the two phenomena were not closely related. Because loudness recruitment is known to be of cochlear origin, these findings support the contention that presbycusis entails some cellular degeneration of more central parts of the auditory system.

The weight of recent research corroborates the statement of Hinchcliffe (1962) that "changes in the brain are primarily responsible for the overall audiologic picture of presbycusis." We must look beyond the cochlea to understand the hearing problems of the elderly. This is easier said than done. Adequate diagnostic tools are lacking at present or have not as yet been applied to the hearing of the aged. Without better understanding and assessment of the parameters underlying the decreased auditory discrimination, development of appropriate rehabilitation procedures is impeded. The state of the art at the moment generally involves application of the same components of rehabilitation as employed with other etiologies. The fact that the aging experience increased distortion of speech in quiet even with mild impairment of sensitivity, display difficulty with the temporal aspect of audition, and experience more pronounced breakdown of auditory reception and processing in the presence of competing signals, testifies to the need for the development of appropriate evaluation and rehabilitation procedures for this population.

Psychosocial Aspects

The impact of hearing loss on psychosocial adjustment is a controversial subject. Much has been written on the subect, but there is little compelling evidence that hearing impairment, particularly that occurring in adult life, produces personality changes or mental illness. Clinical experience suggests that hearing-impaired adults make reasonable adjustments to the limitations imposed by hearing loss, although the process is enhanced by sensitive professional management. The development of hearing loss necessitates adjustments in interpersonal relationships, vocational activities and social participation. The expenditure of extra effort and visual vigilance is required in following the conversation of others; anxiety may be increased as a result of fear of misunderstanding; embarrassment may occur as a result of callous comments by normally hearing people; personal safety of hearing-impaired aging individuals may be jeopardized. In addition, impaired hearing becomes a factor in major decisions of life, such as choosing or changing vocations, marriage, or retirement plans; working-age adults may worry about making costly mistakes, measuring up to job demands, or meeting criteria for advancement; and, dependency on others may be increased (as a result of difficulty communicating on the telephone and in other situations).

The impact of required modifications of behavior on personality and social adjustment must be of concern to professionals serving the hearing impaired but the conclusion that hearing loss results in pathological behavior should be avoided. Published comments and research conclusions must be carefully interpreted because similarity between most subjects studied and the group under discussion here cannot always be ascertained. The typical hearing-impaired adult experienced normal or near normal hearing for many years; the hearing loss developed slowly over time and hearing can be used to some extent in interactions with others. It is unlikely that conclusions drawn from study of the congenitally deaf, the severely to profoundly impaired, or those with sudden traumatic severe hearing losses can be generalized to all hearing-impaired people.

Personality. A review of the writings of hearing-impaired people and the published opinions of experts concerning personality characteristics of hearing-impaired adults reveals inconsistencies (Welles, 1932; Barker, Wright, Meyerson, and Gonick, 1953). Hearing-impaired adults have been described as dependent, introverted, fearful, having a sense of inferiority, supersensitive, brooding, bitter, having a persecution complex, suspicious, listless, apathetic, egocentric, and selfish.

Other authors report few of these psychological manifestations. Pintner, Eisenson, and Stanton (1946) reviewed the early studies and concluded that the results of personality testing with the hearing impaired indicate that, as a group, they are not very different from the normally hearing; most of the studies finding them slightly more introverted and neurotic. Meyerson (1953) reviewed the writings on psychology of hearing loss and the divergent views on personaltiy characteristics of hearing impaired adults, finding that some authors concluded they have a "unique psychology" while others found no difference between normally hearing and hearing-impaired people. Unfortunately, little is known about the hearing loss characteristics and other pertinent history of people serving as subjects in most of the studies.

Ramsdell (1978 and earlier editions) reported that it is common for the hearing-impaired adult to experience depression and to tend toward paranoid reactions. Based on observations of and experiences with young servicemen who had experienced relatively sudden onset of traumatic hearing impairments during World War II, he described three psychological levels of hearing: the symbolic level where hearing is used to comprehend language, the signal or warning level where sound serves to alert us, and the primitive level where sound serves as the auditory background in all aspects of daily living. Ramsdell concluded that the depression that is characteristic of the hearing impaired and deaf occurs as a result of disruption of their hearing at the primitive level. He stated that deafness produces a psychological impairment more basic and more severe than the difficulty in communication.

Published research supporting the contention of Ramsdell is lacking, in spite of statements indicating increasing support for the theory (Ramsdell, 1978). Meyerson (1953) questioned the validity of the Ramsdell theory, because its logical results are not evidenced in most studies. All hearing-impaired people are not depressed and suspicious and, when present, the severity of these feelings does not appear to increase with amount of hearing impairment. Newby (1972), however, supported Ramsdell's theory, claiming that hearing loss often produces maladjustment which frequently consititues the greatest handicap associated with the loss. The Ramsdell theory cannot be accepted as a universal statement because, for example, it appears to run counter to an often observed phenomenon among the aging population. Many of these people seem comfortable with the peace and quiet provided by mild to moderate reductions in hearing level. They usually do not seek rehabilitation until the hearing loss is severe enough to interfere with speech reception and many resist the use of amplification because it entails readjustment to hearing low-level environmental sounds. They seem to regard hearing again at the primitive level as the intrusion of unwanted background noise rather than an essential ingredient in normal homeostasis. With presbycusics in particular the Ramsdell theory does not appear generally applicable, although contentions on both sides of the issue remain to be investigated.

Welles (1932), Pintner (1933) and Pintner, Fusfeld and Brunschwig (1937) employed the *Bernreuter Personality Inventory,* (Bernreuter, undated), a paper-and-pencil test of questionable validity (Meyerson, 1953), to investigate the psychological problems of the hearing-impaired adult. These three studies concluded that the hearing impaired (some of whom were deaf) were slightly more neurotic, more introverted, and less dominant than normally hearing people. Paper-and-pencil tests, including the Bernreuter, have been questioned as suitable for comparing the handicapped with the nondisabled because of differences in interpretive significance of test items which alters the validity depending on the comparability of the life situations of the tested individuals and those of the standardization groups (Barker, Wright, Meyerson, and Gonick, 1953). For example, it is doubtful that the same diagnostic significance can be attached to the responses of two people, one with hearing impairment and one with normal hearing, who prefer to "stay home and read a book" rather than "attend a party," when asked to select their preference. Although descriptions of their behavior are the same, it is grossly inappropriate to conclude that both of them are introverted without determining the influence of the hearing loss on the choice.

Myklebust (1960a) has written about the personality and emotional adjustment of hearing-impaired as well as deaf adults who were deaf from early life. He hypothesized that losses up to 45 dB produce impaired awareness and environmental detachment but that restricted socialization can be alleviated by getting closer to the speaker or by wearing amplification. He suggested that hearing losses between 45 and 65 dB clearly affect social intercourse and that background-foreground use of hearing is not possible. The use of amplification by this group is essential for conversation but limited in effectiveness to one person or small group situations; as a result they experience considerable detachment and seek social relationships with similarly impaired people. He suggested a classification of behaviors based on age of onset, while cautioning that other factors such as degree of loss must be considered. Hearing loss occurring in early to middle adulthood may affect marital adjustment, occupational status, choice of friends and social group, and may lead to development of "characteristic attitudes" based on sensory deprivation. Loss occurring in later life (after 60) may be a significant factor in increased withdrawal and communicative isolation precipitating anxiety and depression. Lack of employment, feelings of being useless and unwanted, and the need for self-care assistance would also contribute to poor adjustment and social isolation.

To test some of these hypotheses, Myklebust (1960b) studied emotional adjustment of hearing-impaired adults using the *Minnesota Multiphasic Personality Inventory* (MMPI) (Hathaway and McKinley, 1943). The subjects were 44 men and

83 women receiving services from a hearing society. The mean age was 45, mean age at onset was 22, and the mean hearing loss was 67 dB (ASA, 1951). (Incidentally, 50 percent of the subjects reported that hearing aids provided an unsatisfactory amount of benefit. Further clarification was not provided; we can only speculate as to reasons.) Myklebust found that the males had high scores on the *Depression, Schizophrenia,* and *Hypomania* scales while females had high scores on the *Interest, Schizophrenia, Hysteria,* and *Hypomania* scales. The females showed less emotional maladjustment that did the males. Based on comparisons with a group of congenitally deaf adults, age of onset and severity of hearing loss, in addition to sex, appeared to be significant factors influencing emotional adjustment. Myklebust found that (1) use of a hearing aid was associated with better adjustment; (2) the subjects did not show evidence of being suspicious; (3) married women were better adjusted than single or divorced women; (4) the better adjusted females were older; and (5) higher educational attainment was associated with better adjustment. The results could be interpreted to suggest personality changes associated with emotional maladjustment occurring as a result of sensory deprivation due to impaired hearing. Myklebust, however, questioned the validity of interpreting the MMPI findings in terms of norms for normally hearing people. He pointed out that high *Schizophrenia* scores might be a measure of anticipated isolation resulting from hearing loss rather than indicative of mental illness. He concluded, for example, "that deafness, particularly when profound and from early life, imposes a characteristic restriction on personality but does not cause mental illness" (p. 158). His research probably should not be interpreted (especially in light of the caution he expressed) as evidence of increased incidence of emotional maladjustment in hearing-impaired adults. Even if that conclusion were accepted its generality should be limited because his sample consisted of subjects with early onset, severe hearing loss.

After reviewing the literature, Goetzinger (1972) concluded that hearing-impaired adults show no more than mild deviation in personality characteristics. He stated that although hearing loss can have an adverse effect on personality and emotional and social adjustment, prevalence of psychosis is no greater in the hearing-impaired group than in the larger population, and the existing psychiatric conditions exhibit the same characteristics in both groups.

Hardick (1964) studied the self-concept of 105 hearing-impaired adults between the ages of 26 and 87 and compared them to a control group of 54 normally hearing adults matched to an appropriate member of the experimental group in terms of age, sex, and amount of formal education. The instrument consisted of semantic differential scales (Osgood, Succi, and Tannenbaum, 1961) evaluating the following concepts: *Myself, Friends, My Happiest Self, Myself with a Hearing Aid, Myself in the Future, People of Authority, and Myself and Failure*. Each concept was judged on three independent dimensions (determined by factor analysis) labeled *Capability, Genuineness,* and *Toughness*. Hardick concluded that the presence of a hearing loss severe enough to interfere with communication tended to make the adult feel less capable at present and in the future. This was interpreted to be a realistic observation based on the communication problems imposed by hearing impairment and the barrier it imposed to full participation in social and vocational pursuits. Hardick also concluded that (1) hearing-impaired adults do not differ in self-regard from normally hearing adults; (2) they do not differ from normally hearing adults in attitude toward friends, hearing loss, strangers, hearing aids, and failure; (3) amount of hearing loss does not appear to be an important variable in terms of altering self-concept; and (4) self-concept varies as a function of age and sex, with most positive self-concepts occurring in women and people over the age of 60.

To summarize what we regard as generally true about the effect of hearing loss on personality structure the study by Shontz (1977) will be cited. He completed an extensive review of the literature on many forms of physical disability and personality. He tested two hypotheses that seem to dominate professional thinking: that somatic disability is associated with particular forms of personality and that the effects on personality are proportional to the severity of the disability. Shontz concluded that neither hypothesis is supported in the research literature. His findings indicated that basic personality structure is remarkably stable and any disorganization that occurs is generally transient; however, all disabling conditions are likely to produce a degree of depression and mourning. Priorities need to be reassessed, interests may change, and social participation may be reduced or altered, but in most cases the basic personality structure seems resilient enough to withstand the assault and remain intact.

The impact may be more severe for those elderly individuals who can no longer assume responsibility for themselves. Some of them undergo personality changes as a result of cortical deterioration (Mead, 1962; Birren, Imus, and Windle, 1959) or as a result of loss of independence or isolation from family and friends. Willeford (1978) has spoken of procrastination and lack of motivation in the geriatric population as significant barriers to rehabilitation that may be related to personality changes associated with aging, as well as sociological factors and to general states of health and well-being. Although personality changes can occur independently of hearing status, it is presumed that hearing impairment would be a significant factor in time of onset, nature, and severity of changes. The reader is referred to Birren (1959, 1964a and b) and Birren, Imus, and Windle (1959) for a more extensive discussion of the effects of aging on the individual.

Social. The presence of a hearing loss might be expected to result in modifications in social behavior. Little research, however, has been directed to this important topic. Myklebust (1960b) has made some comments based on the study of 127 hearing-impaired adults described earlier. Although the results are meaningful for a population with certain hearing loss characteristics caution must be exercised in generalizing them as representative of all subgroups of hearing-impaired adults. His subject group was identified as (1) having a mean age of onset of 22, (2) an average loss of 67 dB, and (3) consisting of a large proportion (50 percent) of people who had never married. The subjects reported increased stress in everyday life; dependence on family members for assistance with messages, obtaining employment, and maintaining friends; increased social isolation; the need for association with other hearing-impaired individuals because it was difficult to maintain primary identification with the normally hearing; and increased concern about obtaining and holding employment. They sought employment and hobbies that did not require good hearing or communication. They de-emphasized companions and group participation, engaging in a form of withdrawal that Myklebust referred to as "perhaps realistic." According to him the most striking revelation was that very few hearing-impaired people maintained friendships established prior to acquiring the hearing loss.

Oyer and Paolucci (1970) found that hearing-impaired homemakers participated less than half as much in outside organizations and meetings as normally hearing homemakers. They also placed more emphasis on the home as a place where family members belonged, in contrast to emphasis of normally hearing homemakers on the home as a place to entertain friends. Hearing loss did not seem to produce significantly greater marital tension, although tension tended to increase with the severity of the hearing loss.

Hildreth and Oyer (1976) investigated the relationship between social participation and self-concept in 30 hearing-impaired adults. They concluded that there were no significant differences in self-concept among high, medium, and low social participators. More than half of the hearing-impaired subjects reported that they would prefer marrying someone with a hearing loss.

Powers and Powers (1978) reported the results of a longitudinal survey of social consequences associated with hearing loss in the elderly. The study consisted of interviews in 1960 with people 60 years of age and older and re-interviews of as many as possible in 1971. The responses of 226 individuals were summarized in the paper. Predicated on the assertions of Ramsdell (1978 and earlier editions) and Newby (1972), they presumed that there would be some disruptions in life-style and mental outlook caused by hearing loss in later life. Powers and Powers concluded that elderly people with hearing loss do not experience disruptions in their social existence or any other problems of adjustment different from their normally hearing contemporaries. Approximately 20 percent of the hearing-impaired sample reported feelings of loneliness; however, 33 percent of those with good hearing reported the same feelings. The authors investigated activities that provided great satisfaction to the respondents, involvement in organizations and frequency of out-of-house trips, social interactions, and feelings of loneliness. In no instance did they find evidence that elderly persons with hearing difficulty experienced unusual social or psychological problems. Their conclusions would have greater significance if hearing loss data had been available; the sample was dichotomized into hearing loss and normally hearing groups on the basis of self-report. It is conceivable that a proportion of the normally hearing group were, in fact, hearing impaired by commonly accepted criteria. If this were true, it would make the self-identified hearing loss group appear more similar to normally hearing people of the same age than actual conditions warrant. Their conclusions, tentative though they are, reinforce the clinical observation that moderate hearing impairments of gradual onset do not produce dramatic psychological problems or traumatic social upheavals in the life-style of most mature adults.

Reactions to Impairment and Adjustment. It is frequently stated that hearing loss is a nonvisible condition that contributes to the existence of a unique psychology of hearing impairment with the implication that there are emotional ramifications that are different from those associated with other disabilities or debilitating health conditions. The hearing impaired as a group are often characterized as withdrawn and neurotic, unusually resistant to acknowledging the presence of impairment, reluctant about seeking assistance, and poorly motivated to obtain rehabilitation. Research evidence, however, is lacking to support any contention that the hearing impaired are more ''unique'' in these respects than other impaired groups. Review of the general literature on disability reveals commonality regarding reactions to physical impairment. Hearing-impaired adults are a cross section of society displaying the same range of attitudes, personality variations, social behaviors, and reactions to adversity as are evident in the larger society. Physical disabilities and serious health problems have psychological ramifications, of course, but human reactions and adjustment processes to these conditions are quite similar. Becasue the psychology of hearing impairment is often treated separately from other disabling conditions in the literature, clinicians may not be aware of the similarities that contribute to the generally accepted, but untrue, notion that hearing impairment is unique in its effects.

Psychological reactions to illness can be classified into 10 major categories, one or more of which is likely to characterize a patient's response to becoming sick (Blum, 1960). The reactions are depression and self-rejection, fear, counterphobia, anxiety, frustration and anger, withdrawal or apathy, exaggeration of symptoms, regression, dependency, and self-centeredness. Enelow and Swisher (1972) have suggested additional descriptive terms including helplessness, inability to accept warmth or tenderness, denial, and projection (paranoid behavior). Initial reactions to disability embody the classical psychological defense mechanisms: regression, repression, isolation, projection, withdrawal, denial, reaction formation, self-rejection, and sublimation. There are no data available to indicate that these reactions are any more prevalent, severe, or persistent in hearing-impaired people than they are among those losing their vision, those adjusting to amputation of an extremity, or those having to cope with life-threatening conditions. Therapeutic approaches to rehabilitation may differ depending on the specific physical limitations, and each disabling condition imposes unique alterations in life-style. Psychological reactions, however, are basically the same, and the methods employed to help the patient work through these reactions to the point of acceptance and motivation to seek solutions are similar.

Rousey (1971) reported that the two defenses most likely used by the hearing impaired are projection and denial, and that the most commonly observed effects manifested by the hearing impaired are mourning, pain, and mortification.

Pollack (1978) reported that the most commonly seen defense mechanisms in the hearing-impaired adult are denial, projection, and withdrawal. He defines denial in the usual way: refusing to acknowledge the existence of hearing loss and communication difficulty. Projection, he claims, can be manifested in two ways when hearing loss is involved. Basically, projection is the distortion of perceptions of external stimuli and is observed in hearing-impaired people who blame others for their communication deficiencies; they may claim their hearing is good but other people do not talk like they used to. Pollack claims that another distortion of reality occurs through loss of ability to detect suprasegmental cues that provide nuances of meaning and emotion resulting in misinterpretation. He defines withdrawal as avoiding contact for fear of being thought stupid, rude, or inattentive.

Care should be exercised in assuming that withdrawal is an abnormal or undesirable characteristic of the hearing impaired. Withdrawal from participation in social activities may be a realistic behavior if little benefit is derived from it. One of the healthiest adjustments a hearing-impaired person makes is to substitute an activity that provides satisfaction and success for one that produces frustration and negligible success. Research and clinical reports that characterize the hearing impaired as "withdrawn" without further clarification do them a disservice. Hearing-impaired people make many adjustments in their interactions with the environment. They may avoid cocktail parties or attending the theater, but rewarding substitute activities are often developed. Too often hearing-impaired people are described only in terms of activities they no longer engage in. Describing the behavior as withdrawal provides an insufficient label at best and may indicate the naivete of professionals regarding logical adjustments to hearing loss. Withdrawal can be a problem for the hearing-impaired individual and for others in close association if it is more extensive than the hearing loss warrants or leads to brooding. The clinician should be alert to this possibility and address the matter, if permitted by the client, during the rehabilitation process.

Denial, procrastination, and lack of motivation are commonly observed behaviors especially during early stages of impairment or disease or with mild conditions. Many people delay a visit to the physician because of fear that suspicions will be confirmed. Less threatening alternative explanations of symptoms may be accepted until events prove them fallacious or until the individual is ready to accept the obvious. Many find it difficult to accept the aging process and for a time deny the existence of changing health status because of unwillingness to accept them as the natural consequence of living. Vision care professionals report that people procrastinate about visual examinations and delay obtaining bifocals, for example, until long after it has become obvious they are needed. Dembo, Ladieu, and Wright (1948) reported that visually impaired servicemen who had difficulty accepting their losses were found to engage in ineffective adjustment behaviors such as rejection of help, avoidance of discussion of their handicap, or acting as if the impairment did not exist. Nathanson, Bergman, and Gordon (1977) reported that 28 percent of 100 consecutive cases of hemiplegia exhibited denial. A study by Gray, Reinhardt, and Ward (1977) attempted to test the assumption that unwillingness or inability to accept impairment was a major reason why cardiovascular patients are rehabilitated less often than other disabled individuals. They concluded that denial occurred more frequently in these patients than in other disability groups and that they tended to be less willing to accept the illness realistically. They also demonstrated that cardiac patients entering a rehabilitation program oriented toward acceptance of impairment were rehabilitated at the same rate as other severely impaired persons.

It is possible that persons with hearing impairment procrastinate about seeking remedial services longer than persons with other types of impairment because hearing loss is not a visible condition. It is doubtful, however, that this assumption deserves the attention it has received. There are many other reasons why hearing-impaired people are not receiving needed services. Rehabilitation programs are not well publicized and comprehensive programs are not widely available. Oyer and Hodgson (1977) reported that the present service delivery system is fragmented and composed of competing components. Health care professionals often give conflicting or poor counseling (''A hearing aid will not help your kind of loss''; ''You do not have enough hearing loss to wear an aid—learn lipreading''; ''See an audiologist for selection of a hearing aid''; ''Go to the hearing aid dealer, he knows all about hearing aids''). Clients can become confused and terminate the search for assistance. According to government reports (Bureau of Consumer Protection, 1978), the traditional hearing aid delivery system has a poor public image. Associated professionals, including speech-language pathologists and audiologists, have not developed the necessary public education programs to improve that image.

Final Comments on Psychosocial Aspects of Hearing Impairment. It is not possible to make general statements about the psychosocial impact of hearing loss that apply to all individuals independent of age of onset, severity of loss, or nature of the origin of the loss. All too often, however, this has happened in the past. For the vast majority of hearing-impaired adults we cannot subscribe to the notion that undesirable personality changes are involved or that they adjust to their impairment in any ways different from others sustaining diverse impairments due to physical damage, degeneration, or debilitating health conditions.

Hearing-impaired clients are likely to present one or more of the reactions to illness or physical impairment previously discussed when they are first seen in the audiological facility. However, some may have already worked their way through these reactions and arrived at some level of acceptance. The sensitive clinician will ascertain the client's situation during the intake interview process or in the counseling session concluding the initial appointment. Initial reactions to impairment are not necessarily permanent states; however, unless the audiologist is sensitive to their presence and their amenability to change, given time or counseling, they may pose significant barriers to successful rehabilitation. Complete success will not be achieved with all clients, but no health care discipline achieves 100 percent success in terms of patient acceptance of the diagnosed condition or recommended therapies that do not promise cure or full restoration of function. For a rehabilitation program to be successful it must assist the hearing-impaired person to acknowledge the presence of the impairment and accept the condition and its ramifications. Hearing professionals should be aware that these are common reactions to illness or disability, expect the behavior to occur, and develop approaches that aid the client in adjustment. Clinicians might also examine their own attitudes and determine whether they provide assistance to clients in developing acceptance rather than engaging in a form of professional *projection,* wherein the hearing impaired are criticized for not doing what is expected or not behaving like "good" clients should.

ASSESSMENT OF HEARING-IMPAIRED ADULTS

The process of rehabilitating the hearing-impaired adult begins with a careful assessment of the communication deficit, the amount and scope of the handicap, and the attitudes of the clients and their close associates. Rehabilitation will be less successful if the sensory deficit is not acknowledged and accepted, or if the client or family and friends have unrealistic expectations of the benefits to be derived. This section discusses dimensions of assessment and their importance to rehabilitation. Commonly used tests for basic hearing assessment and discussion of all approaches to hearing aid recommendations is beyond the scope of this text. The reader is referred to Katz (1978), Rose (1978), Pollack (1975), and Hodgson and Skinner (1977) for a discussion of the theory, administration, and interpretation of audiological tests used in hearing assessment and hearing aid selection.

This discussion assumes that the audiologist is directly involved in the determination of need for rehabilitative services and the delivery of all or most of the recommended procedures. If an audiologist is not so involved, either because of the nature of the employment setting or lack of interest in this aspect of audiology, referral should be made to a rehabilitation-oriented audiological facility at the conclusion of the diagnostic workup and required medical management. The rehabilitation-oriented audiologist should be involved in the dispensing of amplification devices or have developed a hearing aid delivery system permitting professional management of all phases. It is not possible to deliver suitable and appropriate rehabilitative services if decisions regarding the use of amplification are made elsewhere. One reason why civilian audiologic habilitation services have never achieved the success of military or Veterans Administration programs is that the audiologist has not been intimately involved in all aspects of the rehabilitation program. Assuming responsibility for audiologic rehabilitation entails acceptance of accountability, which leads to a growth of professional expertise.

Interviewing Hearing-Impaired Adults

Evaluation of hearing for rehabilitative purposes begins with an interview. In most cases this is the first contact between the hearing-impaired person and the audiologist. The client may be alone or accompanied by another member of the family. During the interview case-history information will be obtained of importance in the choice of tests to be employed, the necessity for medical referral, and in determining rehabilitative needs. The case history should provide information in the following areas: (1) history of medical or surgical attention, (2) a summary of general health status, (3) the effect of the hearing loss on educational progress and achievement and vocational performance (whichever is appropriate), (4) the incidence of hearing loss in the family, (5) social and interpersonal difficulties in communication occurring as a result of the hearing loss, (6) nonmedical rehabilitative services previously obtained, and (7) client attitudes toward the psychosocial consequences of the hearing loss and the use of amplification.

The exact makeup of the case-history form will be determined by the orientation of the employment setting and the staff. Some facilities use an extensive question-answer type format that is completed by the audiologist during the interview process, while others take notes within the broad categories previously enumerated that are summarized in a written report. Other facilities require the client or someone associated with the client to complete a case-history questionnaire prior to the appointment. No matter how the case-history facts are obtained, the process should be supplemented by personal interview. It is by means of the interview that insight is obtained into the major concerns of the client, the acceptance or denial of the problem by the client or family, and any significant barriers to rehabilitation that need to be overcome. It also serves as the mechanism through which the audiologist can be identified as a professional who is genuinely interested in the problems associated with hearing loss and its rehabilitation. Sincere interest in all aspects of hearing loss and a willingness to listen to dimensions of the problem not directly related to the audiogram should be evident to the client. As this interest is communicated to the client, identification with the audiologist is increased, thereby providing the rapport necessary to motivate the client to follow audiologic recommendations. The interview, then, is an important component of the assessment process and will determine, to a great extent, the success of rehabilitative efforts.

The Open-Ended Interview. The establishment of a desirable clinical relationship is most readily accomplished through use of an open-ended interview technique, quite similar to the approach employed by many psychologists and psychiatrists. After comfortably greeting and seating the client in an informal but reasonably private environment, the interview is initiated by the statement "Tell me about your hearing problem." Opening the interview with an invitation to talk is helpful in building rapport, developing insight about the relative importance of concerns either in terms of the order of presentation or emphasis, at the same time being the vehicle for informal gathering of much case-history information. Most hearing-impaired individuals have great need to talk about their hearing loss, the impact on their lives, and their concerns and fears. They have many questions about these matters and would like them answered. All relevant case-history information may not be provided without the interjection of questions by the interviewer, but the client will usually touch on most of the important areas listed previously. If more information is desired the interviewer can steer the conversation by remarks such as "Tell me more about the hearing loss in your family."

The interview should be a two-person conversation with most of the talking done by the client. The audiologist makes comments or asks questions to elicit more information or to clarify points. The audiologist may take notes as the client talks or may fill in the blank spaces on an already prepared form. Through an open-ended interview or informal conversation the required case-history information relative to time of onset, family history, previous treatment, and other topics can be elicited. To avoid omission of important items, beginning clinicians might prepare questions, for example, that will elicit information about the effect of the hearing loss on employment status, activities of daily living, family relationships, social interactions, the practice of religion, emotional status, and attitudes about hearing aids.

Determining client attitudes is particularly important. Reactions to previous experience with hearing aids, otologic management, or audiological services may be relevant to current attitudes and pertinent to counseling strategy. Negative reactions to previous experience with amplification can delay acceptance of further attempts to find suitable hearing aids or otherwise complicate adjustment. Based on previous advice the client may feel that no hearing aid will help, or that learning to read lips will be a primary solution to communication problems. The nature of the advice and the client's degree of acceptance of it are important in determining management strategy. Acceptance of the clinician's habilitative plan may depend on awareness of the existence of such attitudes, their source, and strength. Facts and attitudes about previous management can be elicited by direct question if not volunteered. Emotional reactions to the hearing loss including level of acceptance of the impairment may have to be determined indirectly through analysis of interview content and behavioral observation.

Although the family may be interviewed as a unit initially, it is suggested that they be interviewed separately at some point. Independent interviews permit determination of the degree of congruence of information and attitudes provided by the parties. The existence of family friction and conflicts related to the impairment, or discrepant attitudes about it, may be made apparent by this process, when not observable through joint interviewing. Information gained provides valuable material supporting the need for rehabilitation as well as specific content of the program.

The Authoritarian Interview. Rosenberg (1972) concluded that the open-ended interview just described "is rarely well suited to the practice of audiology." He recommended the authoritarian approach commonly used by the medical profession, because it provides the maximum amount of information in the minimum amount of time. Perhaps it does, but it does not allay fears or encourage discussion of related effects of the hearing problem. Through the process of responding to factual questions the client may have the impression that matters tangential to a direct response are unwelcome. There may be times and employment settings in which the authoritarian approach to interviewing makes the most sense. It is an undesirable approach to employ in a rehabilitation-oriented setting because it limits information obtained to questions asked. It also tends to inhibit development of the perception of the audiologist as someone interested in rehabilitation in the broadest sense.

The Problem-Oriented Record. Enelow and Swisher (1972) have argued that the traditional medical model for interviewing is inadequate in that it is symptom oriented and not designed to treat the whole person. They advocate the open-ended interview and the use of the problem-oriented record. Although Enelow and Swisher are physicians and their book is written for practicing physicians and medical students, applications of the problem-oriented record to speech-language pathology and audiology have been made (Bouchard and Shane, 1977). The problem-oriented record is a means whereby records are organized in a standardized manner facilitating objective and subjective data collection and the formulation of goals and treatment plans. A list of client problems is formulated out of the data base that consists of case-history information, present complaints, life situation, and the results of all evaluations. A management plan is then developed encompassing all active problems. A major advantage of this approach is that it serves to remind the clinician that hearing loss has dimensions beyond differential diagnosis or difficulty hearing speech. The open-ended interview provides an efficient mechanism through which the audiologist obtains vital case-history information, develops hypotheses to be tested through audiologic evaluation procedures, and establishes a friendly professional rapport. The establishment of this relationship is critical to the successful completion of rehabilitative procedures.

Communication Deficit

Inadequate reception of speech is the primary communication deficit of adventitiously hearing-impaired adults. The problems in reception stem from reductions in loudness, the presence of distortion introduced by the defective auditory system, and reductions in redundancy due to external conditions. The reduction in sensation level, the presence of cochlear distortion, and the possible presence of central deterioration combine to reduce the audibility of acoustic cues that result in discrimination loss for conversational speech. Unfavorable listening conditions, including the presence of environmental noise and high reverberation, further compromise auditory discrimination. Listening to low sensation level, distorted speech signals is a difficult task that is compounded by the presence of competing signals.

Fortunately, there are several parameters to oral communication that can contribute to the total number of cues available. The most important parameter is the acoustic signal, which provides frequency, intensity, temporal, coarticulatory, and suprasegmental cues. This signal can be augmented by visual information that can provide useful supplemental information. The known rules of language usage and probabilities of word order and occurrence can also contribute to the information available in speech. Finally, oral communication has an environmental or contextual parameter that can be used to predict probable conversational utterances.

Auditory. The auditory communication deficit is measured as part of the routine assessment of hearing. The deficit may be defined in terms of monaural speech reception thresholds (SRT), thresholds of discomfort, and measures of auditory discrimination at one or more sensation levels. It should also consist of an SRT and discrimination score obtained through a loudspeaker in a sound field, with the discrimination test administered at a normal conversational intensity level. In most clinical situations, a hearing level of 50 dB for discrimination testing should be acceptable if sound-field audiometric zero is calibrated to 12 to 14 dB SPL and assuming conversational speech to be a level of 65 dB SPL (Wilber, 1978).

Speech Reception Thresholds. The SRT provides useful supplemental information about the severity of the hearing loss and the need for rehabilitation, although it can be misleading if considered alone. For example, an SRT of 20 dB could be interpreted as indicative of hearing within the normal range, but if accompanied by a discrimination score of 76 percent the interpretation would be quite different. The importance attached to loss of communication ability varies from individual to individual. The same 45 dB hearing loss may seem catastrophic to a sales representative, but a mere nuisance to the babysitter of five noisy, active children. The decibel difference between the SRT and threshold of discomfort describes the range of potentially useful residual hearing.

Speech Discrimination Scores. Discrimination scores, in percent, are an important estimate of suprathreshold hearing deficit. They provide information about the amount of loss, the similarity of the two ears, comparative performance of hearing aids, and the amount of benefit derived from amplification. A variety of stimulus materials may be used to obtain speech discrimination scores, including phonetically balanced monosyllabic word lists, meaningful sentences, synthetic sentences or sentence tests incorporating variations in predictability due to linguistic factors. These stimuli are described in Chapter 2 along with a discussion of their questionable validity as predictors of communicative handicap. The relations between discrimination test scores and difficulty understanding conversational speech have not been demonstrated. Nevertheless, they provide comparative information that can be used to describe any hearing loss. To determine the effects of a given discrimination score on an individual, the clinician must listen carefully as the client talks about the difficulties experienced in communicating. In the absence of more valid predictors, the client's comments are essential to judging the degree and importance of the communication deficit.

Discrimination testing should be accomplished in the presence of noise or competing speech as well as in the quiet environment of a sound-treated room. Scores obtained under these conditions are often more closely related to the client's impression of communication deficit. The need for testing auditory discrimination in noise cannot be overstressed. The satisfactory rehabilitation of the hearing impaired, particularly the elderly, cannot be accomplished without knowing how well or poorly the client can hear in a noisy environment. Because older people appear to have a heightened aversion to amplification if it means exposure to noise levels reasonably well tolerated by younger individuals, information about speech perception in noise is important to the choice of an appropriate hearing aid and earmold, or to whether or not a hearing aid should be recommended at all (Olsen, 1970).

There are problems associated with the use of noise in discrimination testing that may explain why this test condition is not universally employed. The reliability of such testing has been questioned (Shore, Bilger, and Hirsh, 1960); it may add materially to the length of the evaluation; and there are unresolved questions as to the type of noise to be employed, the presentation levels, and the signal-to-noise ratio to be used. Until more definitive data are available, it is suggested that audiometer-produced speech noise or recorded multispeaker connected discourse be employed as the background noise. This testing should be conducted in the sound field at a level producing a 0 to +10 signal-to-noise ratio.

The questionable predictive ability of currently employed discrimination materials and the lack of consistency in the way they are presented during hearing assessment argue against the use of arbitrary guidelines in the selection of amplification. Examples of conventional wisdom often quoted as rules for hearing aid selection are as follows:

1. Place the hearing aid in the ear with the best discrimination.
2. Place the hearing aid in the ear with the flattest audiometric curve.
3. Place the hearing aid in the ear with the highest discomfort level.
4. Place the hearing aid in the ear with the poorest pure tone thresholds unless the loss in the better ear exceeds 60 dB.

5. Mild hearing losses cannot benefit from amplification.
6. Hearing aids are of no benefit to clients with sensorineural hearing loss.
7. Hearing aids provide no benefit for clients with poor discrimination for speech.

Millin (1975) has reviewed many of these "rules" or "axioms" and concluded that they are untested hypotheses. Predictive validity of discrimination testing materials is not a central issue in all of the above points, but they are included to illustrate another point. The clinician must keep an open mind about all aspects of amplification, as unfettered as possible by unproven assumptions and biases that preclude imagination, innovation, and creativity. Tests of auditory communication deficits provide useful objective baseline data which can be used in conjunction with the more subjective, but perhaps equally important, information provided by the client. The experienced clinician does not ignore nor discard subjective reports by the client simply because they are not supported by objective test scores.

Auditory-Visual. The testing of combined auditory-visual perception should be an important part of any assessment for rehabilitation purposes. As long as amplification systems provide limited benefits, rehabilitation of the hearing impaired cannot be planned without knowledge of the effects of the interaction of visual and auditory cues. The use of such testing is informative to the client as well and may serve an important need by educating them about the existence and the value of rehabilitative services other than the use of a hearing aid.

Auditory-visual testing is accomplished by allowing the client to lipread and listen to speech simultaneously. This is usually accomplished in a face-to-face situation or through the use of videotapes. A discussion of the materials that can be used can be found in Chapters 2 and 3. Although most of the materials suggested have not been designed for combined auditory-visual use nor validated when presented this way, the information obtained can be used (1) to describe the communication deficit, (2) to validate client comments about the degree of handicap, (3) in the evaluation and selection of appropriate amplification (Dodds and Harford, 1968), (4) to determine whether remedial services beyond the recommendation of a hearing aid should be considered, (5) to demonstrate to the client and family the importance of combining auditory and visual cues for the maximal understanding of communication, (6) to motivate the client to participate in therapy activities when they are indicated, and (7) to demonstrate the importance of good vision to individuals sustaining hearing impairment.

Expression. As a rule, people who develop hearing loss in adulthood do not experience difficulty expressing themselves. Sometimes, however, hearing impairment in adulthood can result in defective speech. When changes in speech production do occur, it is because the auditory feedback by which speech is usually monitored is reduced or absent. The specific problems that occur are related to the degree and pattern of the hearing impairment. A severe loss of hearing in the high frequencies, for example, may result in distortions of certain consonants, while a severe to profound loss of hearing across all frequencies is likely to cause changes in voice quality and articulation of many vowels and consonants. Generally speaking, the more severe the hearing loss, the greater the changes in speech. These changes do not occur suddenly, however; they develop slowly over a period of time and changes often occur so slowly as to be almost imperceptible to those who communicate with the hearing-impaired person daily.

The following list gives the most common characteristics of defective speech resulting from acquired hearing loss.

1. Distorted production of consonants, especially affricates, sibilants, and glides such as **ch, s,** and **r.**
2. Inappropriate vocal intensity (too loud or too soft) and failure to modify intensity in different situations.
3. Omission of unstressed word endings or function words (such as **-ed, 's, is,** or **has**).

When hearing loss is severe, the following deviations may also occur.

1. Neutralization of vowels, resulting in poor distinction between similar vowels, such as **-i-** and **ee.**
2. Intonation patterns that do not vary much with different sentence patterns and that are somewhat flat and monotonous.
3. Inappropriate stress on syllables and words.

To the listener these latter changes are perceived as indistinct, "hollow-sounding" speech that seems too rapid and generally blurred. The muffled quality may result from changes in resonance caused by altered tongue and jaw movements during speech, resulting from efforts to monitor speech production in the absence of auditory feedback. They occur only when the acquired hearing loss is severe and usually involve retraction of the tongue and exaggerated movements of the mandible.

Little is known about the exact characteristics of adventitiously hearing-impaired speakers or the rate at which deterioration of speech occurs after hearing is lost. Research has not been reported for subjects of this kind, but clinical experience indicates that both rate and extent of the changes observed vary among individuals and are related to the following factors.

1. Degree of hearing loss. This factor has already been mentioned but bears repeating because it is the single most important determiner of the effects of acquired hearing loss on speech. People who experience a mild or moderate loss rarely exhibit significant changes in speech, with the exception of a tendency to speak louder. People who develop severe or profound hearing impairments almost always exhibit distorted speech as described above. The determining factor is the efficacy of auditory feedback, both its physical limitations and the use made of residual hearing by the individual involved. As a result, the use of amplification is important to maintaining normal speech patterns.

2. Audiometric pattern of the hearing loss. Useful hearing across a broad range of frequencies provides much redundant information that can be used for perception of the speech of others and monitoring of our own. Hearing loss in any frequency region limits redundancy and affects hearing for speech differentially. The complex interactions that occur in connected speech make it impossible to define precisely the effects of hearing loss at a single frequency or on a single phoneme. Certain general statements can be made, however. For example, severe hearing loss in the frequencies above 1500 Hz will affect perception and subsequent production of consonants whose major energy occurs above 1500 to 2000 Hz. These include **th, s, ch, k, f, v, t,** and **z.** The same high frequency loss will not adversely affect pitch, intensity, rhythm, vowel articulation, or consonants whose energy is concentrated in the low or middle frequencies. Low and middle frequency hearing provides information about fundamental frequency and vowel formants and transitions that make monitoring of these facets of speech possible.

Generally speaking, a severe or profound loss of hearing across frequencies, including low frequencies, reduces redundancy of auditory information to such an extent that frequency, intensity, articulation of vowels and consonants, and speech rhythm will be affected eventually.

3. Age of onset of the loss. The degree to which speech production is affected is related to age of onset, but the exact nature of the relationship has not been investigated. An adult undoubtedly has more firmly established speech habits than a young child, but no data exist that make it possible to mkae definite prognostic statements. Experience indicates that children who are deafened as preschoolers sometimes become unintelligible speakers and may cease to use speech altogether unless remedial efforts are prompt and intensive. Such drastic changes in speech do not occur in deafened adults, who usually remain intelligible although inexperienced listeners may have difficulty understanding them at times. Less severe hearing losses also result in fewer changes in the speech of adults than children, but the differences, if any, between young adults and older ones are unknown.

Because changes in speech usually do not occur unless the hearing loss is severe, less than 10 percent of the adult population is likely to exhibit the speech problems described above. Therefore, assessment of speech is not a routine part of the evaluation of hearing-impaired adults. Careful observation of speech during the interview will usually provide the evidence needed to decide if further evaluation is necessary. Use of inappropriate intensity levels can usually be remedied by the use of amplification. Many adults who have had hearing losses for a long time are surprised at how loudly they speak when they listen to themselves while wearing a hearing aid. It only takes one or two sentences before the voice is lowered in intensity and monitored effectively through audition.

Articulation tests or analysis of recorded speech samples will allow the clinician to describe the characteristics of the adults' speech. It is important to determine whether speech was normal before the advent of the hearing loss in order to assess the effects of hearing impairment on the individual's speech. Speech problems such as frontal lisps, stuttering, or pronounced hypernasality, cannot be attributed to acquired loss.

Hearing Handicap. Clinicians have long been aware of the need for some effective means of assessing the handicap imposed by hearing impairment. Hearing *impairment* is usually described by measures of hearing, such as the loss of sensitivity indicated by threshold shift and loss of acuity as measured by suprathreshold discrimination tests. Hearing *handicap* refers to the disadvantages experienced by the individual in activities of daily life that derive from the hearing impairment, but not necessarily solely determined by the *amount* of impairment. Handicap also differs from disability, a term reserved for the real, assumed, or probable inability of the individual to remain employed as a consequence of permanent impairment (American Medical Association, 1961).

There have been attempts to derive categories of handicap directly from degrees of impairment. Attempts to summarize most forms of human behavior are usually frustrating and misleading because they tend to describe only the average situation. Attempts to derive single-number estimates of impairment or handicap cannot take into account all of the factors contributing to the deficit in the individual case. Such is the situation in describing the effects of hearing loss on communication. Table 12.1 (taken from Davis, 1978) shows categories of hearing loss derived from the 1960–1962 National Health Survey and the 1962–1963 Health Interview Survey (Gentile, Schein, and Haase, 1963). This classification system predicts degree of handicap by using pure tone averages as a measure of the ability to understand speech in a quiet environment. Unfortunately, this table gives the impression that hearing losses up to an average of 40 dB produce only marginal, perhaps inconsequential problems. It tends to oversimplify the situation by ignoring the harmful effects of reduced (less positive) signal-to-noise ratios (see Chapter 4) on speech discrimination and does not even consider variations in suprathreshold discrimination ability. Caution should be exercised interpreting the "degree of handicap" and "ability to understand speech" labels. Many people with average hearing losses between 25 and 40 dB would take exception to a description of their problem as "difficulty only with faint speech," and those with hearing losses of less than 25 dB often complain of significant hearing problems, especially in noise. Rather than rigidly applying descriptors of this type to determine rehabilitative needs, the clinician should ascertain from the client the specific effects of the loss.

We have stressed the importance of determining the client's reaction to the hearing loss and the importance of ascertaining those areas of communication that present the greatest difficulty. Anecdotal reports of handicap provide useful information about rehabilitative needs, while giving the hearing-impaired individual an

Table 12.1 Classes of Hearing Handicap[a]

Hearing Threshold Level dB (ISO)	*Class*	*Degree of Handicap*	*Average Hearing Threshold Level for 500, 1000, and 2000 Hz in the Better Ear*[b]		*Ability to Understand Speech*
			More than	*Not More Than*	
25	A	Not significant		25 dB (ISO)	No significant difficulty with faint speech
40	B	Slight handicap	25 dB (ISO)	40 dB	Difficulty only with faint speech
55	C	Mild handicap	40 dB	55 dB	Frequent difficulty with normal speech
70	D	Marked handicap	55 dB	70 dB	Frequent difficulty with loud speech
90	E	Severe handicap	70 dB	90 dB	Can understand only shouted or amplified speech
	F	Extreme handicap	90 dB		Usually cannot understand even amplified speech

[a] From Hallowell Davis and S. Richard Silverman (eds.), *Hearing and Deafness,* 4th ed. Copyright © 1978, 1970, 1960, copyright 1947 by Holt, Rinehart and Winston. Reprinted by permission of Holt, Rinehart and Winston.

[b] Whenever the average for the poorer ear is 25 dB or more greater than that of the better ear in this frequency range, 5 dB is added to the average for the better ear. This adjusted average determines the degree and class of handicap. For example, if a person's average hearing-threshold level for 500, 1000, and 2000 Hz is 37 dB in one ear and 62 dB or more in the other his or her adjusted average hearing-threshold level is 42 dB and his or her handicap is Class C instead of Class B.

opportunity to talk with a sympathetic person about related problems. Anecdotal material, however, does not lend itself to comparisons from person to person or for measuring the effectiveness of a therapy program. Objective and quantifiable measures are needed to assess handicap in the individual case, to accomplish research on the relationships between impairment and other variables influencing the degree of handicap, and for determining the need for and effectiveness of therapeutic treatment. High, Fairbanks, and Glorig (1964) have indicated that these research needs are probably greatest for individuals sustaining moderate degrees of hearing loss, a large proportion of individuals in the adult hearing-impaired group under consideration.

Impairment can be measured rather precisely, with results reported in dB (SRT, threshold of discomfort, stapedial reflex thresholds) or percent loss of discrimination. The handicapping effects of a given impairment are not so easily ascertained or quantified. Clinical experience indicates that the amount of handicap is influenced by personality factors, the importance of communication in the vocational setting, avocational interests, family structure, ability to use lipreading as a supplement to acoustic cues, and other variables. Basing hearing aid recommendations, for example, solely on measures of impairment might lead to inappropriate recommendations in equivocal cases if changing the handicapping effects of the loss is the purpose of hearing aid use. For example, it might be difficult to justify the recommendation of a hearing aid for all individuals with a 30 dB hearing loss if measures of impairment were used as the primary criteria. It is possible, however, that significant positive changes in *handicap* could occur with amplification even though there are only minimal changes in the aided measures of *impairment*.

In spite of the recognized need in audiology for a valid instrument to assess hearing handicap, no commonly accepted instrument has yet been developed. Many of the proposed measures of handicap have been criticized for being too narrow in scope, including items more correlated to loss of sensitivity than to loss of discrimination, using self-assessment scales susceptible to falsification, or being derived solely from measures of impairment. One or more of these objections apply to all of the measures to be discussed. The ideal instrument should provide a summary of how handicapped the individual is as a result of a given amount of hearing impairment, by providing the following information: (1) an estimate of communication difficulties in various settings, (2) the effect of hearing loss on vocational performance and security, (3) changes that have occurred in daily living activities, (4) how future goals and plans have been modified, (5) personal attitudes about hearing loss and hearing aids, (6) emotional reactions to the hearing loss, and (7) an estimate of the personal importance of noncommunicative aspects, such as reduced ability to hear environmental sounds, localization problems, and reactions to tinnitus. The test should be easy to administer, objective, and quantifiable. It should be sensitive to changes in attitude or behavior, and it must be reliable and demonstrate good face validity. The test will probably have to be a questionnaire of the self-assessment type because it is difficult to obtain more direct measures of some observations and reactions. With these comments in mind, a review of presently available measures of handicap will be undertaken.

Hearing Handicap Scale. High, Fairbanks, and Glorig (1964) developed the *Hearing Handicap Scale* (HHS), a self-assessment procedure. They defined handicap as "any disadvantage in the activities of everyday living which derives from hearing impairment." Two equivalent forms consisting of 20 items each were developed (see Appendix A). Subjects responded to each item by selecting one of five responses along a continuum from "almost always" to "almost never" with the middle position represented by "sometimes" The authors administered the measurement items to 50 hearing-impaired adults along with a battery of audiological tests including pure tone thresholds, speech reception threshold, and discrimination tests employing two different monosyllabic word lists.

The *HHS* has been criticized because it is too narrow in scope (it does not deal with vocational problems or attitudes) and because the items seem more related to hearing sensitivity than to discrimination problems (Giolas, 1970). The last comment reflects the fact that many professionals expect a test of handicap to correlate highly with discrimination score. They have been perplexed to discover that the *HHS* correlates with measures of threshold ($r = .70$) and poorest with measures of discrimination ($r = -.24$). Because the appropriateness of monosyllabic word lists for discrimination testing is questionable, the low correlation between discrimination test scores and the *HHS* may result more from the poor validity of the PB lists than the *HHS* itself. Subjects may have responded to *HHS* items on the basis of their ability to participate in conversations or follow continuous discourse. These activities may not be predicted well by a score on a hearing test consisting of monosyllabic words.

High, Fairbanks, and Glorig (1964) concluded that loss of sensitivity is apparently a major determinant of amount of handicap, a conclusion that is suspect unless we assume that the *HHS* is a valid test of handicap. Evidence supporting this conclusion is available from Koniditsiotis (1971) who correlated audiological test scores with observations of actual performance of subjects in communication situations. She concluded that actual performance was better predicted by SRT than by suprathreshold discrimination scores for monosyllabic words.

A major limitation of the *HHS* would appear to be its narrow scope rather than its poor correlation with measures of auditory discrimination. Questions are limited to the ability to hear and carry on conversations; the scale does not sample other aspects of daily living. A major advantage to the *HHS* is the fact that it evolved from rigorous developmental procedures and has been subjected to further research (Blumenfeld, Bergman, and Millner, 1969; Speaks, Jerger, and Trammel, 1970; Peters, 1974).

Peters (1974) investigated the relationship between audiologic measures and the *HHS*. His findings have a bearing on the criticism of the *HHS* that falsification of responses can occur easily. Peters hypothesized that increased impairment, as revealed by audiological tests, would produce greater self-estimated handicap. He further postulated that if self-assessed handicap was not found to be different from estimates made by the spouse, this would indicate that respondents provided honest appraisals. He administered the *HHS* to hearing-impaired males and their wives. Peters found that greater impairment was associated with increases in self-reported handicap, and he found no significant difference between independent ratings provided by the subject and spouse, which were highly correlated ($r = .80$). These results lend credibility to the *HHS* and indicate that, although falsification of responses can occur, subjects tend to provide honest reports. Peters also found higher correlations between self-assessed handicap and discrimination scores and somewhat lower correlations between threshold measures and self-assessed handicap than reported by High, Fairbanks, and Glorig (1964).

Schow and Tannahill (1977) have provided useful information regarding classification of *HHS* scores. They administered the test to 50 subjects with varying degrees of hearing loss including some with normal hearing. The normally hearing subjects obtained a mean *HHS* socre of 7.8 percent; those with an average HL between 11 and 25 dB showed a mean score of 25.6 percent; and those with average HL's worse than 27 dB obtained a mean score of 54.3 percent. Their classification system is shown in Table 12.2. Because their sample of hearing loss subjects was small and no individual had a pure tone threshold (500, 1000, or 2000 Hz) loss greater than 65 dB, the classification system shown is regarded as a tentative guideline at present.

Tannahill (1979) administered the *HHS* to 24 hearing-impaired adults before and after a one-month trial with hearing aids and found it useful for assessing benefit in daily listening experiences. He also reported that reductions in handicap as measured by the *HHS* were more highly correlated with improvements in auditory discrimination at conversational level than improvements in SRT. He concluded

Table 12.2 Classification of Handicap Based on Percentage Score on the Hearing Handicap Scale[a]

Category	*Range of Percentage Scores*
No handicap	0–20
Slight hearing handicap	21–40
Mild–moderate hearing handicap	41–70
Severe hearing handicap	71–100

[a] From R. Schow and J. Tannahill, Hearing handicapped scores and categories for Ss with normal and impaired hearing sensitivity, *J. Amer. Audiol. Society*. Baltimore: Williams and Wilkins, Co., © 1977.

that improvement in SRT in cases of mild loss or high frequency loss was less important than increases in discrimination.

These studies indicate that the *HHS* has reasonable validity as an estimate of handicap because *HHS* scores reflect decreases in the ability to discriminate speech. Therefore, the *HHS* can be used to estimate degree of handicap, although it may be narrower in scope than desirable.

Hearing Measurement Scale. Noble and Atherley (1970) refined the *Hearing Measurement Scale* (*HMS*) for assessing the degree of handicap caused by hearing loss of cochlear origin due to noise exposure. Through several experimental procedures they developed a 42-item test divided into seven sections: I, Speech Hearing; II, Acuity for Non-speech Sound; III, Localization; IV, Emotional Response; V, Speech Distortion; VI, Tinnitus; and VII, Personal Opinion. Each section has a weighted score with a possible maximum score of 226. The scale is designed to be administered in an interview situation. Responses are quantified after the conclusion of the interview according to scoring criteria developed by the authors. The manual of instructions must be read in order to administer and score the test, but these instructions are only available from the principal author (see Appendix B for *HMS* items and address).

Noble and Atherley conducted three preliminary studies in which the original pool of items and modified forms of the test were administered to 114 subjects whose hearing impairment was caused primarily by exposure to noise. Reliability data on the final form of the test were obtained from 27 subjects with occupationally caused noise-induced hearing loss and a final study involving 46 men with noise-induced hearing loss was done to determine relationships between reported handicap and various audiological measures of impairment. The authors reported high correlations between hearing-threshold measures and Speech Hearing (I), Acuity for Non-speech Sound (II), and Localization (III). Discrimination scores correlated highest with Distortion of Speech Sounds (V). The authors contended that the obtained correlations with audiologic measures of hearing impairment supported the validity of the *HMS*. They attributed the fact that measures of SRT seemed to be a better predictor of handicap than discrimination scores to the auditory discrimination necessary to achieve the 50 percent correct identification required for an SRT. These authors even hypothesized that a 50 percent correct identification requirement for SRT may be a more valid measure of everyday hearing capacity than suprathreshold discrimination for monosyllabic words.

The *HMS* appears to satisfy the requirements for an acceptable measure of hearing handicap. Its chief limitation is the amount of clinician time required to complete the interview (between 10 and 40 minutes). The authors indicated that the *HMS* could be modified to be given as a paper-and-pencil task and has been recently published in that format (Noble, 1979). Even though the test was developed specifically for use with working-age adults having noise-induced sensorineural hearing loss, there is evidence that it is equally useful with other adults or other etiologies (McCartney, Maurer, and Sorenson, 1976). The instrument has been subjected to rigorous study and deserves to be considered, at the moment, as a primary tool for determining the amount of handicap exhibited by hearing-impaired adults.

Social Hearing Handicap Index. Ewertsen and Birk-Nielsen (1973) developed the *Social Hearing Handicap Index (SHHI)* (see Appendix C). This scale was developed because of the need to measure psychological, vocational, and family aspects of hearing loss not available through knowledge of audiometric test results. Their questionnaire is quite similar to that of High, Fairbanks, and Glorig (1964), but consists of only one 21-item form. The primary difference between the *SHHI* and the *HHS* is the method of obtaining answers from the hearing-impaired patient. Ewertsen and Birk-Nielsen felt that the multiple choice format of the *HHS* would tend to produce superficial and random answers, while a free-response mode, such as the interview technique used with the *HMS,* would make responses difficult to score. To avoid these problems they wrote all items in the form of questions that could be answered either "yes" or "no." Uncertain responses should be enclosed in parentheses. If the respondent is unfamiliar with a given situation or cannot remember the amount of difficulty associated with it, the response can be "I do not know."

The 21 questions sample conversational situations with one person in quiet as well as in noisy surroundings, group conversation, capacity to communicate effectively over the telephone, and understand speech via radio or television. Questions are written in such a way that some answers must be "yes" and others must be "no" if handicap exists. If answers indicate handicap they are given 2 points, if the answer is in parentheses it is given 1 point and the "don't know" answer receives 0 points. The maximum handicap score (h) is 42. A decimal system Social Handicap Index score (the score is referred to as the SHI by the authors rather than *SHHI)* is derived by the formula: SHI $= (h/42) \times 100$. This produces a scale from 0 to 100, where 0 means no handicap and 100 means maximum handicap.

Although the *SHHI* is a self-report scale and economical of professional time, it consists of only one form and thus does not lend itself to repeated administration over short time intervals. In addition, it is subject to the same criticism as the *HHS*; it is narrow in scope because it is limited to the assessment of problems in hearing speech. Ewertsen and Birk-Nielsen (1973) reported administration of the *SHHI* to 198 hearing-impaired adults. Results indicated that the SHI is related to the quantity of hearing impairment, but it also produces a measure independent of the SRT. For example, of 123 subjects with mild hearing impairments (30 to 45 dB) 81 of them experienced serious social handicap, producing SHI scores between 75 to 100 percent. This instrument is used in a hearing rehabilitation center in Denmark and the authors plan to publish further data when 1000 patients have been evaluated before and reevaluated after rehabilitation procedures.

The Denver Scales. The *Denver Scale of Communication Function* (Alpiner, Chevrette, Glascoe, Metz, and Olsen, 1974) and the *Denver Scale of Communication Function for Senior Citizens Living in Retirement Centers* (Zarnoch and Alpiner, 1976) have recently appeared in print (Alpiner, 1975; Alpiner, 1978), but all of the developmental aspects and subsequent reliability studies mentioned by Alpiner are unpublished at this time. The *Denver Scale of Communication Function* (see Appendix D) is a self-assessment device involving 25 statements to which the subject responds along a seven-point continuum from "agree" to "disagree." *The Denver Scale for Senior Citizens Living in Retirement Centers* consists of seven basic questions with two to eight subquestions, all of which are answered "yes" or "no." It is administered in an interview situation. Alpiner (1978, p. 32) reported that the *Denver Scale of Communication Function* assesses "communication function" relative to "family, self, social-vocational, and general communication experience." *The Denver Scale of Communication Function for Senior Citizens Living in Retirement Centers* focuses on the unique characteristics of life in such a facility and altered family relationships. Examination of both scales indicates that they are designed to determine attitudes and reactions to the hearing loss and communication difficulties rather than ascertaining specific types of hearing and communication problems. The Denver scale most appropriate for a specific client might be a useful adjunct to an instrument of the *HHS* type, because together they might provide data not sampled by either one alone. The Denver scales may ultimately prove useful but at the moment they must be categorized as unstandardized questionnaires.

Profile Questionnaires for Home, School, Social, and Occupational Environments. Sanders (1975) has proposed four profile questionnaires for rating communicative performance in the home, school, social, and occupational environments. Each questionnaire (see Appendix E) consists of six to nine statements to which the respondent chooses one of four answers from "little or no difficulty" to "great difficulty." The items are much like those in the *HHS* or the *SHHI,* in that difficulty experienced in communication is assessed rather than attitudes or reactions.

Sanders proposed an interesting concept for scoring that enables the respondent to weight the significance of the response. The four possible responses to each item are given a numerical value of $+2$ to -2. Each item has a subpart that requires the subject to indicate how often the situation occurs, with the possible choices being "seldom," "often," or "very often." These responses carry a weight of 1, 2, and 3. Thus, if a respondent indicates having "great difficulty" (-2) when sitting and talking with friends in a quiet room and further indicates that this occurs "very often" (3) the total score on the item ($-2 \times 3 = -6$) is quite different from that of a subject who gives the same initial response but indicates that it "seldom" (1) happens. It is an interesting approach to weighting answers based on frequency and severity of experiences, but its reliability and validity are undetermined at present.

According to Sanders, the printed questionnaires are examples of appropriate scales that have not yet been standardized. He reported that his questionnaires can be used in a complementary fashion with the Denver scales.

Hearing Attitude Scale. Another scale worthy of mention has been in existence since World War II, but apparently has not been subjected to further study nor widespread clinical use. It is the *Bronfenbrenner Hearing Attitude Scale* and is most readily found in a book by Levine (1960). It consists of 100 statements to which the respondent chooses an ''agree'' or ''disagree'' response. Its purpose is to determine attitudes of hearing-impaired people in such areas as self-appraisal, depression, overoptimism, tension, reaction to rehabilitation, job worry, sensitivity, cover-up, withdrawal, and eccentric reactions. No data have been published regarding this test but it was standardized on several hundred military personnel suffering varying degrees of hearing impairment.

Hearing Performance Inventory. The most recent scale developed is the *Hearing Perfromance Inventory (HPI)* (Giolas, Owens, Lamb, and Schubert, 1979). The authors believed that previous attempts failed to ''assess comprehensively and accurately the hearing-impaired listener's response to a variety of listening situations'' and that other scales had ''not been subjected to appropriate item analysis'' (p. 169). The originally published *HPI* (Experimental Form II) consists of 158 items in a self-assessment paradigm requiring one of six possible answers: *practically always, frequently, about half the time, occasionally, almost never,* or *does not apply*. Inventory items were divided into six sections on the basis of content: (1) understanding speech, (2) intensity, (3) response to auditory failure, (4) social, (5) personal, and (6) occupational. An original pool of 289 items was administered to 220 hearing-impaired people with the results subjected to item analysis. A further revision of the *HPI* was accomplished after administeration of Experimental Form II to 164 subjects exhibiting a wide range of hearing loss (Lamb, Owens, Schubert, and Giolas, 1979). The revised form is presented in Appendix F. It consists of 90 items divided into the same six sections.

Even though few data are available regarding this instrument preliminary examination suggests that it is more comprehensive than other scales and might be the most useful tool available. Its self-report nature continues to be a limitation, particularly for use in matters involving compensation, but this should not be considered a major flaw influencing research or clinical use in habilitation. The *HPI,* like other scales, will only have limited meaning until normative data are available; clinical researchers are encouraged to participate in gathering relevant data concerning its use.

Summary. At the moment it would appear that only the *Hearing Measurement Scale* and the *Hearing Performance Inventory* have the potential for meeting most of the conditions proposed for an adequate instrument for assessing handicap. They should receive major consideration as tools for assessing the handicapping effects of hearing loss. An advantage of these two instruments is that the items are divided into sections that permit the development of individual profiles that may be useful in the habilitation process. The *HPI* in particular offers rich research possibilities because of its broad scope and the ease with which it can be quantified.

The *Hearing Handicap Scale* can also be used with confidence although its greatest deficiency is that it does not sample attitudes or reactions. It might be used in conjunction with the *Denver Scale of Communication Function* after investigation of the reliability and validity of the latter.

No data are available for any of the handicap scales with regard to how responses might be used to develop a rehabilitation or counseling program. Comparison of scores before and after treatment have not been reported except for the study involving the *HHS* reported by Tannahill (1979). Until it can be domonstrated that these tests are useful in developing individualized management plans and assessing post-treatment change, they should be used with caution. The need for repeated measurement suggests the necessity for equivalent alternative forms and most of the proposed tests do not meet that criterion.

REFERENCES

Alpiner, J., Hearing aid selection for adults. In M. Pollack (Ed.), *Amplification for the Hearing Impaired*. New York: Grune and Stratton, 1975.

Alpiner, J. (Ed.), *Handbook of Adult Rehabilitative Audiology*. Baltimore: Williams and Wilkins Co., 1978.

Alpiner, J., Chevrette, W., Glascoe, G., Metz, M., and Olsen, B., *The Denver Scale of Communication Function*. Unpublished study, University of Denver, 1974.

AMA Committee on Medical Rating of Physical Impairment, Guides to the evaluation of permanent impairment, *J. Amer. Med. Assoc.*, 168, 475–488, 1958.

Anonymous, Twenty-third annual facts and figures, *Hearing Aid J.*, 31, 6, 1977.

Antonelli, A., Auditory processing disorders in problems with hearing aid fitting in old age, *Audiology*, 17, 27–31, 1978.

Barker, R., Wright, B., Meyerson, L., and Gonick, M., *Adjustment to Physical Handicap and Illness: A Survey of the Social Psychology of Physique and Disability*. New York: Bulletin 55, Social Science Research Council, 1953.

Bergman, M., Hearing and aging: Implications of recent research findings, *Audiology*, 10, 164–171, 1971.

Bernreuter, R., *The Personality Inventory*. Palo Alto, CA: Stanford University Press, undated.

Birren, J. (Ed.), *Handbook of Aging in the Individual*. Chicago: University of Chicago Press, 1959.

Birren, J., *The Psychology of Aging*. Englewood Cliffs, NJ: Prentice-Hall, 1964a.

Birren, J. (Ed.), *Relations of Development and Aging*. Springfield, IL: Charles C Thomas, 1964b.

Birren, J., Imus, H., and Windle, W. (Eds.), *The Process of Aging in the Nervous System*. Springfield, IL: Charles C Thomas, 1959.

Blum, R. H., *The Management of the Doctor-Patient Relationship*. New York: McGraw-Hill, 1960.

Blumenfeld, V., Bergman, M., and Millner, E., Speech discrimination in an aging population, *J. Speech Hearing Res.*, 12, 210–217, 1969.

Bocca, E. and Calearo, C., Central hearing processes. In J. Jerger (Ed.), *Modern Developments in Audiology*. New York: Academic Press, 1963.

Bouchard, M. and Shane, H., Use of the problem-oriented medical record in the speech and hearing profession, *Asha*, 19, 157–159, 1977.

Brandy, W. and Studebaker, G., Audiological management of environmental noise. In D. Rose (Ed.), *Audiological Assessment*, 2nd edition. Englewood Cliffs, NJ: Prentice-Hall, Inc., 1978.

Bureau of Consumer Protection, *Hearing Aid Industry Staff Report: Final Report to the FTC and Proposed Trade Regulation Rule* (16 CFR, Part 440). Washington, Federal Trade Commission, 1978.

Corso, J., Age and sex differences in pure tone thresholds, *Arch. Otolaryngol.*, 77, 385–405, 1963a.

Corso, J., Aging and auditory thresholds in men and women, *Arch. Environmental Health*, 6, 350–356, 1963a.

Davis, H., Hearing handicap, standards for hearing, and medical legal rules. In H. Davis and S. Silverman (Eds.), *Hearing and Deafness*, 4th edition. New York: Holt, Rinehart and Winston, 1978.

Dembo, T., Ladieu, G., and Wright, B., *Adjustment to Misfortune: A Study in Social-Emotional Relationships Between Injured and Noninjured People*. Final Report to the Army Medical Research and Development Board, Office of the Surgeon General, War Department, April 1948.

Dodds, E. and Harford, E., Application of a lipreading test in a hearing aid evaluation. *J. Speech Hearing Dis.*, 33, 167–173, 1968.

Enelow, A. and Swisher, S., *Interviewing and Patient Care*. New York: Oxford University Press, 1972.

Ewertsen, H. and Birk-Nielsen, H., Social Hearing Handicap Index, *Audiology*, 12, 180–187, 1973.

Fairbanks, G., *Voice and Articulation Drillbook*. New York: Harper, 1940.

Gaeth, J., A study of phonemic regression associated with hearing loss, Ph.D. Dissertation, Northwestern University, 1948.

Garstecki, D. and Mulac, A., Effects of test material and competing message on speech discrimination, *J. Aud. Res.*, 14, 171–178, 1974.

Gentile, A., Schein, J., and Haase, K. (Eds.), *Characteristics of Persons with Impaired Hearing: United States, July 1962-June 1963*. Washington: National Center for Health Statistics (Series 10, No. 35), 1963.

Giolas, T. C., The measurement of hearing handicap: A point of view, *MAICO Audiol. Library Series*, 8, 6, 1970.

Giolas, T., Owens, E., Lamb, S., and Schubert, E., Hearing performance inventory, *J. Speech Hearing Dis.*, 44, 169–195, 1979.

Glorig, A., *Noise and Your Ear*. New York: Grune and Stratton, 1958.

Glorig, A. and Roberts, J., Hearing levels of adults by age and sex, United States 1960–1962, *Public Health Service Publication, N 1000-Series*, Washington, D. C., 1965.

Goetzinger, C. P., The psychology of hearing impairment. In J. Katz (Ed.), *Handbook of Clinical Audiology,* 1st edition. Baltimore: Williams and Wilkins Co., 1972.

Goetzinger, C., Proud, G., Dirks, D., and Embrey, J., A study of hearing in advanced age, *Arch. Otolaryngol.,* 73, 662–674, 1961.

Goetzinger, C. and Rousey, C., Hearing problems in later life, *Medical Times,* 771–780, June 1959.

Gray, R., Reinhardt, A., and Ward, J., Psychosocial factors involved in the rehabilitation of persons with cardiovascular diseases. In J. Stubbins (Ed.), *Social and Psychological Aspects of Disability.* Baltimore: University Park Press, 1977.

Harbert, F., Young, I., and Menduke, H., Audiologic findings in presbycusis, *J. Aud. Res.,* 6, 297–312, 1966.

Hardick, E., *Presbycusis, Recruitment, and Tinnitus.* Research Report to U.S. Department of Labor (Contract No. J-9-E-8-0190, 1978–9), 1979.

Hardick, E., The self concept of hard of hearing adults as measured by the semantic differential technique, Ph.D. Dissertation, Michigan State University, 1964.

Hathaway, S. and McKinley, J., *The Minnesota Multiphasic Personality Inventory,* revised edition. New York: The Psychological Corporation, 1943.

Henderson, D., Hamernik, R., Dosanjh, D., and Mills, J. (Eds.), *Effects of Noise on Hearing.* New York: Raven Press, 1976.

High, W., Fairbanks, G., and Glorig, A., Scale for self assessment of hearing handicap, *J. Speech Hearing Dis.,* 29, 215–230, 1964.

Hildreth, G. and Oyer, E., Social participation factors related to the family life of hard of hearing unmarried adults, *J. Acad. Rehab. Audiol.,* 9, 48–57, 1976.

Hinchcliffe, R., The anatomical locus of presbycusis, *J. Speech Hearing Dis.,* 27, 301–310, 1962.

Hodgson, W. and Skinner, P. (Eds.), *Hearing Aid Assessment and Use in Audiological Habilitation.* Baltimore: Williams and Wilkins Co., 1977.

Humes, L., Schwartz, D., and Bess, F., Two experiments on subtle mid-frequency hearing loss and its influence on word discrimination in noise-exposed listeners, *Audiology,* 18, 303–319, 1979.

Jerger, J., Audiological findings in aging, *Adv. Oto-Rhino-Laryngology,* 20, 115–124, 1973.

Jerger, J., Shedd, J., and Harford, E., On the detection of extremely small changes in sound intensity, *Arch Otolaryngol.,* 69, 200–211, 1959.

Katz, J. (Ed.), *Handbook of Clinical Audiology,* 2nd edition. Baltimore: Williams and Wilkins Co., 1978.

Koniditsiotis, C., The use of hearing tests to provide information about the extent to which an individual's hearing loss handicaps him, *MAICO Audiol. Library Series,* 9, 10, 1972.

Konig, E., Pitch discrimination and age, *Acta Oto-Laryngologica,* 48, 475–489, 1957.

Konkle, D., Beasley, D., and Bess, F., Intelligibility of time altered speech in relation to chronological aging, *J. Speech Hearing Res.,* 20, 108–115, 1977.

Lamb, S., Owens, E., Schubert, E., and Giolas, T., *Hearing Performance Inventory, Revised Form.* Unpublished document, July 1979.

Levine, E., *The Psychology of Deafness.* New York: Columbia University Press, 1960.

Lipscomb, D. (Ed.), *Noise and Audiology.* Baltimore: University Park Press, 1978.

Maas, R., Industrial noise and hearing conservation. In J. Katz (Ed.), *Handbook of Clinical Audiology.* Baltimore: Williams and Wilkins Co., 1972.

Marston, L. and Goetzinger, C., A comparison of sensitized words and sentences for distinguishing non-peripheral auditory changes as a function of aging, *Cortex,* 8, 213–223, 1972.

McCartney, J., Maurer, J., and Sorenson, F., A comparison of the Hearing Handicap Scale and the Hearing Measurement Scale with audiometric measures on a geriatric population, *J. Aud. Res.,* 16, 51–58, 1976.

Mead, B., Emotional struggles in adjusting to old age, *Post Graduate Medicine,* 31, 156–160, 1962.

Melrose, J., Welch, O., and Luterman, D., Auditory responses in selected elderly men, *J. Geront.,* 18, 267–270, 1963.

Meyerson, L., Somatopsychological significance of impaired hearing. In R. Barker (Ed.), *Adjustment to Physical Handicap and Illness: A Survey of the Social Psychology of Physique and Disability.* New York: Bulletin 55, Social Science Research Council, 1953.

Millin, J., Practical and philosophical considerations. In M. Pollack (Ed.), *Amplification for the Hearing Impaired.* New York: Grune and Stratton, 1975.

Myklebust, H., *The Psychology of Deafness: Sensory Deprivation, Learning and Adjustment.* New York: Grune and Stratton, 1960a.

Myklebust, J., The psychological effects of deafness, *Amer. Ann. Deaf,* 105, 372–385, 1960b.

Nathanson, M., Bergman, P., and Gordon, G., Denial of illness: Its occurrence in one hundred consecutive cases of hemiplegia. In J. Stubbins (Ed.), *Social and Psychological Aspects of Disability.* Baltimore: University Park Press, 1977.

National Center for Health Statistics, *Characteristics of Persons with Impaired Hearing: United States, July 1962, June 1963.* Bethesda, MD: Department of Health, Education and Welfare, 1967.

Newby, H., *Audiology,* 3rd edition. New York: Appleton-Century-Crofts, 1972.

Noble, W., *Assessment of Impaired Hearing.* New York: Academic Press, 1978.

Noble, W., The Hearing Measurement Scale as a paper-pencil form: Preliminary results, *J. Amer. Aud. Soc.,* 5, 95–106, 1979.

Noble, W. and Atherley, G., The Hearing Measurement Scale: A questionnaire for the assessment of auditory disability, *J. Aud. Res.,* 10, 229–250, 1970.

Olsen, I., Discrimination of auditory information as related to aging, *J. Geront.,* 20, 394–397, 1965.

Olsen, W., Presbycusis and hearing aid use, *J. Acad. Rehab. Audiol.,* 3, 34–41, 1970.

Olsen, W. and Matkin, N., Differential audiology. In D. Rose (Ed.), *Audiological Assessment,* 2nd edition. Englewood Cliffs, NJ: Prentice-Hall, Inc., 1978.

Osgood, C., Suci, G., and Tannenbaum, P., *The Measurement of Meaning.* Urbana: University of Illinois Press, 1961.

Oyer, E. and Paolucci, B., Homemakers' hearing losses and family integration, *J. Home Economics,* 62, 257–262, 1970.

Oyer, H. and Hodgson, W., Aural rehabilitation through amplification. In W. Hodgson and P. Skinner (Eds.), *Hearing Aid Assessment and Use in Audiologic Habilitation.* Baltimore: Williams and Wilkins Co., 1977.

Pestalozza, G. and Shore, I., Clinical evaluation of presbycusis on the basis of different tests of auditory function, *Laryngoscope,* 65, 1136–1163, 1955.

Peters, G., The relationship between some measures of hearing loss and self-assessment of hearing handicap, Ph.D. Dissertation, Wayne State University, 1974.

Pintner, R., Emotional stability of the hard of hearing, *J. Gen. Psych.,* 43, 293–311, 1933.

Pintner, R., Eisenson, J., and Stanton, M., *The Psychology of the Physically Handicapped.* New York: F. S. Crofts, 1946.

Pintner, R., Fusfeld, I., and Brunschwig, L., Personality tests of deaf adults, *J. Gen. Psych.,* 51, 305–327, 1937.

Pollack, M. (Ed.), *Amplification for the Hearing Impaired.* New York: Grune and Stratton, 1975.

Pollack, M., The remediation process: Psychological and counseling aspects. In J. Alpiner (Ed.), *Handbook of Adult Rehabilitative Audiology.* Baltimore: Williams and Wilkins Co., 1978.

Powers, J. and Powers, E., Hearing problems of elderly persons: Social consequences and prevalence, *Asha,* 20, 79–83, 1978.

Ramsdell, D., The psychology of the hard of hearing and the deafened adult. In H. Davis and S. Silverman (Eds.), *Hearing and Deafness,* 4th edition. New York: Holt, Rinehart and Winston, 1978.

Rose, D. (Ed.), *Audiological Assessment,* 2nd edition. Englewood Cliffs, NJ: Prentice-Hall, Inc., 1978.

Rosenberg, P., Case history: The first test. In J. Katz (Ed.), *Handbook of Clinical Audiology.* Baltimore: Williams and Wilkins Co., 1972.

Rousey, C., Psychological reactions to hearing loss, *J. Speech Hearing Dis.,* 36, 382–389, 1971.

Sanders, D., Hearing aid orientiation and counseling. In M. Pollack (Ed.), *Amplification for the Hearing Impaired.* New York: Grune and Stratton, 1975.

Schow, R. and Tannahill, J., Hearing handicap scores and categories for subjects with normal and impaired hearing sensitivity, *J. Amer. Aud. Soc.,* 3, 134–319, 1977.

Schuknecht, H., Further observations on the pathology of presbycusis, *Arch. Otolaryngol.,* 80, 369–382, 1964.

Shontz, F., Physical disability and personality: Theory and recent research. In J. Stubbins (Ed.), *Social and Psychological Aspects of Disability.* Baltimore: University Park Press, 1977.

Shore, I., Bilger, R., and Hirsh, I., Hearing aid evaluation: Reliability of repeated measurements, *J. Speech Hearing Dis.,* 25, 152–170, 1960.

Smith, R. and Prather, W., Phoneme discrimination in older persons under varying signal-to-noise conditions, *J. Speech Hearing Res.,* 14, 630–638, 1971.

Spahr, R., 1971 White House Conference on Aging, *Asha,* 13, 14–17, 1971.

Speaks, C., Jerger, J., and Trammell, J., Comparison of sentence identification and conventional speech discrimination scores, *J. Speech Hearing Res.,* 13, 755–767, 1970.

Subcommittee on Human Communication and Its Disorders, *Human Communication and Its Disorders: An Overview.* Bethesda, MD: National Institutes of Health, Public Health Service, Department of Health, Education and Welfare, 1969.

Suter, A., The ability of mildly hearing-impaired individuals to discriminate speech in noise, Ph.D. Dissertation, University of Maryland, 1977.

Tannahill, J., The Hearing Handicap Scale as a measure of hearing aid benefit, *J. Speech Hearing Dis.,* 44, 91–99, 1979.

Tiven, M., *Older Americans: Special Handling Required*. Washington, D. C.: National Council on the Aging, 1971.

Ward, W., Fleer, R., and Glorig, A., Characteristics of hearing losses produced by gun fire and steady noise, *J. Aud. Res.,* 1, 325–356, 1961.

Welles, H., The measurement of certain aspects of personality among hard-of-hearing adults, *Teachers College Contributions to Education, No. 545*. New York: Columbia University, 1932.

Wilber, L., Calibration: Pure-tone, speech and noise signal. In J. Katz (Ed.), *Handbook of Clinical Auidology,* 2nd edition. Baltimore: Williams and Wilkins Co., 1978.

Willeford, J., The geriatric patient. In D. Rose (Ed.), *Audiological Assessment*. Englewood Cliffs, NJ: Prentice-Hall, Inc., 1971.

Willeford, J., The geriatric patient. In D. Rose (Ed.), *Audiological Assessment,* 2nd edition. Englewood Cliffs, NJ: Prentice-Hall, Inc., 1978.

Zarnoch, J. and Alpiner, J., *The Denver Scale of Communication Function for Senior Citizens Living in Retirement Centers*. Unpublished study, University of Denver, 1976.

APPENDIX A
Hearing Handicap Scale

The items contained in Forms A and B are listed below. The client's response to each item is recorded on the following scale:

______Almost always
______Usually
______Sometimes
______Rarely
______Almost never

FORM A

1. If you are 6 to 12 feet from the loudspeaker of a radio do you understand speech well?
2. Can you carry on a telephone conversation without difficulty?
3. If you are 6 to 12 feet away from a television set, do you understand most of what is said?
4. Can you carry on a conversation with one other person when you are on a noisy street corner?
5. Do you hear all right when you are in a street car, airplane, bus, or train?
6. If there are noises from other voices, typewriters, traffic, music, etc., can you understand when someone speaks to you?
7. Can you understand a person when you are seated beside him and cannot see his face?

From W. High, Fairbanks, G., and Glorig, A., Scale for self assessment of hearing handicap (Forms A and B), *J. Speech Hearing Dis.,* 29, 3, 1964.

8. Can you understand if someone speaks to you while you are chewing crisp foods, such as potato chips or celery?
9. Can you carry on a conversation with one other person when you are in a noisy place, such as a restaurant or at a party?
10. Can you understand if someone speaks to you in a whisper and you cannot see his face?
11. When you talk with a bus driver, waiter, ticket salesman, etc., can you understand all right?
12. Can you carry on a conversation if you are seated across the room from someone who speaks in a normal tone of voice?
13. Can you understand women when they talk?
14. Can you carry on a conversation with one other person when you are out-of-doors and it is reasonably quiet?
15. When you are in a meeting or at a large dinner table, would you know the speaker was talking if you could not see his lips moving?
16. Can you follow the conversation when you are at a large dinner table or in a meeting with a small group?
17. If you are seated under the balcony of a theater or auditorium, can you hear well enough to follow what is going on?
18. When you are in a large formal gathering (a church, lodge, lecture hall, etc.) can you hear what is said when the speaker does not use a microphone.
19. Can you hear the telephone ring when you are in the room where it is located?
20. Can you hear warning signals, such as automobile horns, railway crossing bells, or emergency vehicle sirens?

FORM B

1. When you are listening to the radio or watching television, can you hear adequately when the volume is comfortable for most other people?
2. Can you carry on a conversation with one other person when you are riding in an automobile with the windows closed?
3. Can you carry on a conversation with one other person when you are riding in an automobile with the windows open?
4. Can you carry on a conversation with one other person if there is a radio or television in the same room playing at normal loudness?
5. Can you hear when someone calls to you from another room?
6. Can you understand when someone speaks to you from another room?
7. When you buy something in a store, do you easily understand the clerk?
8. Can you carry on a conversation with someone who does not speak as loudly as most people?
9. Can you tell if a person is talking when you are seated beside him and cannot see his face?
10. When you ask someone for directions, do you understand what he says?
11. If you are within three or four feet of a person who speaks in a normal tone of voice (assume you are facing one another), can you hear everything he says?

12. Do you recognize the voices of speakers when you don't see them?
13. When you are introduced to someone, can you understand the name the first time it is spoken?
14. Can you hear adequately when you are conversing with more than one person?
15. If you are in an audience, such as in a church or theater and you are seated near the front, can you understand most of what is said?
16. Can you carry on everyday conversations with members of your family without difficulty?
17. If you are in an audience, such as in a church or theater and you are seated near the rear, can you understand most of what is said?
18. When you are in a large formal gathering (a church, lodge, lecture hall, etc.) can you hear what is said when the speaker does use a microphone?
19. Can you hear the telephone ring when you are in the next room?
20. Can you hear night sounds, such as distant trains, bells, dogs barking, trucks passing, and so forth?

APPENDIX B
The Hearing Measurement Scale

This scale is designed for administration in an interview situation only. The items are listed here for reference only. The instruction manual for administration and scoring is only available from Dr. W. G. Noble, Department of Psychology, University of New England, Armidale, N.S.E. 2351, Australia.

SECTION I SPEECH HEARING

1. Do you ever have difficulty hearing in the conversation when you're with one other person when you're at home?
2. Do you ever have difficulty hearing in the conversation when you're with one other person outside?
3. Do you ever have difficulty in group conversation at home?
4. Do you ever have difficulty in group conversation outside?
5. Do you ever have difficulty hearing conversation at work?

5a. Is this due to your hearing, due to the noise or a bit of both?

6. Do you ever have difficulty hearing the speaker at a public gathering?
7. Can you always hear what's being said in a TV program?
8. Can you always hear what's being said in TV news?
9. Can you always hear what's being said in a radio program?
10. Can you always hear what's being said in radio news?
11. Do you ever have difficulty hearing what's said in a film at the cinema?

From W. Noble, *Assessment of Impaired Hearing*. New York: Academic Press, 1978. Reproduced with permission of author and publisher.

SECTION II ACUITY FOR NONSPEECH SOUND

12. Do you have any pets at home? (Type ______) Can you hear it when it ______ (barks, mews, etc.)?
13. Can you hear it when someone rings the doorbell or knocks on the door?
14. Can you hear a motor horn in the street when you're outside?
15. The sound of footsteps outside when you're inside?
16. The sound of the door opening when you're inside that room?
17. Can you hear the clock ticking in the room?
18. The tap running when you turn it on?
19. Water boiling in a pan when you're in the kitchen?

SECTION III LOCALIZATION

20. When you hear the sound of people talking and they're in another room would you be able to tell whereabouts this sound was coming from?
21. If you're with a group of people and someone you can't see starts to speak would you be able to tell where that person was sitting?
22. If you hear a motor horn or a bell can you always tell which direction it's sounding?
23. Do you ever turn your head the wrong way when someone calls to you?
24. Can you usually tell, from the sound, how far away a person is when he calls you?
25. Have you ever noticed outside that a car you thought, by its sound, was far away turned out to be much closer in fact?
26. Outside, do you always move out of the way of something coming up from behind, for instance a car, a trolley, or someone walking faster?

SECTION IV REACTION TO HANDICAP

27. Do you think you are more irritable than other people or less so?
28. Do you ever give the wrong answer to someone because you've misheard them?
29. When you do this, do you treat it lightly or do you get upset?
30. How does the other person react? Does he get irritated or make little of it?
31. Do you think people are tolerant in this way or do they make fun of you?
32. Do you ever get bothered or upset if you are unable to follow a conversation?
33. Do you ever get the feeling of being cut off from things because of difficulty in hearing?
33a. Does this feeling upset you at all?

SECTION V SPEECH DISTORTION

34. Do you find that people fail to speak clearly?
35. What about speakers on TV or radio? Do they fail to speak clearly?
36. Do you ever have difficulty, in everyday conversation, understanding what someone is saying even though you can hear what's being said?

SECTION VI TINNITUS

37. Do you ever get a noise in your ears or in your head?
37a. to 37e. A series of items on nature and incidence of tinnitus.
38. Does it ever stop you sleeping?
39. Does it upset you?

SECTION VII PERSONAL OPINION OF HEARING LOSS

40. Do you think your hearing is normal?
41. Do you think any difficulty with your hearing is particularly serious?
42. Does any difficulty with your hearing restrict your social or personal life?
42a. to 42f. A series of items on temporary threshold shift, specifically for those with chronic acoustic trauma, on the relative importance of eyesight over hearing and on other difficult hearing situations not mentioned in the interview.

APPENDIX C
Social Hearing Handicap Index

Appropriate answers are ''yes'' or ''no.'' If response is uncertain it should be enclosed in ( ). If the client has never experienced the situation the response should be ''I don't know.''

1. If you are sitting opposite a person at a distance of about 1 meter, will you be able to understand everything if the person speaks in a normal tone of voice?
2. Do you have problems in understanding when members of the family are gathered together?
3. Is it difficult for you to hear in the kitchen when the water is running?
4. Do you find it difficult to hear what the shop assistant says to you?
5. Is it difficult for you to carry on a telephone conversation?
6. Can you follow the conversation when you are talking to several persons?
7. Is it difficult for you to follow a conversation at a tea table with several persons?
8. Can you hear most of what is said when sitting at the back of a lecture room, a theatre, or a church?
9. Can you carry on a conversation with someone sitting at the other end of the room and speaking in a normal tone of voice?
10. Can you hear the radio well when it is set at normal volume?
11. Can you carry on a conversation easily in a car, tram, train or bus?
12. Can you carry on a conversation easily at the dinner table at home?
13. Do you understand what is said to you when there is noise from other voices, typewriters, traffic, music?

From H. Ewertsen and H. Birk-Nielsen (1973). Reprinted with permission.

14. Do you recognize a person by his voice?
15. Is it difficult for you to hear people speaking on TV when it is not turned up?
16. Is it difficult for you to follow a conversation at a large dinner table?
17. Can you carry on a conversation with someone when the radio or TV is not turned up?
18. Is it difficult for you to carry on a conversation with someone in a busy street?
19. Is it difficult for you to understand what is said to you from an adjoining room?
20. Can you carry on a conversation with a person where there is noise, for instance at a restaurant or at a party?
21. Do you often misunderstand other people's conversation?

APPENDIX D
The Denver Scale of Communication Function

The following questionnaire was designed to evaluate your communication ability as you view it. You are asked to judge or scale each statement in the following manner.

If you judge the statement to be *very closely related* to either extreme, please place your check mark as follows:

Agree __X__ _____ _____ _____ _____ _____ _____ Disagree

or

Agree _____ _____ _____ _____ _____ _____ __X__ Disagree

If you judge the statement to be *closely related* to either end of the scale, please mark as follows:

Agree _____ __X__ _____ _____ _____ _____ _____ Disagree

or

Agree _____ _____ _____ _____ _____ __X__ _____ Disagree

If you judge the statement to be only slightly related to either end of the scale, please mark as follows:

Agree _____ _____ __X__ _____ _____ _____ _____ Disagree

or

Agree _____ _____ _____ _____ __X__ _____ _____ Disagree

If you consider the statement to be irrelevant or unassociated to your communication situation, please mark as follows:

Agree _____ _____ _____ __X__ _____ _____ _____ Disagree

From Alpiner, J. G. (Ed.), Evaluation of communication function, *Handbook of Adult Rehabilitative Audiology,* The Williams and Wilkins Company, 1978. Reproduced by permission.

PLEASE NOTE: Check a scale for every statement.
Put only one checkmark on each scale.
Make a separate judgment for each statement.
ALSO: You may comment on each statement in the space provided.

1. The members of my family are annoyed with my loss of hearing.

Agree ______ ______ ______ ______ ______ ______ ______ Disagree
Comments:

2. The members of my family sometimes leave me out of conversations or discussions.

Agree ______ ______ ______ ______ ______ ______ ______ Disagree
Comments:

3. Sometimes my family makes decisions for me because I have a hard time following discussions.

Agree ______ ______ ______ ______ ______ ______ ______ Disagree
Comments:

4. My family becomes annoyed when I ask them to repeat what was said because I did not hear them.

Agree ______ ______ ______ ______ ______ ______ ______ Disagree
Comments:

5. I am not an ''outgoing'' person because I have a hearing loss.

Agree ______ ______ ______ ______ ______ ______ ______ Disagree
Comments:

6. I now take less of an interest in many things as compared to when I did not have a hearing problem.

Agree ______ ______ ______ ______ ______ ______ ______ Disagree
Comments:

7. Other people do not realize how frustrated I get when I cannot hear or understand.

Agree ______ ______ ______ ______ ______ ______ ______ Disagree
Comments:

8. People sometimes avoid me because of my hearing loss.

Agree ______ ______ ______ ______ ______ ______ ______ Disagree
Comments:

9. I am not a calm person because of my hearing loss.

Agree ______ ______ ______ ______ ______ ______ ______ Disagree
Comments:

10. I tend to be negative about life in general because of my hearing loss.

Agree ______ ______ ______ ______ ______ ______ ______ Disagree
Comments:

11. I do not socialize as much as I did before I began to lose my hearing.

Agree ______ ______ ______ ______ ______ ______ ______ Disagree
Comments:

12. Since I have trouble hearing, I do not like to go places with friends.

Agree ______ ______ ______ ______ ______ ______ ______ Disagree
Comments:

13. Since I have trouble hearing, I hesitate to meet new people.

Agree ______ ______ ______ ______ ______ ______ ______ Disagree
Comments:

14. I do not enjoy my job as much as I did before I began to lose my hearing.

Agree ______ ______ ______ ______ ______ ______ ______ Disagree
Comments:

15. Other people do not understand what it is like to have a hearing loss.

Agree ______ ______ ______ ______ ______ ______ ______ Disagree
Comments:

16. Because I have difficulty understanding what is said to me, I sometimes answer questions wrong.

Agree ______ ______ ______ ______ ______ ______ ______ Disagree
Comments:

17. I do not feel relaxed in a communicative situation.

Agree ______ ______ ______ ______ ______ ______ ______ Disagree
Comments:

18. I do not feel comfortable in most communication situations.

Agree ______ ______ ______ ______ ______ ______ ______ Disagree
Comments:

19. Conversations in a noisy room prevent me from attempting to communicate with others.

Agree ______ ______ ______ ______ ______ ______ ______ Disagree
Comments:

20. I am not comfortable having to speak in a group situation.

Agree ______ ______ ______ ______ ______ ______ ______ Disagree
Comments:

21. In general, I do not find listening relaxing.

Agree ______ ______ ______ ______ ______ ______ ______ Disagree
Comments:

22. I feel threatened by many communication situations due to difficulty hearing.

Agree ______ ______ ______ ______ ______ ______ ______ Disagree
Comments:

23. I seldom watch other people's facial expressions when talking to them.

Agree ______ ______ ______ ______ ______ ______ ______ Disagree
Comments:

24. I hesitate to ask people to repeat if I do not understand them the first time they speak.

Agree ______ ______ ______ ______ ______ ______ ______ Disagree
Comments:

25. Because I have difficulty understanding what is said to me, I sometimes make comments that do not fit into the conversation.

Agree ______ ______ ______ ______ ______ ______ ______ Disagree
Comments:

APPENDIX E
Profile Questionnaire for Rating Communicative Performance

The items contained in three profiles (Home, Occupation, Social) are listed below.

The client's response to each item is recorded on the following scales:

From D. A. Sanders, Hearing aid orientation and counseling. In M. C. Pollack (Ed.), *Amplification for the Hearing Impaired*. Grune and Stratton, 1975. Reprinted by permission of Grune and Stratton, Inc. and the author.

+2	+1	−1	−2
little or no difficulty in understanding	some difficulty (but not a lot)	a fair amount of difficulty (quite a lot)	great difficulty in understanding

This happens

1	2	3
seldom	often	very often

HOME ENVIRONMENT

1. In my living room, when I can see the speaker's face, I have
2. If I am talking with a person in my living room or family room while the television, radio, or record player is on, I have
3. In a quiet room in my house, if I cannot see the speaker's face I have
4. If someone in my home speaks to me from another room on the same floor, I experience
5. If someone calls me from upstairs when I am downstairs, or from the window when I am in the garden, I will experience
6. Understanding people at the dinner table gives me
7. When I sit talking with friends in a quiet room I have
8. Listening to the radio, record player, or watching TV gives me
9. When I use the phone at home, I have

OCCUPATIONAL ENVIRONMENT

1. In talking with someone in the room where I work, I have
2. When I am in a room at work where there is noise, I have
3. When I am at a meeting with a small group of people, around a table in a fairly quiet room, I have
4. If I have to take notes by dictation in a fairly quiet room, I have
5. If I have to make notes at a meeting, I have
6. If I have to use the phone at work, I have

SOCIAL ENVIRONMENT

1. If we are entertaining a group of friends, understanding someone against the background of others talking gives me
2. If we are playing cards, understanding my partner gives me
3. When I am at the theater or the movies, I have
4. In church, when the minister gives the sermon, I have
5. Following the conversation when we eat out, I have
6. In the car, I find that understanding what people are saying gives me
7. When I am outside talking with someone, I have

APPENDIX F
Hearing Performance Inventory Revised Form

INSTRUCTIONS

We are interested in knowing how your hearing problem has affected your daily living. Below you will find a series of questions that describe a variety of everyday listening situations and ask you to judge how much difficulty you would have hearing in these situations.

Some of the questions ask you to judge how well you can understand what people are saying when their voices are loud enough. The term *understand* means hearing the words a person is saying clearly enough to be able to participate in the conversation. Other questions ask whether you can hear enough of a particular sound (doorbell, speech, etc.) to be aware of its presence. Other questions concern occupational, social or personal situations. Still others ask what you *do* when you miss something. Always assume you are interested in what is being said.

To answer each question, you are asked to check the phrase that best describes how often you experience the situation being described:

Practically always . . . .(or always)
Frequently . . . .(about three-quarters of the time)
About half the time
Occasionally . . . .(about a quarter of the time)
Almost never . . . .(or never)

For example, if you can understand what a person is saying on the telephone about 100 percent of the time, then you should check *practically always*. On the other hand, if you can understand almost nothing of what a person is saying on the telephone, then you should check *almost never*. If you can understand what a person is saying on the telephone about 50 percent of the time, then you should check *about half the time*.

Your answers to the questions should describe your present hearing ability as it is on the average rather than from a single instance.

If you wear a hearing aid in the situation described, answer the question accordingly.

Please check one, and only one, phrase for each question. You should check *Does not apply* only if you have not experienced a particular situation or one similar to it.

Questions that appear identical do differ in at least one important detail. Please read each question carefully before checking the appropriate phrase.

We know that people talk differently. Some mumble, others talk too fast, and others talk without moving their lips very much. Please answer the questions according to the way *most* people talk to you.

If the question does not specify whether the person speaking is male or female, answer according to which sex you have the most difficulty hearing.

From S. Lamb, E. Owens, E. Schubert, and T. Giolas, 1979. Hearing Performance Inventory, Revised Form. Unpublished document. Reprinted with permission.

Asterisks on the score sheet are for scoring purposes and should be ignored.

1. You are watching your favorite news program on television. Can you understand the news reporter (female) when her voice is loud enough for you?
2. You are reading in a room with music or noise in the background. Can you hear a person calling you from another room?
3. You are with a male friend or family member in a fairly quiet room. Can you understand him when his voice is loud enough for you and you can see his face?
4. Can you hear an airplane in the sky when others around you can hear it?
5. You are watching a drama or movie on television. Can you understand what is being said when the speaker's voice is loud enough for you and there is music in the background?
6. Can you understand what a woman is saying on the telephone when her voice is loud enough for you?
7. You are at a restaurant and you hear only a portion of something the waitress/waiter said. Do you repeat the portion when asking him/her for a repetition?
8. You are with a child (6 to 10 years old) in a fairly quiet room. Can you understand the child when his/her voice is loud enough for you and you can see his/her face?
9. You are the driver in an automobile with several friends or family members. One or more of the windows are open. Can you understand the passenger behind you when his/her voice is loud enough for you?
10. You are at a restaurant and there is background noise such as music or a crowd of people. Can you understand the waiter/waitress when his/her voice is loud enough for you and you can see his/her face?
11. You are talking with a close friend. When you miss something important that was said, do you immediately adjust your hearing aid to help you hear better?
12. You are with five or six strangers at a gathering of more than 20 people and there is background noise such as music or a crowd of people. One person talks at a time. When you are aware of the subject, can you understand what is being said when the speaker's voice is loud enough for you and you can see his/her face?
13. You are at a play or movie, or listening to a speech. When you miss something important that was said, do you ask the person with you?
14. You are with a child (6 to 10 years old) and several people are talking nearby. Can you understand the child when his/her voice is loud enough for you and you can see his/her face?
15. You are playing cards, monopoly or some similar game with several people and there is background noise such as music or a crowd of people. Can you understand what a friend or family member is saying to you when his/her voice is loud enough for you and you can see his/her face?
16. Does your hearing problem discourage you from attending lectures?
17. You are talking with five or six friends. When you miss something that was said, do you ask the person talking to repeat it?
18. You are in an auditorium listening to a lecturer (female) who is using a microphone. Can you understand what she is saying when her voice is loud enough for you and you can see her face?
19. Can you hear water running in another room when others around you can hear it?

20. You are with a friend or family member and you hear only a portion of what was said. Do you repeat that portion when asking him/her for a repetition?

21. You are at a party or gathering of less than 10 people and the room is fairly quiet. Can you understand what a friend or family member is saying to you when his/her voice is loud enough for you, but you can *not* see his/her face?

22. Does your hearing problem lower your self-confidence?

23. You are in a fairly quiet room with five or six strangers. One person talks at a time. When you are aware of the subject, can you understand what is being said when the speaker's voice is loud enough for you, but you can *not* see his/her face?

24. You are with five or six friends or family members at a gathering of more than 20 people and several people are talking near by. One person talks at a time and the subject of conversation changes from time to time. Can you understand what is being said when the speaker's voice is loud enough for you and you can see his/her face?

25. When an announcement is given over a public address system in a bus station or airport, is it *loud enough* for you to hear?

26. You are talking with a stranger. When you miss something important that was said, do you ask for it to be repeated?

27. You are talking with a friend or family member. When you miss something that was said, do you pretend you understood?

28. You are at a fairly quiet restaurant. Can you understand the waiter/waitress when his/her voice is loud enough for you and you can see his/her face?

29. You are seated with five or six strangers around a table or in a living room. Often two persons are talking at once and one person frequently interrupts another. When you miss something important that was said, do you pretend you understood?

30. You are playing cards, Monopoly or some similar game and the room is fairly quiet. The subject of conversation changes from time to time. Can you understand what is being said when the speaker's voice is loud enough for you, but you can *not* see his/her face?

31. You are at a party or gathering of less than 10 people and the room is fairly quiet. Can you understand what a friend or family member is saying to you when his/her voice is loud enough for you and you can see his/her face?

32. Does your hearing problem discourage you from going to concerts?

33. Do you find that children (6 to 10 years old) speak loudly enough for you?

34. When an announcement is given over a public address system in a bus station or airport, can you understand what is being said when the speaker's voice is loud enough for you?

35. You are seated with five or six strangers around a table or in a living room. Often two persons are talking at once and one person frequently interrupts another. Can you understand what is being said when the speaker's voice is loud enough for you and you can see his/her face?

36. You are seated with five or six friends around a table or in a living room. Often two persons are talking at once and one person frequently interrupts another. When you miss something that was said, do you ask the person talking to repeat it?

37. You are with a female stranger in a fairly quiet room. Can you understand her when her voice is loud enough for you and you can see her face?

38. You are with a stranger and there is background noise such as music or a crowd of people. Can you understand the person when his/her voice is loud enough for you, but you can *not* see his/her face?
39. Does your hearing problem tend to make you impatient?
40. You are talking with five or six strangers. When you miss something important that was said, do you let the person talking know—at least one time—that you have a hearing problem?
41. You are at a party or gathering of less than 10 people and several people are talking near by. Can you understand what a friend or family member (female) is saying to you when her voice is loud enough for you and you can see her face?
42. Does your hearing problem discourage you from going to plays?
43. You are having dinner with five or six friends and you hear only a portion of what was said. Do you repeat that portion when asking the speaker for a repetition?
44. You are at a restaurant with a friend or family member and there is background noise such as music or a crowd of people. Can you understand the person when his/her voice is loud enough for you and you can see his/her face?
45. When you have difficulty understanding a person who speaks quite rapidly, do you ask him/her to speak more slowly?
46. You are talking to a woman sitting in a ticket or information booth and it is fairly noisy. She is giving directions or information. Can you understand her when her voice is loud enough for you and you can see her face?
47. You are having dinner with five or six friends. When you miss something important that was said, do you ask the person talking to repeat it?
48. When others are listening to speech on the television or radio, is it loud enough for you?
49. Does your hearing problem discourage you from going to the movies?
50. You are riding in an automobile with several friends or family members. One or more of the windows are open and you are sitting in the front seat. Can you understand the driver when his/her voice is loud enough for you and you can see his/her face?
51. You are at home watching television or listening to the radio. Can you hear the doorbell ring when it is located in the same room?
52. You are in a fairly quiet room talking with five or six strangers. One person talks at a time and the subject of conversation changes from time to time. Can you understand what is being said when the speaker's voice is loud enough for you and you can see his/her face?
53. You are seated with five or six friends or family members around a table or in a living room. Often two persons are talking at once and one person frequently interrupts another. When you miss something important that was said, do you remind the person talking, at least once, that you have a hearing problem?
54. You are attending a stage play. Can you understand what the actors/actresses are saying when their voices are loud enough for you and you can see their faces?
55. You are with a friend or family member in a fairly quiet room. Can you understand him/her when his/her voice is loud enough for you, but you can *not* see his/her face?

56. A person is talking to you from a distance of no more than six feet. There is music or noise in the background. Would you be aware that he/she is talking if you did not see his/her face?

57. You are having dinner with five or six friends or family members at home and there is background noise such as music or a crowd of people. Can you understand what is being said when the speaker's voice is loud enough for you, but you can *not* see his/her face?

58. When you have difficulty understanding a person with a pipe, toothpick or similar object in his/her mouth, do you ask him/her to remove the object?

59. You are the driver in an automobile with several friends or family members. The windows are closed. Can you understand the passenger behind you when his/her voice is loud enough for you?

60. When you have difficulty understanding a person because he is holding his hand in front of his mouth, do you ask him to lower his hand?

61. You are at a party or gathering of more than 20 people and there is background noise such as music or a crowd of people. Can you understand what a stranger is saying to you when his/her voice is loud enough for you and you can see his/her face?

62. Do you feel that others cannot understand what it is to have a hearing problem?

63. You are at a movie. Can you understand what the actors/actresses are saying when their voices are loud enough for you and you can see their faces?

64. You are talking with five or six strangers. When you miss something important that was said, do you ask the person talking to repeat it?

65. You are at a party or gathering of more than 20 people and several people are talking near by. Can you understand what a friend or family member (male) is saying to you when his voice is loud enough for you and you can see his face?

66. You are in a fairly quiet room. Can you carry on a conversation with a man in another room if his voice is loud enough for you?

67. You are with a male friend or family member and several people are talking near by. Can you understand him when his voice is loud enough for you and you can see his face?

68. You are with five or six friends or family members. One person talks at a time. When you miss something important that was said, do you pretend you understood?

69. You are watching a drama or movie on television. Can you understand what is being said when the speaker's voice is loud enough for you and there is no music in the background?

70. You are with five or six friends or family members and there is background noise such as music or a crowd of people. One person talks at a time. When you are aware of the subject, can you understand what is being said when the speaker's voice is loud enough for you, but you can *not* see his/her face?

71. You are at a lecture. If you have difficulty hearing what is being said, do you move to a place where you can hear better?

72. Does your hearing problem tend to make you feel nervous or tense?

73. You are with a female stranger and there is background noise such as traffic, music, or a crowd of people. Can you understand her when her voice is loud enough for you and you can see her face?

74. You are in a quiet place and the person seated on the side of your better ear whispers to you. Can you hear the whisper?

75. You are at a small social gathering. If you have difficulty hearing what is being said, do you move to a place where you can hear better?

OCCUPATIONAL ITEMS

76. You are with a male co-worker at work in a fairly quiet room. Can you understand him when his voice is loud enough for you and you can see his face?

77. You are with five or six co-workers at work. One person talks at a time. When you miss something important that was said, do you pretend you understand?

78. Does your hearing problem interfere with helping or instructing others on the job?

79. You are with a female co-worker at work and there is background noise such as traffic, music, or a crowd of people. Can you understand her when her voice is loud enough for you and you can see her face?

80. You are with a co-worker at work and you hear only a portion of what was said. Do you repeat that portion when asking the speaker for a repetition?

81. You are talking with a co-worker at work. When you miss something important that was said, do you ask for it to be repeated?

82. You are talking with your employer (foreman, supervisor, etc.) and several people are talking near by. Can you understand him/her when his/her voice is loud enough for you and you can see his/her face?

83. You are with a female co-worker at work in a fairly quiet room. Can you understand her when her voice is loud enough for you and you can see her face?

84. You are talking with a co-worker or employer. When you miss something important that was said, do you remind him/her that you have a hearing problem?

85. You are in a fairly quiet room at work with five or six co-workers. One person talks at a time and the subject of conversation changes from time to time. Can you understand what is being said when the speaker's voice is loud enough for you and you can see his/her face?

86. Does your hearing problem interfere with learning the duties of a new job easily?

87. You are seated with five or six co-workers around a table at work. Often two persons are talking at once and one person frequently interrupts another. Can you understand what is being said when the speaker's voice is loud enough for you and you can see his/her face?

88. You are talking with a co-worker at work. When you miss something important that was said, do you pretend you understood?

89. You are with a male co-worker at work and there is background noise such as traffic, music, or a crowd of people. Can you understand him when his voice is loud enough for you and you can see his face?

90. You are talking with a co-worker at work. When you miss something that was said, do you immediately adjust your hearing aid to help you hear better?

Item Categories	Item Numbers
Understanding speech	
With visual cues	1, 3, 5, 8, 10, 12, 14, 15, 18, 24, 28, 31, 35, 37, 41, 44, 46, 50, 52, 54, 61, 63, 65, 67, 69, 73
With no visual cues	6, 9, 21, 23, 30, 34, 38, 55, 57, 59, 66, 70
Intensity	2, 4, 19, 25, 33, 48, 51, 56, 74
Response to auditory failure	7, 11, 13, 17, 20, 26, 27, 29, 36, 40, 43, 45, 47, 53, 58, 60, 64, 68, 71, 75
Personal	16, 22, 32, 39, 42, 49, 62, 72
Social	9, 12, 15, 17, 21, 23, 24, 29, 30, 31, 35, 36, 40, 41, 43, 47, 50, 52, 53, 57, 59, 61, 64, 65, 68, 70, 75
Occupational	
Understanding speech with visual cues	76, 79, 82, 83, 85, 87, 89
Response to auditory failure	77, 80, 81, 84, 88, 90
Personal	78, 86

CHAPTER 13

Rehabilitation Programs for Adults

I. Basic Components of Rehabilitation
- **A.** Selection of Amplification
- **B.** Improvement of Speech Reception Through Auditory and Visual Input
- **C.** Facilitating Adjustment to Impairment

II. Delivery of Services to Special Populations
- **A.** Age-Related Factors that Influence Rehabilitation
- **B.** Reaching the Elderly

III. Approaches to Rehabilitation
- **A.** Behavior Modification Approach
- **B.** Military Aural Rehabilitation Programs
- **C.** Analytic Approach
- **D.** Verbotonal Method
- **E.** Communication Effectiveness Program

The development of effective audiologic rehabilitation programs for adults involves two major tasks. Procedures must be planned that will minimize the communication and adjustment problems discussed in Chapter 12, and the service delivery system must allow outreach to adults who may not be willing or able to participate in traditional, clinic-based habilitation. The purpose of this chapter is to describe the basic components of audiologic rehabilitation programs for adults, to discuss briefly some of the ways they are currently used, and to present a detailed model for an outreach rehabilitation program.

BASIC COMPONENTS OF REHABILITATION

As discussed in Chapter 12, adults who lose some of their hearing experience three major difficulties. They no longer hear speech clearly, they must communicate through a combination of visual and auditory effort, and they must make adjustments in their social or vocational lives and in their view of themselves. Because of these three difficulties, adults usually undergo certain psychological adjustments. The purpose of rehabilitation is to improve communication and ease the adjustments that must be made. Because rehabilitation procedures do not usually restore communication skills to normal levels, it is essential that clinicians be aware of and address adjustment problems directly. To be most effective, treatment programs must be tailored to the needs of individuals as much as possible, but several basic components should be included for all clients. The amount of time spent on them will vary according to need.

Selection of Amplification

Helping a hearing-impaired person obtain and learn to use amplification is the most important contribution the audiologist can make to rehabilitation. There is no substitute for audition as the primary means of communication, and every effort should be made to find the optimal combination of hearing aid and earmold for each client. The life-style of the individual should be considered as well as the characteristics of the hearing impairment. The amplification needs of a salesman who uses the telephone to conduct business and those of a trucker are likely to be quite different even if their hearing losses are similar.

Hearing aids are usually selected during individual hearing aid evaluation appointments. A complete assessment of hearing for pure tones and speech is used as a basis for selection of appropriate electroacoustic characteristics of aids to be evaluated. After several measures are made while the client listens to amplified sound, recommendations are usually made about the purchase of a specific aid. In most augiologic facilities, especially those that dispense hearing aids, a brief orientation is conducted during which the individual practices inserting the earmold, changing volume control settings, inserting batteries, cleaning the earmold, and so on. Suggestions may be given for gradually increasing the amount of time the hearing aid is used or for its use in special situations, such as telephone conversations or in concert halls. Alternative types of amplification (telephone amplifiers,

FM auditory trainers) may be discussed. Hearing aid monitoring procedures are provided and follow-up visits are arranged.

For many hearing-impaired adults, the individual hearing aid consultation procedure described above is all that is required for satisfactory rehabilitation. This is particularly true for young or middle aged adults, people with mild to moderate hearing impairments, those with reasonably good speech discrimination skills, and people who have adjusted easily to the view of themselves as hearing impaired.

For others, additional procedures will be needed if they are to develop the best communication skills possible.

Improvement of Speech Reception Through Auditory and Visual Input

After amplification has been selected, some clients continue to experience serious problems understanding speech. For them, training in the discrimination of phonemes, words, or sentences using auditory, visual, or combined auditory-visual information may be indicated. Drill on selected materials and practice making finer and finer discriminations are typical activities used to accomplish this purpose. These activities have traditionally been labeled auditory training and lipreading, and in the past constituted the major portion of programs for adults. Their use is illustrated in the discussion of current rehabilitation programs that follows.

Facilitating Adjustment to Impairment

Sometimes clients have difficulty adjusting to hearing aid use because of unrealistic expectations about rehabilitation or problems in psychological acceptance of the hearing loss and adjustment to the changes it brings to their lives. Any of the defense mechanisms discussed in Chapter 12 may occur in hearing-impaired adults, but the most common are projection and denial. A considerable number of people are seen in audiologic clinics, not because they believe they have a hearing problem, but because someone else does and has insisted that they seek professional help. In some cases the client is correct in the belief that the hearing impairment, if it exists, is not interfering with communication significantly and the problem lies with others. In other cases the individual is denying the hearing loss or projecting the cause of communication breakdowns onto others in the environment.

There is no easy way to quickly identify projection or denial, but evidence of their existence should be noted and viewed as important factors that may influence habilitation adversely.

Use of the Family to Aid Adjustment. Hearing-impaired adults can be assisted in working through these defense mechanisms to an acceptance of the impairment through a combination of counseling and improvement of communication skills. It is important that normally hearing members of the family or friends be included in the treatment program. The audiologist will use information from all informants to determine the extent to which these or other defense mechanisms are present, whether or not the communication needs of the client differ from family expectations, and how best to manage these problems for a given individual. If the audiologist is insensitive to the possibility that adjustment problems exist, alienation may result and recommendations may be rejected.

Acceptance of the need for habilitation may be fostered through a variety of procedures. Sometimes the interpretation of test results as they relate to the difficulty they impose on *all* participants in communication may be helpful. Discussing how family members may modify their speaking habits to enhance understanding, as well as steps that the client may take, can help alleviate the perception that the full responsibility for the success of communication rests with the client alone.

Permitting the client to experience amplification at the conclusion of the audiologic assessment is another technique that may prove helpful. This preevaluation trial of an appropriately chosen hearing aid can provide unmistakable evidence of impaired hearing, demonstrate the potential benefits of a hearing aid, and help to dispel preconceived negative feelings about amplification.

The task of improving receptive communication skills and changing attitudes requires considerable effort on the part of hearing-impaired people. It is important that the normally hearing people with whom they communicate understand as well as possible the consequences of hearing loss. It is frustrating to recommend a hearing aid for a client and to provide the necessary counseling, only to have acceptance of the aid or rehabilitative services weakened by a well-meaning but uninformed family member. For example, people often assume that a hearing aid will restore hearing to normal. If the hearing aid does not meet these expectations, they conclude that it is inappropriate or doesn't work, or that the user is not wearing it properly or is failing to "listen." Criticisms of this nature may result in insecurity, doubt, or feelings of guilt that are unwarranted. Therefore, family members should be included in counseling sessions in which the general nature of communication and hearing aids are discussed.

In addition to participating in counseling, family and friends can be actively involved in individual or group remediation. They should have the opportunity to observe the benefits and limitations of amplification firsthand. This can occur through observation in test situations and through actual use of a hearing aid in quiet and in background noise. They can also participate in lipreading or combined auditory-visual activities, as well as attitude or behavior modification discussions.

Hearing-impaired people need to engage less in such defeating behaviors as bluffing, avoiding, self-deprecation, and feeling guilty over communication failures. By the same token normally hearing people need to know that certain of their own behaviors may not be conducive to good communication or the mental health of the hearing impaired. It is often helpful for them to examine their tendencies to avoid communication with the hearing impaired because it is too frustrating, to leave hearing-impaired people out of conversations, or to engage in conversations in their behalf. These types of behaviors can be modified through open communication among normally hearing and hearing impaired people, which is particularly fruitful when accomplished in groups. There is something more convincing about the same complaints when they are expressed by a stranger rather than a spouse.

Counseling parents of hearing-impaired children is accepted widely as an important aspect of habilitation because of the influential role they play in a child's development. Counseling is also important for people in close association with hearing-impaired adults. Wright (1975) summarized the major psychosocial factors negatively influencing adjustment of physically impaired people. She discussed the influence of well-meaning people and the role they play in determining whether the handicapped adopt *coping* or *succumbing* behavior. *Succumbing* emphasizes the negative aspects of impairment with little attention devoted to meaningful adaptation. *Coping* stresses adaptation and constructive involvement. Clinicians can influence family behavior to improve communication, alter environmental barriers, and assist the hearing impaired to develop a *coping* orientation. Family and friends must understand that hearing aids, while very useful, do not restore normal hearing; that sound distortion and the presence of ambient noise make it unlikely that complete understanding of all messages will occur; that lipreading, while providing important supplemental information, will not result in normal reception under most circumstances; that improvement of their own speaking skills and the communication environment would be helpful; and that their own attitudes and expectations can influence whether *coping* or *succumbing* behavior is adopted by the hearing-impaired person.

Audiologists know that hearing aids, lipreading, and auditory training will not restore normal communicative function for a large proportion of hearing-impaired clients. It is important that other people become aware of the limitations of rehabilitation as well as its substantial benefits. The program should increase the sensitivity of family members and friends to the problems imposed by hearing impairment and suggest constructive behaviors to improve communication and promote adjustment.

DELIVERY OF SERVICES TO SPECIAL POPULATIONS

There are two major groups of adults who usually participate in audiologic rehabilitation programs. One of these is composed of young or middle-aged adults, most of whom seek out services because the hearing impairment interferes with some aspect of their lives enough to motivate them to look for remediation. In most cases the hearing loss is having adverse effects on employment, educational, or social activities. Because many productive years lie ahead, the need for rehabilitation is obvious to members of this group. Furthermore, its members are healthy and energetic enough to pursue solutions to their needs through unfamiliar and sometimes circuitous routes. Many of these clients are served adequately by hearing aid consultation, orientation, and follow-up services, which are held at an audiologic facility on an individual appointment basis. Those who require more extensive treatment can arrange for it at the time of or subsequent to hearing aid fitting.

The second group consists primarily of individuals who are of retirement age or older. The aging process involves difficulties that complicate most aspects of life and force changes in life-style. Declining health, reduced mobility, loss of friends or relatives, loss of independence, and a feeling of being unimportant all contribute to a psychological state that may impose a severe barrier to the rehabilitation of hearing loss.

Age-Related Factors That Influence Rehabilitation

There are four general factors related to the aging process itself that may prevent an elderly person from seeking relevant services or participating in them when they are made available.

1. Declining physical health, which may include life-threatening conditions, assumes primary importance for many elderly persons. When people live with pain or chronic illness, they have reduced strength and endurance. Survival and comfort are of greater importance than less immediate concerns, such as the ability to communicate optimally.

2. The extent to which basic needs are satisfied is an important determinant of attitude toward rehabilitative services. There are two types of basic needs that influence life-style: physical needs and emotional ones. Physical needs include adequate food, housing, and transportation, in addition to matters of health. Satisfaction of these needs requires financial security, a serious problem for the majority of elderly people. When there is not enough money available to buy food or pay taxes and utility bills, the purchase of a hearing aid assumes a rather low priority. Emotional needs are met by affectionate relationships, the ability to participate in interests, and the feeling of being needed or respected. The ways in which these needs are fulfilled change throughout life. The elderly must adapt to social isolation brought about by death or geographic separation from loved ones and contemporaries. The ability to participate in activities declines, influencing the degree of satisfaction they provide. If emotional needs are not met, the individual may become depressed and lose interest in maintaining social interactions. The depression and sense of isolation are difficult for many people to overcome, resulting in a lack of desire to rejoin or increase participation in the community.

3. The gradual change in mental capacity associated with the aging process reduces the effectiveness of rehabilitation even if it is accepted. Reductions in awareness, logic, and memory are all factors that must be taken into account when interacting with elderly clients. The reduced ability to handle sensory input, including the visual and auditory components of speech, limits the achievement of rehabilitation goals. The introduction of amplified ambient noise may result in auditory distractions so severe that they limit the effectiveness of amplification and produce anxiety, confusion, and fatigue.

4. Changes in personality are often associated with the aging process, but they are probably more closely related to disease than old age itself. The elderly may become introverted and unmotivated to participate in communication (Alpiner, 1978).

Although the aging process has predictable effects on people, the degree to which the effects are handicapping varies widely. Elderly people who are potential candidates for rehabilitation services fall into three major groups. Members of the first group enjoy good health and are able to maintain a life-style in the mainstream of society. They live alone or with members of their families and are active in the affairs of the community. These individuals usually maintain social interaction with friends and family. Although they may be somewhat limited in mobility and financial resources, these elderly people usually seek necessary professional services and are willing to participate in rehabilitation programs.

The second group consists of those individuals who possess most of the features of the first group but are limited in their ability to use available services because of deteriorating health or severe financial problems. This group is less likely to seek out professional services but will participate in programs if they can be made convenient to them. For example, residents of retirement centers are more likely to participate in rehabilitation when it is provided at the retirement center than when they must travel to an audiologic facility (Harless and Rupp, 1972).

The third group consists of residents of nursing homes or extended care facilities. This group presents unique problems in rehabilitation because many of its members have serious physical or mental health problems. Those who do not are often poorly motivated to participate in a rehabilitation program because of the nature of the environment. Personal interactions among residents may be reduced because of health factors and because no one encourages residents to participate in activities or develop new friends. It is not uncommon to see elderly people in these environments sitting in close proximity to each other for long periods of time without engaging in any form of communication. Living in a residential care facility involves a significant departure from earlier life-styles and epitomizes the emotional isolation that accompanies aging.

Reaching the Elderly

Delivery of services to each of the subgroups of the geriatric population requires different strategies. The first group of individuals is capable of obtaining available services provided in the community, although only a small proportion do so. Better public relations are necessary if elderly adults are to know about and participate in rehabilitation programs held at speech and hearing clinics or hospitals (Davis, 1980).

For the other two groups of elderly people, an audiologic outreach program may be necessary. Descriptions of outreach programs have been provided by Harless and Rupp (1972), McCartney, Maurer, and Sorenson (1974), Colton and O'Neill (1976), Hull and Traynor (1977), Hull, (1978), and Alpiner (1978). Both hearing testing and remedial services are provided where the elderly clients live (either retirement centers or nursing homes) or at senior citizen centers where they gather for meals or recreation. Although it is less convenient for audiologists to provide rehabilitation in these settings, it may be the only way to ensure that services are available to those who need them.

Even when outreach programs are available, other factors may interfere with an individual's motivation to participate in them. Interviewing prospective clients and their families will yield important information regarding the desire or need for audiologic services. In many cases services are desired more by family members than by the elderly persons themselves, who may be comfortable living in a world of reduced sound, communicating as effectively as they want to in most circumstances. The need to communicate may change with age, so all deviations from normal hearing may not require intervention. It is important that family members understand the normal changes that occur with age so that they do not insist on a level of functioning equal to that of a young adult. With the help of appropriate counseling, families can often improve the environment in which communication occurs enough to relieve some of the tensions that may exist. For some elderly people this type of counseling and modification of the environment are all that are necessary for improving communication performance. For others, the willingness of family members to take some responsibility for the success of communication increases their motivation to participate in rehabilitative measures.

Developing Programs for the Elderly. Most treatment programs used with elderly populations involve the same type of habilitation activities that are offered to younger clients. The central auditory dysfunction associated with presbycusis and presbyopia suggests that significant improvements in auditory and visual reception through auditory training and lipreading may not occur, but data are unavailable as evidence to argue either for or against such procedures. Amplification appears to be the major means for improving communication and general awareness of the environment, but its benefits are likely to be limited.

Being able to predict who will accept and use amplification and who will not is helpful in planning habilitation programs for the elderly. *The Feasibility Scale for Predicting Hearing Aid Use* (Rupp, Higgins, and Maurer, 1977) was designed for this purpose. The scale involves assessment of eleven areas of prognostic significance (see Table 13.1). The 11 factors are assessed on a 0- to 5-point scale and multiplied by a weighting factor. For example, *self-referral* under item 1 (Motivation and Mode of Referral) would be assigned an assessment value of 5 while *family referral* would be given a value of 0. More detailed instructions for assessing the various factors and assigning scores is contained in the original article. The authors

Table 13.1 Feasibility Scale for Predicting Hearing Aid Use[a]

Prognostic Factors/Descriptions (continuum, high to low)	*Assessment 5-High: 0-Low*	*Weight*	*Weight Score (Possible)*	*Actual*
1. Motivation and referral (self . . . family)	5 4 3 2 1 0	× 4	(20)	______
2. Self-assessment of listening difficulties (realistic . . . denial)	5 4 3 2 1 0	× 2	(10)	______
3. Verbalization as to "fault" of communication difficulties (self-caused . . . projection)	5 4 3 2 1 0	× 1	(5)	______
4. Magnitude of loss: amplification results.				
A. Shift in spondaic threshold: ______	5 4 3 2 1 0	× 1	(5)	______
B. Discrimination in quiet: ______ at ______ dB HTL	5 4 3 2 1 0	× 1	(5)	______
C. Discrimination in noise: ______ at ______ dB HTL	5 4 3 2 1 0	× 1	(5)	______
5. Informal verbalizations during hearing aid evaluation Re: quality of sound, mold, size (acceptable . . . awful)	5 4 3 2 1 0	× 1	(5)	______
6. Flexibility and adaptability versus senility (relates outwardly . . . self)	5 4 3 2 1 0	× 2	(10)	______
7. Age: 95 90 85 80 75 70 65 (0 1 2 3 4 5)	5 4 3 2 1 0	× 1.5	(7.5)	______
8. Manual hand, finger dexterity, and general mobility (good . . . limited)	5 4 3 2 1 0	× 1.5	(7.5)	______
9. Visual ability (adequate with glasses . . . limited)	5 4 3 2 1 0	× 1	(5)	______

(continued)

Table 13.1—*continued*

Prognostic Factors/Descriptions (continuum, high to low)	*Assessment 5-High: 0-Low*	*Weight*	*Weight Score (Possible) Actual*
10. Financial resources (adequate . . . very limited)	5 4 3 2 1 0	× 1	(7.5) ______
11. Significant other person to assist individual (available . . . none)	5 4 3 2 1 0	× 1.5	(7.5) ______
12. Other factors, please cite	?	?	?
Client ______	FSPHAU: Very limited	0 to 40%	
Age ______	Limited	41 to 60%	
Date ______	Equivocal	61 to 75%	
Audiologist ______	Positive	76 to 100%	[ ] % Total Score

[a] R. Rupp, J. Higgins, and J. Maurer, A feasibility scale for predicting hearing aid use (FSPHAU) with older individuals, *J. Acad. Rehab. Audiol.*, 11, 33–45, 1978. Reprinted with permission.

reported that the use of the scale is helpful in identifying the client requiring more services than usual, including more extensive counseling or an alternative program to improve receptive communication. Although little documentation of its validity is available, the scale may be helpful as a guide for selecting candidates for hearing aid consultation or a more extensive habilitation program.

Inservice Training of Nursing Home Personnel. Management of geriatric clients who live in residential care facilities often depends on the use of nursing home staff to carry out the rehabilitation program (Hull, 1978). Elderly residents are dependent on the staff for assistance in handling prosthetic devices (including hearing aids), controlling background noise, and arranging the environment so that they can participate in communication with others. Without some assistance from audiologists, nursing home staff lack the specific knowledge of hearing loss, its effects on communication, and the role of amplification that will enable them to encourage and facilitate communication attempts. Therefore, staff members should be trained to monitor and troubleshoot hearing aids and encourage their use. They should also be taught to develop their own communication skills that will facilitate auditory and visual reception of speech by nursing home residents.

To be successful, programs for nursing home residents must encourage communication and stimulate the development or continuation of interpersonal relationships. The audiologist should be as concerned about developing or maintaining an environment in which communication *can* occur, as with techniques for improving the communication abilities of the clients themselves. The time spent providing inservice training to nursing staff is usually quite beneficial to the residents being served.

APPROACHES TO REHABILITATION

There are several types of programs currently in use with adults that consist of a combination of the basic components just described. Each type of program emphasizes one or more of the components. Four programs are discussed below; the first three are described briefly to illustrate how the various components of rehabilitation can be combined to form quite different programs. The fourth is a program used and recommended by the authors; it is described in detail.

Behavior Modification Approach

Fleming (1972) described a program used with groups of hearing-impaired adults in a Veterans Administration hospital. The program is designed to foster more effective communication without emphasis on the traditional components of lipreading or auditory training. With the help of an audiologist, each client determines specific situations in which communication breaks down. They then make contracts with themselves and with the group to accomplish certain goals during a specified period of time. Examples of some contracts are as follows.

1. To make better use of the hearing aid in telephone communication.
2. To reduce personal embarrassment associated with wearing a hearing aid.
3. To cope with teenaged children in the family who say "skip it" when not heard by the hearing-impaired parent.
4. To improve ability to interact in multiperson conversations, including manipulating the environment to advantage.

At the end of each week members of the group are required to determine the extent to which their contracts have been accomplished and to generate new contracts for themselves. In addition, group activities are structured to provide emotional support for hearing-impaired members learning to cope with their impairment. For example, situations are contrived to illustrate that normally hearing people also have communication difficulty under certain circumstances, must ask for repetition, or acknowledge that they did not hear or were not listening. Every attempt is made to provide supportive assistance with the intention of reducing blame or guilt and developing coping attitudes rather than permitting hearing loss to become an excuse for performance that is not consistent with potential. The professional staff involved in group management consists of audiologists and psychologists. Family members are encouraged to participate along with the client, and individuals are permitted to continue in the program for as long as they wish.

The emphasis in this program is on adjustment to the hearing impairment. Use of amplification is not stressed, although it is encouraged. Assertiveness training is an integral part of the contract system, while activities involving practice in visual or auditory reception of speech are minimized.

Military Aural Rehabilitation Programs

Sedge, Walden, and Montgomery (1978) described a two-week residential program for army personnel who are sent to Walter Reed Army Hospital for treatment of significant hearing impairment. The major components of the program are a comprehensive evaluation of rehabilitation needs and a unique approach to improving combined auditory-visual speech reception.

Following a hearing aid evaluation and fitting, a rehabilitation evaluation is conducted that assesses speech perception and production status, awareness of the need to alter behavior in communication situations in order to assume control over the listening environment, and adjustment problems related to the communication handicap.

Speech perception is evaluated by testing auditory, visual, and auditory-visual performance. The auditory and visual materials consist of CV nonsense syllables used to determine auditory confusions and the number of consonant groups that can be distinguished visually (Walden, Prosek, and Worthington, 1974). The auditory-visual test consists of sentences presented in the presence of a competing signal to obtain a measure of everyday receptive communication ability. Speech production is evaluated to determine adequacy of articulation, voice quality, and use of prosodic features.

Interviews, self-assessment inventories (such as those described in Chapter 12), and observations of communication behavior are used to determine how well the client can control environmental conditions and whether or not adjustment problems exist. Of particular interest is the degree to which the client is aware of and adjusted to the problems associated with hearing loss.

The results of this evaluation are used to choose procedures for individual rehabilitation sessions. In addition, group and individual training (involving lectures, demonstrations, and discussions) is provided to assist the individual in learning to use amplification and to modify communication strategies to permit better interactions with others.

Training in speech perception constitutes an important part of the program. It consists of watching and listening to sentences presented by videotape. The audio portion of the signal is directed to a voice-activated switch permitting the high-intensity sounds to be transmitted while gating out low-intensity components. The switch is adjustable so that dependence on visual cues for understanding can be decreased or increased as the message is made more or less audible. This appears to be a promising technique for training clients to combine the visual cues associated with high-frequency, low-intensity consonant sounds with the auditory cues provided by low-frequency, high-intensity vowels and consonants. Montgomery (1977) reported that such training can produce as much as 18 percent improvement in sentence recognition following several hours of individual practice. This program combines drills that require auditory-visual perception with activities designed to foster adjustment to the hearing loss.

Analytic Approach

Recent developments in the analysis of distinctive features associated with speech signals have been incorporated into rehabilitation strategies designed to improve speech reception. The research of Hutton (1960), Erber (1972), Binnie, Montgomery, and Jackson (1974), Walden, Prosek, and Worthington (1974), and Binnie (1976) has suggested that a phonetic analysis of the auditory and visual confusions made by hearing-impaired observers can be used to identify specific training needs and to plan appropriate therapy. Instead of lipreading activities that involve determining the meaning of the message, visual training consists of teaching clients to categorize speech sounds into viseme groups and to analyze speech signals accordingly. The client's auditory confusions of phonemes are used to develop drill materials for practicing auditory discrimination. The complexity of the training stimuli gradually increases from syllables to sentences.

Materials such as the *Semi-Diagnostic Test* (Hutton, Curry, and Armstrong, 1959), *Modified Rhyme Test* (Kreul, Nixon, Kryter, Bell, and Lang, 1968), *California Consonant Test* (Owens and Schubert, 1977), or the Larsen materials for auditory training (Davis and Silverman, 1963) are used to determine auditory confusions. Viseme confusions are evaluated by a screening test developed by Binnie, Jackson, and Montgomery (1976) or some similar technique based on other viseme classifications (see Chapter 3).

This analytic approach to rehabilitation is similar to the early programs that stressed lipreading and auditory training drills with noncontextual speech materials. It differs from the military aural rehabilitation program described above because it does not include structured activities designed to improve the client's ability to control communication situations or foster adjustment to the hearing loss. This type of program is often used in military hospitals as well as in other audiologic settings.

Verbotonal Method

The rationale and procedures of the verbotonal method are discussed in Chapter 2. Its use with adults at the New York League for the Hard of Hearing was described by Santore (1978), who reported that the method "provided for (1) extensive diagnosis of the variables related to auditory perception; (2) remediation of auditory perceptual errors; (3) preparation of the patient for amplification; and (4) selection of amplification according to demonstrated needs'' (p. 34).

The Verbotonal method is used with three groups of hearing-impaired adults: those with poor discrimination, those with good discrimination but difficulty functioning in many listening situations, and those unable to adjust to amplification. The clients are scheduled for individual therapy consisting of two sessions per week for as long as three months. A detailed analysis of hearing is completed, including testing with sentences and monosyllabic words. Conventional PB word lists and *tonality lists,* made up of monosyllabic words organized on the basis of their frequency characteristics, are employed. One tonality list consists of 25 words that are recognizable on the basis of low-frequency components, such as the word ''wood.'' Four other lists represent *low-mid, mid, mid-high,* and *high* frequencies. An example of a high-frequency word is ''cease.''

Phonemic confusions and the effects of distance, speed of presentation, rhythm, length of sentences, and the effects of noise on discrimination are obtained for each subject. The SUVAG 1 and 2 auditory training units are used to determine the *optimal field of hearing,* which defines the frequency range through which reception of speech is clearest and which should be amplified. Clients engage in drills designed to improve auditory speech perception of those speech sounds (low, mid-high, and so on) that are most difficult for the client to hear. At the end of the auditory training period a hearing aid is recommended whose frequency response corresponds as closely as possible to the optimal band of frequencies identified through testing with SUVAG 1 and 2.

Santore reported that noticeable improvement in auditory performance occurred in 71 percent of the subjects with whom the approach has been used. She also reported that 85 percent of the group who had previous unsuccessful experience with hearing aids made excellent adjustment to the recommended amplification. The subjects who benefited least from the approach were over age 65; Santore hypothesized that their continuing difficulties may have been related to a central processing problem.

The verbotonal approach involves the use of equipment that is not readily available to most audiologists. The results reported by Santore (1978) suggest that it may be an effective program for adults if the procedures and equipment can be made available. The emphasis of the method is on improvement of speech perception. Psychological reactions to hearing impairment are apparently not addressed directly.

Communication Effectiveness Program

For those adults who need services beyond selection of a hearing aid and orientation to its use, the most successful programs appear to be those that combine hearing aid management, improvement of communication skills, and counseling. The program described in detail below has evolved (Hardick, 1977) out of several years of trial and error attempts to package activities for adults that accomplish the following objectives: (1) encourage individuals to accept their impairment and rehabilitation, (2) minimize the inadequacies of current clinical strategies for recommending hearing aids, (3) provide assistance in adjustment to amplification and residual hearing loss, (4) encourage improved use of communication cues and manipulation of the environment to advantage, and (5) develop a support system among family and friends that is conducive to maintenance of effective communication and good mental health. It has been used successfully in a variety of communities and with different populations of hearing-impaired adults. Specific activities and discussion topics can be modified according to the needs of the clients to be served.

Characteristics of the Program. The program has the following five distinguishing characteristics that are believed to be essential to its success.

1. The program is organized on a group basis. Most adult clients benefit from participating in group activities, sharing common problems, and discovering through group interactions more satisfactory ways of coping with the problems associated with hearing loss. The group approach gives each client realistic experiences in communicating with others. Groups should be as homogeneous as possible on the basis of degree and duration of hearing loss, age, and socioeconomic status. In some cases heterogeneous groups can work well together and produce surprising results, but clients with severe hearing impairment, multiple handicaps or health conditions, and those with severe language problems are best managed individually or in a separate group. Group size should be kept small, between 4 and 12 clients; the exact number should be determined by the number of clinicians involved and the range of severity of the problems represented. If individualized help is to be provided, more than one clinician will be needed; otherwise clients exhibiting unusual problems must be seen at a different time for individual attention.

2. The program is client centered. The audiologist is interested in the specific problems of each participant, whether or not they are readily quantifiable by an audiometer or other means. Each member of the group usually has at least one significant problem that interferes with acceptance or use of amplification. That problem may be related to characteristics of the hearing loss, psychological factors, family or employment considerations, or some combination of these. Continued attendance and satisfactory progress in the program will not occur unless clients feel their individual concerns are respected and given attention by the audiologist and/or by the group.

3. The program stresses amplification as a primary means of rehabilitation. The major focus of the program is to find an amplification system for each person that improves reception, can be tolerated, and will be worn. For some adults this is a rather straightforward problem; for others it is complicated. Although the contribution of visual information is important, no other single form of remedial assistance provides as much benefit as amplification. Therefore, primary emphasis is placed on improving reception and supplementing it with visual cues. Because they directly affect speech perception, the noise environment and communication patterns in the home or place of employment are taken into account when making suggestions about hearing aid use.

4. The program involves participation of normally hearing friends or relatives. Rehabilitation is enhanced if the client obtains support from members of the family or close friends. Learning to accept and use amplification is a difficult process that is made easier by the assistance and understanding of others. Unless normally hearing people are knowledgeable about the importance and limitations of hearing aids, lipreading, and auditory reception, they may be critical of communication efforts and offer advice that seems sensible to the layman but is ill founded.

The normally hearing friends and relatives of the clients participate in all phases of the program. They experience amplification, take part in lipreading and listening activities, and contribute to group discussions. Participation facilitates their understanding of hearing loss while hearing-impaired clients gain insight about the severity of their own problems as they compare their performance to that of the normally hearing group members. In addition, hearing-impaired people often lose sight of the fact that normally hearing people do not always communicate effectively either.

Large age differences between the client and the participating relative (or other normally hearing people being used as a reference) will produce differences in performance on many tasks because of the age effect as well as the hearing loss. This may be undesirable for some clients but can be helpful in demonstrating some of the common problems encountered when attempting to use visual cues or communicate in noise.

5. The program is short term in duration. Rehabilitation programs for most adults should average about 12 to 20 hours of group meetings. Scheduling one two-hour session per week for 6 to 10 weeks permits learning to be spread out over an appreciable period with sufficient time between sessions to complete outside assignments and practice techniques. Other schedules (two one or two hour sessions per week, for example) may be equally effective.

As soon as certain objectives (to be enumerated later) have been achieved, the program should be terminated. Because complete restoration of communicative function is not likely to occur no matter how much therapy is provided, the program should be terminated at the end of a specified period of time. Because this is not likely to be true for the group as a whole, individuals may be referred for further individual services or for participation in another group. Those clients who enjoy the social aspects of group participation and wish to continue for that purpose may be referred to facilities offering programs of that type.

Maintaining an Ongoing Group Rehabilitation Program. The heterogeneity of hearing-impaired clients poses a problem to the development and maintenance of appropriate group rehabilitation programs. The advantages of group management are strong enough, however, to warrant attempts to provide this type of therapy to a wide variety of adult clients. Neither creating instantaneous groups nor delaying therapy until enough clients are available to form a group is a satisfactory way to provide an effective rehabilitation program. The following guidelines are suggested for developing and maintaining an ongoing rehabilitative program for hearing-impaired people whose needs cannot be met by hearing aid selection and orientation alone. Attracting participants, integrating clients from different sources, scheduling, and funding will be discussed.

Attracting Participants. Clients enter group programs from two major sources: referral from audiologists or directly from the relatively untapped but large pool of hearing-impaired adults that exists in every community. The latter group consists of people who may or may not be aware of their hearing impairments and who, either because they are unaware of the services that exist or because it has not occurred to them, have not sought audiological services. If this population can be attracted, a flow of participants is assured. Some relevant questions to be answered are (1) How is this nonclinical population recruited?, (2) In what ways do they differ from audiologist-referred participants?

A successful technique for gaining access to the pool of hearing-impaired adults in a community is by establishing a relationship with the area or community agency on aging or directly with centers serving the health, recreational, or social needs of older people. A relationship can be established by offering hearing screening services several times a year at convenient locations where other needs of this population are being met, such as at congregate meal sites. The agency on aging or the community center will usually provide all publicity and the use of a facility for these activities. The hearing screening, which may be part of a multifaceted health screening program, is followed by individual consultations in which hearing test results are reviewed and recommendations made. If a client has obvious difficulty communicating, expresses concern about it, or exhibits significant hearing loss, participation in the group program is suggested. Complete audiological and otological examinations need not be a prerequisite for enrollment, because many potential participants will not follow such recommendations initially.

The orientation and activities of the program are described to potential participants and they are encouraged to join the group to obtain information about hearing and communication, gain experience with amplification, and improve their ability to communicate. General information about the time and place of meetings is provided; more precise information is detailed by letter to those who express interest.

Experience suggests that approximately one-half of those who have their hearing screened under these circumstances are candidates for the rehabilitation program. A single screening may provide enough potential participants for several future groups. Because most of the people who come to have their hearing screened have not previously committed themselves to exploring rehabilitation, they are usually in no hurry and are willing to wait for services, if necessary. Many of them are amenable to being scheduled for groups as much as six months in advance. If they want more immediate attention than can be provided in the group program, they can be referred to an audiologic facility. Many of the people contacted in this fashion are members of that group commonly identified in the literature as unmotivated. This may not be the case. Many of them have mild hearing impairments that present problems only under certain circumstances. Others have not viewed themselves as having a hearing impairment severe enough to warrant rehabilitation. One value of a program spread out over a period of weeks is that it provides time for the client to evaluate the amount of assistance provided by amplification and to experience a gradual change of attitude if it is warranted.

Figure 13.1 summarizes the two service delivery options: the conventional individual hearing-aid consultation and the group audiologic rehabilitation approach. On the left side of the figure the hearing-aid consultation events are outlined, with clients entering the system through some form of referral (professional, agency, self, or peer). The group program is diagrammed on the right, showing the several methods of entry, including referral from the conventional model, if warranted.

If possible a group should be in session at most times during the year, so that when one group terminates another begins within a week or two. Having several

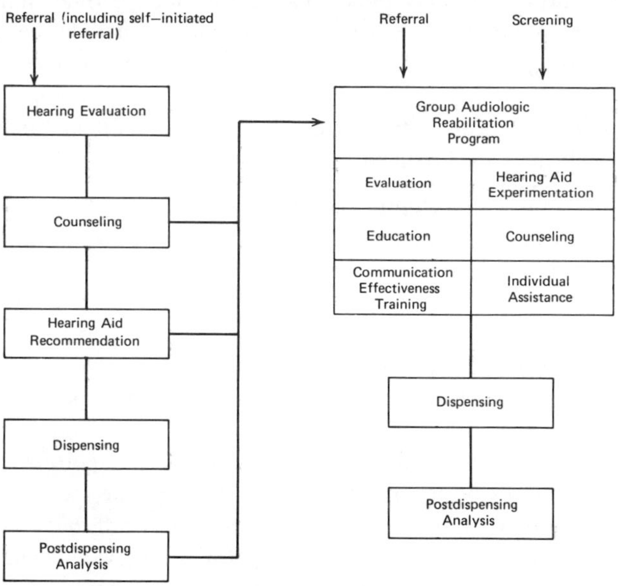

Figure 13.1. Block diagram of a service delivery system showing the interface between a group habilitation program and conventional hearing aid consultation approach.

groups per year makes it possible to channel individual referrals from the audiologic facility into a program with minimal delay.

Integrating clients from different sources. The first meeting of the group is usually attended only by those entering by the outside referral or screening route; that is, those participants for whom complete audiological workups are not yet available. The first session is devoted to activities designed to develop warm, informal social and professional relationships among the participants and staff; to review the purposes, activities and costs of the remaining sessions; and to set the stage for subsequent meetings. The participants are informed that complete audiological workups, case histories, and evaluations of handicap need to be obtained for a definitive analysis of their communication problems. Clients are scheduled for an evaluation, including the taking of earmold impressions of one or both ears. Clients are also informed that they will need to see a physician and have their candidacy for amplification verified by signature. The additional costs that will be involved if a hearing aid is purchased are explained. As a result of this orientation, participants usually have completed audiological workups by the second session. It is usually at this point that clients who are referred from conventional hearing aid and consultation programs join the group.

Scheduling Group Sessions. The program outlined in the remainder of this chapter requires 6 to 10 two-hour sessions scheduled over several weeks. Sessions can be offered during the day, in the evening, or on weekends. It is suggested that they be held during the normal workday rather than during leisure time, unless there are compelling reasons not to do so. Most clients are able to schedule sessions into their work week by making minimal alteration of their schedules, revising the workday, or leaving work early. Interestingly enough, many retired people have as much difficulty scheduling sessions as those who work because of the number of different activities in which they are involved.

Financial Support for Rehabilitation Services. The matter of financing rehabilitation is often of concern. The importance of the issue varies according to the nature and mission of the facility or individual offering the service. A small fee per session may be charged, but expenses may be covered by hearing aid dispensing fees or the sessions may be considered a business investment and offered free.

The program described here was developed within a university whose mission is education, research, and the development of innovative approaches to service delivery. Participants pay for the evaluations, earmolds, medical appointments, and hearing aids, but the weekly sessions are free. It is often as important to demonstrate the need for and benefits of programs as it is to demonstrate their profitability. As the benefits of rehabilitation become more generally known throughout the community, more participants will be willing to pay for the service rendered. What is required now is leadership in providing quality service. Experience shows that half of the hearing aids dispensed by one university that conducts such a group program have been dispensed to individuals who enter through the outreach program. Any approach that can attract the unserved hearing-impaired people in the community by offering high quality, relevant management will realize an increase in financial revenues through its dispensing program.

Objectives of the Program. There are six major objectives that shape the orientation and activities of the program.

1. *To provide information about hearing, hearing loss, and hearing aids.* The participants should develop a basic understanding of the structure and function of the auditory system, the causes and characteristics of common types of hearing loss, the importance of medical examination, and common medical-surgical procedures. Information about different types of hearing aids, how they function, how they can be purchased, their common controls and electroacoustic characteristics, possible accessories, and the importance of periodic service and how it can be obtained should be presented. In addition, participants should know the professional areas of competence and responsibility of audiologists, otologists, hearing aid dealers, speech-language pathologists, and teachers of the hearing impaired. Finally, participants should be familiar with the types of services they might expect from various community agencies. The more sophisticated clients are about these matters the more likely they are to seek otologic examinations and rehabilitation services. They will be less inclined to accept advertising claims for new treatments or hearing aids without question, thus better-informed consumers.

Experience with aging clients, in particular, suggests that one of the reasons they do not pursue rehabilitation is lack of information; they have unrealistic expectations about rehabilitation and a poor understanding of the roles of the various professionals involved. Many are suspicious of the hearing aid dispensing system because of sales techniques, costs that seem unreasonable, and previous experiences of their own or of acquaintances who derive minimal benefit from amplification. With sufficient information the majority develop positive attitudes toward rehabilitation. A 10- to 15-minute presentation on one of these or other topics is presented at each session. Presentations should permit time for questions and group discussion.

2. *To experiment with hearing aid systems and their use in improving communication.* Many of the group members have difficulty realizing significant benefit from amplification. Some have been placed in the group to determine whether or not amplification is beneficial; some already own a hearing aid but are experiencing difficulty in adjusting to it. In any case, experimentation with amplification and coupling systems is a central feature of the program. It is possible that a more optimal system may be found for some hearing aid users, or that experimentation with different forms of amplification will bring about desirable changes in attitude.

Each session includes trial use of a hearing aid. Conventional fittings should be used as well as those that may appear to be inconsistent with preconceived clinical notions of what is most appropriate. For example, a hearing aid that allows the contralateral routing of the signal (CROS) with open earmold might be utilized one week on a client who appears to be a logical candidate for binaural amplification with vented earmolds. A high frequency emphasis aid might be tried on an individual one week, with a full-frequency response instrument used the next. The use of a bone conduction vibrator in place of an air conduction receiver may be explored for individuals sustaining severe or profound losses who have experienced little success with hearing aid use. The purpose is to allow the clients to experiment with amplification in a safe, supportive environment. Although variations in hearing aid type and gain-frequency response characteristics are employed, MPO (or SSPL 90) is held to the lowest level possible.

As soon as possible each client assumes responsibility for preparing the hearing aid for operation, coupling it to the ear, and setting the appropriate controls. Once the hearing aid and earmold chosen for experimentation have been put in place, formal session activities begin. Sometime during each session aided discrimination in quiet, noise, and with combined auditory-visual presentation is evaluated. Stimuli can be presented to the group by use of audio and videotapes played through a suitable amplification system. Good-quality cassette tape recorders and a videotape playback systems employing a television monitor may be employed efficiently. The fact that the sound reproduction qualities of these systems may not be comparable to those of a clinical audiometer in a sound-treated room should not prohibit the activity. One of the purposes is to provide listening and learning experiences for the participants under less than ideal conditions. If the conditions are the same from week to week the derived data can be used for comparative purposes. Therefore, instrumentation should be calibrated periodically to assure equality of presentation level over time. Sound level measurements made at several places in the room will determine uniformity of intensity and provide reasonable estimates of ear level sound pressure level.

The *Modified Rhyme Test* (Kruel, Nixon, Kryter, Bell, Lang, and Schubert, 1968) is useful for group discrimination testing because it is a convenient paper-and-pencil test in a multiple-choice format. Sentence materials should be used for auditory-visual presentation. The *Speech Perception In Noise* (*SPIN*) test (Kalikow, Stevens, and Elliott, 1977) is recommended because it is the most convenient material at present. The *CID Everyday Speech Sentences* (Davis and Silverman, 1978) or the revised CID sentences (Harris, Haines, Kelsey, and Clack, 1961) may be used, but these require more time for administration because the participants must write all of the words understood in the sentence. Videotapes can be presented without sound, without picture, or with varying degrees of sound to demonstrate the importance to communication of combining auditory and visual cues.

Time is also allotted in each session for use of the hearing aid in a common environmental context. Examples include an informal group discussion, listening to music, taking a walk outside, or going to a cafeteria for coffee.

At the conclusion of each session the clients' reactions to the amplification system are solicited. They are asked (1) to compare the aid to any previously worn systems, (2) to comment on the amount of benefit provided in comparison to the unaided situation, (3) whether the aid was convenient to operate, (4) whether it was comfortable, natural, pleasant, and could be tolerated, and (5) whether it was noisy. Reactions are recorded for future reference on a form similar to that shown in Appendix A at the end of this chapter.

If possible, each participant is allowed to wear an appropriate hearing aid for a few days at home and in other social settings. The reaction to this experience is explored in a group discussion the following week. Clients are also asked to describe the amount of time the aid was worn, whether it was a source of embarrassment, and any reactions received from other people.

Eventually this experimentation results in the determination of a hearing aid-earmold arrangement that provides optimal results. As the program draws to a conclusion decisions are made by the clinician in cooperation with each client regarding the specific amplification system to be recommended. Experience has shown that approximately 90 percent of the participants follow through with purchase of the recommended system, a degree of success that is remarkable given the nature of the group. The participants are reevaluated at intervals on the same outpatient basis as those completing a conventional hearing aid selection procedure.

3. *To improve listening skills*. Barker (1971) states that listening is a skill that can be improved. Listening is not the same as hearing; hearing is a physiological process, while listening is a psychological process, involving attending to sounds and messages received by the auditory system. Barker indicates that there are four processes involved in listening: hearing, attending, understanding, and remembering.

There are two factors related to listening and hearing-impaired people that are of consequence to rehabilitation. First, hearing loss makes listening a more difficult task. Hearing-impaired people must attend closely when communicating, this requires increased muscular tension that may be accompanied by an increased level of anxiety. Hearing-impaired people in communication-oriented employment settings often report extreme fatigue at the end of the day, with insufficient energy remaining to engage in social activities in the evening. Because listening is fatiguing, hearing-impaired people become selective listeners in an attempt to conserve energy. Although normally hearing people find it humorous or irritating when Aunt Clara hears some things but not others, Aunt Clara may be engaging in very logical and necessary behavior. Selective listening is appropriate unless it is carried to extremes. A few adults listen only when forced to do so by angry or frustrated speakers; others rely on a normally hearing associate to serve as a communication intermediary. Some marital partners, for example, find themselves serving as interpreters for their hearing-impaired mates, whether this activity is required or not.

Second, improving hearing is often a prerequisite to improving listening behavior. The hearing of some clients, particularly elderly people, is difficult to improve because of the nature of the hearing loss and because of the reduction in hearing sensitivity associated with hearing loss produces a desirable isolation from constant and disturbing ambient noise. Some elderly clients are agitated by background noise even without a hearing aid. Although they want to improve their hearing for communication, they discover that use of amplification to hear speech involves exposure to higher levels of unwanted ambient noise. The immediate reaction is rejection of amplification. The resulting ambivalence toward hearing through a hearing aid must be acknowledged and dealt with. Many individuals, through counseling and listening activities learn to accept amplified ambient noise as an accompaniment to improved speech reception.

It is helpful for hearing-impaired adults to be aware of their listening behavior and the reasons for it in order to minimize antagonizing others or becoming unnecessarily selfish or dependent. Increased awareness makes it possible for them to understand their own behavior, make adjustments, and use selective listening to better advantage. This goal is achieved through group discussion as well as through listening activities. Presentation of recorded environmental sounds and speech provide practice in sound identification while familiarizing participants with the limitations imposed by hearing loss and amplification. Outside assignments are used to encourage improving listening behavior. If hearing-impaired clients can become accustomed to the presence of background sounds and learn to identify them, they will be able to suppress them more effectively and attend to the most meaningful sounds. Reacquaintance with environmental noises is a necessary prerequisite to hearing aid use and an important part of improving listening skills.

4. *To improve the use of visual information to understand speech.* Activities involving lipreading with or without simultaneous auditory cues are used for the following purposes: (1) to demonstrate that people with adequate vision can make use of visual cues to supplement auditory comprehension, (2) to encourage increased visual attention, and (3) to provide participants with suggestions for securing maximum access to these cues.

The orientation is one that Tannahill and Smoski (1978) refer to as the "informational and tutorial counseling" approach, in contrast to a second approach that they label the "practice makes perfect" approach. Lipreading skill is viewed as a complex behavior that individuals seem to exhibit in varying amounts. During the early stages of impaired hearing most people improve their lipreading ability without instruction. Little is really known about this type of linguistic behavior or how to teach it. That people can read lips and benefit significantly is unquestioned, but valid methods of measuring the skill or data demonstrating improvement after training are unavailable.

During the program clients are made aware of the specific contributions that lipreading can make to communication. The degree to which combining auditory and visual cues improves speech reception is discussed and demonstrated. Practice is provided in the use of situational cues and linguistic context as aids to understanding what is said. Lipreading drills are not conducted, but practice using visual cues as an adjunct to auditory cues is stressed.

Lipreading activities can also be used to illustrate the difficulties involved in making use of visual cues. The effects of speaker variables (rapid or slurred speech, for example), environmental factors (distance and lighting), and message characteristics (linguistic complexity and familiarity) are demonstrated. These influences on lipreading are discussed in Chapter 3.

The practice provided during lipreading activities usually does not result in measurable improvement in lipreading performance. The goal of these activities is not to improve lipreading scores, but to familiarize the participants with the supplementary benefits that can be obtained if they are visually alert and to teach them how to make maximum use of the visual information that *is* or can be made available. If this goal is made clear by the clinician, participants enjoy the activities but are under little pressure to improve performance. As they learn about the limitations involved in understanding speech through lipreading, most adults relax, begin to view their level of performance as acceptable, and make better use of it.

Even though pre- and post-test results generally reveal no improvement, most clients report enthusiasm for the activities and increased comfort in communication situations. Many report the impression of improved ability to understand the speech of others, even though formal measures of lipreading ability do not reflect improvement. This is not surprising, because lipreading activities stress the use of situations, combined auditory-visual reception, and context, factors that are not reflected in lipreading tests.

5. *To provide counseling to develop positive attitudes and coping behaviors.* Persons with hearing loss describe remarkably similar experiences and frustrations resulting from their reduced ability to hear. They report embarrassment when they fail to understand what is said and anxiety about wearing a hearing aid. Most of them have had negative experiences with friends, family members, or strangers. They resent being expected to understand in all situations, even though they realize the hearing loss is not apparent to others. Hearing-impaired adults may be reluctant to ask for repetitions or to admit that they have not heard or understood a message. They have vague feelings of isolation and rejection, although these are by no means pathological reactions. Many adults do not readily admit the hearing impairment to others. Instead, they engage in nonproductive behaviors such as pretending to understand messages, avoiding communication situations previously enjoyed (cocktail parties, bridge games, church meetings), or dominating conversations in order to avoid having to listen and risk misunderstandings. They frequently feel guilty for not being able to communicate normally.

Lectures concerning the inappropriateness of these behaviors are usually ineffective in changing them, but guided group discussions are often quite helpful. Group members share experiences, express mutual frustration and concern, and come to realize that their individual experiences are not unique. Gradually, the clinician can elicit suggestions from the group about alternative productive behaviors and encourage them to try them out as class or home assignments.

Clients may need assistance in accepting the natural consequences of hearing impairment, developing assertiveness, cultivating a sense of humor about inevitable communication errors, and developing a "thick skin" to serve as a buffer against inconsiderate attitudes and behaviors of normally hearing people. Those who accept the physical impairment emotionally and intellectually will adopt compensatory behaviors that allow them to function as normally as possible.

Some clinicians include assertiveness training as a part of the group therapy. Role playing difficult situations enables group members to try out new behaviors in the context of familiar experiences. Reactions of other group members, including the normally hearing participants, are usually positive and serve to encourage them to take more control over what happens to them in communicative situations.

The key to success in meeting this goal lies in the clinician's ability to facilitate group discussion. Participants should be the ones who suggest alternate behaviors, discuss their pros and cons, and arrive at a list of mutually agreed upon suggestions for future use. Their sensitivity to inconsiderate statements and behaviors of others may be reduced as a result of the group's empathy and support. If participants can develop a sense of humor about communication errors, or at the least a tolerance for them, their adjustment to the hearing loss will be significantly enhanced.

6. *To provide participants with suggestions for resolving miscellaneous problems.* Hearing-impaired people often present problems that are not adequately resolved by any of the techniques so far discussed. For example, use of a hearing aid may not be helpful in hearing an alarm clock or telephone bell, and it may not satisfactorily resolve telephone communication problems. Alternative solutions to these and other problems are discussed and assistance provided in obtaining necessary instrumentation or services. For example, an alarm clock radio with an appliance outlet can be used in conjunction with an electric light to substitute a visual signal for an auditory alarm. Some hearing-impaired individuals benefit more from the installation of a telephone amplifier than they do from use of the telephone coil in their hearing aids. If loud radio or television sound produces irritation or friction among family members or neighbors, earphones or inserts may be installed that permit direct hearing by the hearing-impaired person without interfering with normal loudspeaker function. This arrangement also diminishes the amount of distracting environmental noise by providing a better signal-to-noise ratio at the ear. The use of a wireless microphone and FM receiver may improve communication in large group situations, such as in church or at home or work when communication must occur across distance or in moderate levels of noise.

Some people, particularly elderly persons living alone, may be concerned about remaining in touch with neighbors and relatives because of their inability to hear the ring of the telephone or doorbell. They may have concerns about personal safety because they cannot detect the presence of intruders or hear warning signals such as fire alarms. There are devices available that can reduce some of these concerns. Louder bells can be installed in telephones, extension bells can be installed in other rooms, and bells can be supplemented with flashing lights. The array of potential problems of hearing-impaired people and their families is quite extensive. The clinician who is interested in rehabilitation can readily extract such problems for consideration, most of which have solutions limited only by the interest and imagination of the clinician or relevant technical personnel. Some of the items alluded to are commercially available, and technical resources exist in most communities for resolution of other problems if the clinician is willing to explore them.

Conducting the Sessions. The objectives reviewed in the previous section can be accomplished in numerous ways and in various organizational structures. The following description of 10 group sessions is based on the experiences of the authors. It assumes that the participants have had minimal previous contact with audiologic rehabilitation or hearing assessment. If group members have completed audiologic workups or participated in previous programs, the makeup of the sessions, particularly the first one or two, can be modified accordingly.

The Staff and the Physical Environment. All materials and instrumentation for the sessions should be arranged and tested in advance to minimize the time spent moving from one activity to another. Ideally, there should be one clinician for every two or three clients, especially during hearing aid selection procedures. A staff meeting should be held prior to each session to review the progress of each client and to plan the sequence of events for the coming session.

The use of visual aids, such as posters, chalkboards, and handouts, is recommended whenever possible to ensure adequate understanding of information or instructions by the participants. Recorded materials should be used if auditory, visual, or combined performance is evaluated. Equipment should be calibrated so approximate levels and signal-to-noise ratios are known.

The group leader should have excellent speaking skills and observe certain basic rules of communication with the hearing impaired. Speech should be produced at a conversational loudness level but a little slower than usual. Mannerisms that detract from efficient communication should be eliminated, such as excessive gestures, facial grimaces, speaking with a cigarette or other object in the mouth, or pacing the room while speaking. The speaker should face the group at all times unless there is a specific reason not to. Lighting in the room should be appropriate with natural and artificial light sources directed on the speaker. Visual distractions behind the speaker should be minimal, and the ambient noise level should be conducive to efficient communication.

The participants should be seated so they can see and hear all other participants. A semicircular seating arrangement is generally satisfactory. Normally hearing participants should sit beside or slightly behind their friends or relatives. It is helpful if a seating chart is developed during the first session so that all measures of communicative performance are made under similar circumstances.

Suggested Outline of Group Sessions

First Session

•The preliminary phases of this session consist of introductory material pertaining to:

1. Introduction of all participants and professional staff.
2. General review of program goals, procedures, and chronology of events.
3. Review of costs, if any.

If complete audiological evaluation data are not available for clients, arrangements must be made for obtaining that information and earmold impressions.

•Screening of visual acuity. This can be done using a Snellen chart or an Orthorater or similar instrumentation, and can be carried out by a staff member or a visual consultant.

Lipreading activities, no matter what their purpose, should not be conducted without knowledge of visual status, which is as essential to lipreading as hearing is to listening. Vision screening also reinforces the need for maintaining optimal visual correction.

•Lecture-discussion. A presentation is made by one of the staff members on the general structure and function of the auditory system. This consists of a brief review of the parts of the ear and how auditory signals progress through the system. The use of wall charts, models, and film strips is helpful. It is important not to overwhelm the clients with scientific terminology or the complexities of the system.

•Auditory-visual discrimination. An activity incorporated into all sessions consists of obtaining auditory and combined auditory-visual discrimination scores for speech presented at typical conversational levels in quiet and against a background of noise. The task also serves to sensitize normally hearing observers to the problem of hearing in noise and the potential contribution of visual cues.

•Outside assignment. As a final activity of this session each participant is given a case history questionnaire and a copy of the *Hearing Performance Inventory* (Lamb, Owens, Schubert and Giolas, 1979; see also Appendix F, Chapter 12), or similar scale, to be completed before the next session.

Second Session

•Provision of amplification. Whether individually fitted amplification systems and personal earmolds are used at this session depends on the interval of time between sessions and the availability of complete audiological data. If necessary, stock earmolds can be used, especially if open earmolds are a practical consideration. During this session clients are familiarized with the general features of amplification, including where the battery is placed and how to insert it, function of switches and controls, connecting the earmold to the hearing aid, and general procedures for placement on the body. Later clients will use this information to assemble, place, and control the specific aid to be used during each session.

•Lecture-discussion. The topic for this session concerns the causes of hearing loss and its effects on hearing for communication. Types of conductive losses are reviewed briefly, but most attention is focused on causes and effects of sensorineural hearing loss, particularly those related to the aging process and noise exposure. Clients should have available their personal clinical file materials; the information presented can be related to their own audiometric test results. Having access to their clinical files seems to heighten the sense of participation, stimulate learning, and permit personal assessment of progress. Documents or letters requiring release should be withheld or appropriate permission obtained.

•Counseling. The third activity of this session consists of the initiation of group counseling through informal dialogue. The goal of this first group conversation is not counseling per se; it is to initiate communication among participants, to use amplification to listen to different speakers and at varying distances, and to become familiar with the speaking mannerisms of group members. This introductory session consists of having each person introduce themselves, giving name, place of birth, describing major events of their lives, and making any comment they wish about their hearing or any matters related to it. The information shared can be a rich source of topics for future consideration.

The group moderator often asks group members to summarize their ability to hear a specific individual. This stimulates discussion of positive and negative communication behaviors, and encourages participants to listen and think critically about common speaking mannerisms. The activity often reveals misunderstandings by the listener that are humorous and can be used to increase tolerance to errors. Laughter is a natural reaction and is encouraged when misunderstandings occur. Instead of being perceived as insensitive, the laughter of other hearing-impaired listeners is interpreted as a shared response to a common occurrence, a laughing *with* rather than *at*. Occasionally, a group member is too sensitive to see the humor involved, but most clients accept their errors and the response to it in a good-natured way. Group members usually display a high degree of sensitivity to each other and modify their responses accordingly.

•Auditory-visual discrimination with amplification. This activity is a repetition of the group speech discrimination testing done during the first session. The same type of materials, listening conditions, and signal-to-noise ratios are employed, using different lists. Results are compared to those obtained without amplification during the first session.

•Outside assignment. A medical release form is provided along with instructions for obtaining the signature of a physician approving their candidacy for amplification. These forms may be completed anytime before the purchase of a hearing aid. Clients are encouraged to consult their family doctors or specialists, and a list of local otologists is provided.

•Subjective reaction to amplification. At the end of the session each participant wearing amplification is asked to record in writing or on a rating scale their reaction to the amplification system worn (see suggested form in Appendix A).

They are encouraged to comment on the amount of help provided by the aid, the quality of sound reproduction, physical comfort, the amount of difficulty in operating the controls, and their reaction to the presence of amplified ambient noise. For many, this is a difficult task at first because they have little basis for comparison. The information obtained is helpful in planning for the next session and for making final recommendations about amplification.

Third Session

•Amplification. The selected amplification system is placed on each client, and the instructions given during the second session are repeated. Clients then practice putting the hearing aid in place.

•Lecture-Discussion. A staff member discusses hearing aids, describing common hearing aid types, components, characteristics, benefits, and limitations.

•Expanding hearing aid experience. The third activity of this session is one that extends the hearing aid experience to new and more complicated situations. Clients leave the quiet therapy room and attempt to communicate in other environments, such as a cafeteria, office, auditorium, or on a busy street.

•Counseling. Upon returning from the preceding activity, group members discuss their experiences briefly. They are then guided into a discussion of their feelings about hearing impairment. This activity begins with a discussion of the communication behaviors of normally hearing people that pose a barrier to interpersonal interactions. This usually produces a lively discussion that provides important insights for both the normally hearing and hearing-impaired group members into their respective communication behaviors. Beginning a discussion of feelings on this neutral ground permits the clients to become familiar with one another and gradually move toward expressing personal feelings openly. The discussion leader should not necessarily limit client responses to the topic of the speech patterns of normally hearing people, but it is best not to push the group members into sensitive discussions before they are ready.

•Auditory-visual discrimination. Evaluation of auditory and auditory-visual discrimination should be accomplished under the previously established conditions. Clients should be seated in the same relative location as during the previous sessions. If changes in seating occur, records should be kept not only of client performance but also of location relative to the loudspeaker.

•Outside assignment. Group members are asked to discuss what they know about their individual hearing losses with another person. An alternate assignment is to discuss with someone the ways in which normally hearing people could improve their communication with hearing-impaired people.

•Subjective reaction to amplification. Before leaving the session, clients record their reactions to the amplification system used during the session and compare it with the experience of the preceding week.

Fourth Session

•Amplification. By now the hearing-impaired client should be able to assume major responsibility for preparing the selected hearing aid for use and putting it in place, with assistance provided as necessary.

•Lecture-discussion. The benefits and limitations of lipreading are presented through a combination of lecture and demonstration. The visual characteristics of English are reviewed and demonstrated, and the speaker, receiver, and environmental factors that contribute to lipreading are reviewed. There are several types of materials that can be used to illustrate the principles discussed. Videotapes using different speakers and messages that vary in familiarity and complexity are very useful. Handouts such as the one shown in Appendix B provide reminders of the type of behavior that will enhance the combined use of auditory and visual clues.

•Lipreading activities. To reinforce the information just presented, activities are introduced that involve the use of situational cues and linguistic context to determine what is said. Common situations are described, then clients attempt to lipread conversations acted out by staff members. Jokes or short anecdotes are presented, followed by punchlines or summary statements that must be lipread. Any activity that allows practice in the use of available information to aid in visual reception of speech will be appropriate.

•Counseling. The counseling activity of this session focuses on behaviors of the hearing impaired that are not conducive to effective communication. The purpose of this discussion is to encourage clients to talk about common ways in which they contribute to their communication problems and to help them evolve suggestions for changing those behaviors. Some of the behaviors involve refusing to admit being hearing impaired; pretending to understand when they don't; and failing to ask for repetitions, reduction of noise levels, or changes in seating that would make listening easier. Role playing is an excellent method by which both coping and succumbing behaviors can be demonstrated. As soon as group members appear comfortable enough, role playing should be introduced and used frequently.

•Auditory-visual discrimination.

•Outside assignment. Several types of assignments are appropriate at this time. Clients may be asked to rate people with whom they communicate often as to their lipreadability and to give reasons for labeling them as easy or difficult to lipread. Groups of sentences containing homophenous words may be provided for home practice. Clients may also be asked to keep a log of the number of times and the situations in which they use maladaptive behaviors such as avoiding communication, bluffing, or relying on others to communicate for them.

•Subjective reaction to amplification.

Fifth Session

•Amplification. As usual this session opens with the fitting of appropriate amplification. The same hearing aid may be used more than once; changes in fitting may involve variations in earmolds or changes in the internal adjustments of the aid. Definite client preferences may begin to emerge at this time.

•Lecture-discussion. This week's talk by the professional staff is on the topic of hearing and listening. It should provide basic information about speech acoustics and the effects of background noise and reverberation on speech intelligibility. The clients are fully aware that the speech they hear is not clear and that noise further reduces their ability to understand. The more they know about why they have difficulty understanding speech, the less they blame themselves for not communicating perfectly. Because there are logical explanations for the difficulties they experience, hearing-impaired individuals develop increased feelings of being in control and fewer feelings of being victimized by strange and poorly understood forces. Information about speech and room acoustics assists clients in learning to manipulate their environments to allow for better reception of speech. Some individuals with mild hearing impairments profit from this type of information to such an extent that the improvement in listening skills that occurs makes the immediate use of amplification unnecessary. Although it does not actually simulate hearing impairment, a recording of filtered speech may be played for normally hearing group members to help them understand the effects of hearing loss better.

•Listening practice. To allow for immediate practice of listening skills, the counseling session is replaced by listening practice. Easy tasks are presented first, such as identification of recorded everyday sounds in noise. Many clients have difficulty with this relatively gross listening task. Recognizing group members' voices, localizing sounds and voices, and following simple instructions given in noise without visual clues are types of activities employed. Analysis of the factors that seemed to influence performance (nature and location of the sounds, for example) completes the listening activity.

•Auditory-visual discrimination.

•Outside assignment. With the assistance of a normally hearing group member, participants are asked to compile a list of sounds they hear but cannot identify during the next week. Lists of soft sounds that are often not heard easily are provided with instructions to listen for them and record how many are heard and under what circumstances.

•Subjective reactions to amplification.

Sixth Session

•Amplification. By now the client should be able to manage hearing aid preparation and placement without assistance.

•Lecture-discussion. The options available for purchasing a hearing aid in the local community are discussed. The differences among options are explained along with their advantages and disadvantages. Price ranges and their relation to "bundled" and "unbundled" costs are presented. Clients are informed of the services that are included in the purchase price under each delivery option. If the price includes only the hearing aid and earmold, clients should be told about potential future costs. Participants are encouraged to "shop around," contacting any dispenser of the recommended aid for information about cost or service that seems relevant. If requested, staff members assist clients in interpreting the information obtained from various sources. Experience indicates that most participants will purchase a hearing aid from the facility that sponsors the group activities, if it dispenses and prices are competitive. Clients should always be made aware of the options available and given the opportunity to choose among them without being pressured.

•Counseling. The discussion of feelings about being hearing impaired is resumed. Clients should also explore their feelings about wearing hearing aids. Those who have used amplification in the past are encouraged to describe their experiences and compare them to experiences within the group. If they have had the opportunity to use a hearing aid outside the group sessions, clients are asked to talk about how they *felt* when doing so.

Attitudes about hearing aid use are often negative, even when the need for using amplification is obvious. One 80-year-old woman who looked and behaved like a much younger person resisted obtaining a hearing aid because "it makes people think I'm 80 years old"! The fact that many people continue to experience frustration and resentment because of poor communication skills even after they learn that a hearing aid will provide significant help, indicates the strength of some of the feelings that inhibit hearing aid use. One of the most important aspects of the group rehabilitation program is the safe environment in which the difficult decisions regarding hearing aid use can be made. Therefore, ample time should be given to discussions of the strong feelings surrounding this issue.

•Auditory-visual discrimination.

•Outside assignment. Group members are asked to observe hearing aid users in public, taking note of their own and other people's reactions to the wearer.

•Subjective reactions to amplification.

Seventh Session

•Amplification. By now it should be relatively clear what the final recommendation regarding amplification is likely to be. The fitting at this session should be a reasonable approximation of what will be recommended, if amplification is to be recommended at all. Clients will be permitted to sign out the hearing aid worn at this session for a few days to wear at home and in other situations. Permitting clients to wear nonpurchased aids for a few days may not be possible in all settings, but use in outside settings is an important and helpful part of the program. Some clinics use loaner aids purchased for this purpose. This is only satisfactory if a relatively wide variety of loaner aids can be kept on hand. None of the clients served by the authors in group programs has ever lost or damaged an aid, so this important feature of the program is strongly recommended.

Clients are encouraged to wear the aid as much as possible and in as many different kinds of settings as can be managed. They are encouraged to listen with and without amplification in various settings to get an estimate of the amount and degree of benefit that may be expected.

•Lecture-discussion. The talk given during this session covers aspects of the care and cleaning of the hearing aid and earmold. Listening check procedures are demonstrated as discussed in Chapter 4. A handout giving step-by-step procedures is also provided.

•Counseling. The focus of the group counseling activity should be determined on the basis of group needs. It is doubtful, for example, that all issues previously introduced have been exhausted. If a new topic is needed, clients are asked to share specific concerns that are related to every day living. Examples of the type of concern that is usually discussed include the inability to hear the doorbell or the telephone ring at night, problems associated with personal safety, difficulty hearing the radio or television at levels that are comfortable for others who are present, concerns about how the hearing loss will affect advancement at work, and similar topics. Suggestions for solving or reducing the problems should be provided by staff *only if* the group demonstrates that it cannot devise solutions. Staff members should have handouts ready that list devices that can be purchased or made to alleviate some of the problems including information provided by telephone and hearing aid accessory companies.

•Auditory-visual discrimination.

•Outside assignment. (See next section.)

•Subjective reaction to amplification. The usual forms are completed at the end of the session and additional forms are provided to be completed during the trial period with the aid. Clients are also asked to keep a record of the amount of time the hearing aid was worn, how comfortable it and the earmold were over an extended period of time, the situations in which it was worn, and any unusual problems that occurred.

Eighth Session

•Amplification. Unless they request a change, clients wear the same hearing aids and earmolds that were used during the preceding week for all remaining sessions.

•Lecture-discussion.

•Counseling. The lecture-discussion period is combined with counseling so that ample time is allowed for discussion of the home-trial experiences. Some of the group members may be discouraged if the hearing aid was not helpful in all situations. Staff and group members should discuss the need for a gradual increase in both the time and the situations in which the hearing aid is worn. The topic of part-time versus full-time use of the hearing aid is frequently introduced by group members. Final resolution is left to each client but they are encouraged to wear the hearing aid regularly, even if it is not always turned on. A handout that summarizes some of the important points made in this and previous discussions is distributed (see Appendix C).

•Unscheduled period. This session can be devoted to any of the previous activities that have proven of interest or value to the group. The most popular ones usually involve lipreading or combined listening and lipreading activities.

•Auditory-visual discrimination.
•Subjective reaction to amplification.

Ninth Session

This session is left unscheduled in preliminary planning so that it can serve whatever purpose is necessary based on progress or the nature of group dynamics. If the group has experienced few complications and rapid progress this session could be the last one offered and the activities of the tenth session presented. On the other hand, more extensive counseling, additional listening or combined auditory-visual practice, or further instruction in the management of hearing aids may be necessary.

Tenth Session

•Amplification. The hearing aid fitting should consist of the hearing aid-earmold combination that is to be recommended. Hearing aids need not be provided for those few clients who have not benefited from or who have rejected their use. In rare cases there may be clients for whom a final decision has not yet been made. They may be seen individually for further hearing aid consultation.

•Lecture-discussion. If clients plan to obtain hearing aids from (or through) the audiologic facility providing the rehabilitation program the professional staff should discuss the details of the dispensing and post-dispensing services offered. The information presented should be included in a detailed handout that describes the services offered, a recommended schedule of clinic visits, the name and address of repair facilities, the name, address, and telephone number of the audiologist who will serve as the clinic contact, and the costs of all services and products, if any.

•Counseling. Clients are asked to evaluate the program and their own progress. This can be handled through discussion, by completion of a questionnaire, or some combination of these approaches. Participants seem to prefer open discussion, so any evaluation forms used should probably be brief and require little writing. Evaluation by the non-hearing-impaired participants should also be obtained, using the same procedures. As always, normally hearing group members are encouraged to participate in the discussions.

•Auditory-visual discrimination. Auditory and auditory-visual discrimination should be evaluated for the final time. This step may be eliminated if all participants have been previously evaluated with the system they are presently wearing. Final recommendations should be made for each participant. If hearing aids are recommended some paper work may have to be completed and appointments for follow-up visits made. If hearing aids are not recommended, but other rehabilitative procedures seem appropriate, they should be discussed until each client understands what is to be done next.

Final Comments

Few of the components of this program are new or innovative. Other authors have described the need for some of the types of activities and instructions that are described above (Carhart, 1947; Di Carlo, 1948; Johnson and Siegenthaler, 1951). Unfortunately, most hearing-impaired adults do not have access to training that includes all of the components described. The success of a program such as this is significantly enhanced when it involves hearing aid dispensing by the audiologists who are involved because services are not fragmented and accountability is a positive feature. Dispensing allows flexible audiologic management of clients whose communication problems are severe or complicated as well as those whose problems are mild. The existence of an ongoing group program that addresses the needs of the more complicated cases or those less likely to seek conventional intervention serves to educate the general hearing-impaired population about goals of rehabilitation. It provides an alternative approach to individual hearing aid consultations; its chief features are that it allows clients to grow at their own pace and provides group encouragement and reinforcement. Although the group program described deemphasizes auditory training and lipreading practice as critical components to significant improvement in communication, it does address these factors in a positive way and permits the clinician considerable latitude with respect to goals and procedures regarding their use.

It is difficult to attach a single identifying label to the program described. It is a group hearing aid selection, hearing aid orientation, communication effectiveness and attitude modification program. Throughout the group discussions, participants are encouraged to analyze their own communication situations, determine the sources of difficulty they experience, and divide those difficulties into two categories: those that can be controlled by the listener and those that cannot. Most adults begin therapy convinced that few factors are under their control. By the end of the group meetings it is obvious that most factors are under the control of the individual who is willing to admit the hearing loss, request necessary assistance (seating changes, requests for repetitions, requests for slower speech), and use amplification intelligently. Factors outside the control of the individual are discussed and put in proper perspective. Ways of controlling the others are suggested and practiced in a supportive atmosphere. The desired result is more effective communication by a more confident and relaxed individual.

Until our understanding of the effects of hearing loss on speech perception is more complete and amplification systems are developed that can compensate better for the hearing that is lost, there will be a need for rehabilitation programs that focus on adjustment to less than optimal hearing. The program described above appears to be successful in achieving that modest goal.

REFERENCES

Alpiner, J. (Ed.), *Handbook of Adult Rehabilitative Audiology*. Baltimore: Williams and Wilkins Co., 1978.

Barker, L., *Listening Behavior*. Englewood Cliffs, NJ: Prentice-Hall, Inc., 1971.

Binnie, C., Relevant aural rehabilitation. In J. Northern (Ed.), *Hearing Disorders*. Boston: Little, Brown and Company, 1976.

Binnie, C., Jackson, P., and Montgomery, A., Visual intelligibility of consonants: A lipreading screening test with implications for aural rehabilitation, *J. Speech Hearing Dis.*, 41, 530–539, 1976.

Binnie, C., Montgomery, A., and Jackson, P., Auditory and visual contributions to the perception of consonants, *J. Speech Hearing Res.*, 17, 619–630, 1974.

Carhart, R., Auditory training. In H. Davis (Ed.), *Hearing and Deafness*. New York: Rinehart, Inc., 1947.

Colton, J. and O'Neill, J., A cooperative outreach program for the elderly, *J. Acad. Rehab. Audiol.*, 9, 38–41, 1976.

Davis, H. and Silverman, S. (Eds.), *Hearing and Deafness*. New York: Holt, Rinehart and Winston, 1963.

Davis, H. and Silverman, S. (Eds.), *Hearing and Deafness*, 4th edition. New York: Holt, Rinehart and Winston, 1978.

Davis, J., Advice from some satisfied customers, *J. Acad. Rehab. Audiol.*, 13, 122–127, 1980.

DiCarlo, L., Auditory training for the adult, *Volta Rev.*, 50, 490–496, 1948.

Erber, N., Auditory, visual and auditory-visual recognition of consonants by children with normal and impaired hearing, *J. Speech Hearing Res.*, 15, 413–422, 1972.

Fleming, M., A total approach to communication therapy, *J. Acad. Rehab. Audiol.*, 5, 28–31, 1972.

Giolas, T., Owens, E., Lamb, S., and Schubert, E., Hearing Performance Inventory, *J. Speech Hearing Dis.*, 44, 169–195, 1979.

Hardick, E., Aural rehabilitational programs for the aged can be successful, *J. Acad. Rehab. Audiol.*, 10, 51–67, 1977.

Harless, E. and Rupp, R., Aural rehabilitation of the elderly, *J. Speech Hearing Dis.*, 37, 267–273, 1972.

Harris, J., Haines, H., Kelsey, P., and Clack, T., The relation between speech intelligibility and the electroacoustic characteristics of low fidelity circuitry, *J. Aud. Res.*, 5, 357–381, 1961.

Hull, R., Assisting the elderly client. In J. Katz (Ed.), *Handbook of Clinical Audiology*, 2nd edition. Baltimore: Williams and Wilkins Co., 1978.

Hull, R. and Traynor, R., Hearing impairment among aging persons in the health care facility: Their diagnosis and rehabilitation, *Amer. Health Care Assoc. J.*, 3, 14–18, 1977.

Hutton, C., A diagnostic approach to combined techniques in aural rehabilitation, *J. Speech Hearing Dis.*, 25, 267–272, 1960.

Hutton, C., Curry, E., and Armstrong, M., Semidiagnostic test materials for aural rehabilitation, *J. Speech Hearing Dis.*, 24, 319–329, 1959.

Johnson, A. and Siegenthaler, B., A clinical auditory training program, *J. Speech Hearing Dis.*, 16, 35–39, 1951.

Kalikow, D., Stevens, K., and Elliott, L., Development of a test of speech intelligibility in noise using sentence materials with controlled word predictability, *J. Acoust. Soc. Am.*, 61, 1337–1351, 1977.

Kreul, E., Nixon, J., Kryter, K., Bell, D., Lang, J., and Schubert, E., A proposed clinical test of speech discrimination, *J. Speech Hearing Res.,* 11, 536–552, 1968.

Lamb, S., Owens, E., Schubert, E., and Giolas, T., *Hearing Performance Inventory, Revised Form*. Unpublished document, July 1979. (See also T. Giolas et al., 1979.)

McCartney, J., Maurer, J., and Sorenson, F., A mobile audiology service for the elderly: A preliminary report, *J. Acad. Rehab. Audiol.,* 7, 25–36, 1974.

Montgomery, A., Assessment of a new auditory visual integration technique. Paper presented at the Annual Convention of the American Speech and Hearing Association, Chicago, 1977.

Owens, E. and Schubert, E., Development of the California Consonant Test, *J. Speech Hearing Res.,* 20, 463–474, 1977.

Rupp, R., Higgins, J., and Mauer, J., A feasibility scale for predicting hearing aid use (FSPHAU) with older individuals, *J. Acad. Rehab. Audiol.,* 10, 81–104, 1977.

Santore, F., The Verbotonal aural rehabilitation program with hearing impaired adults: A five-year summary report, *J. Acad. Rehab. Audiol.,* 11, 33–45, 1978.

Sedge, R., Walden, B., and Montgomery, A., *Aural Rehabilitation for Individuals with High Frequency Hearing Loss*. Unpublished manuscript, 1978.

Tannahill, J. and Smoski, W., Introduction to aural rehabilitation. In J. Katz (Ed.), *Handbook of Clinical Audiology,* 2nd edition. Baltimore: Williams and Wilkins Co., 1978.

Walden, B., Prosek, R., and Worthington, D., Predicting audio-visual consonant recognition performance of hearing impaired adults, *J. Speech Hearing Res.,* 17, 270–278, 1974.

Wright, B., Social-psychological leads to enhance rehabilitation effectiveness, *Rehab. Couns. Bull.,* 214–223, (June) 1975.

APPENDIX A
Subjective Reaction to Amplification

Name ____

Date ____

Amount of Time Used ________________________________
(hours per day)

INSTRUCTIONS

Place an X in the space which best describes your reaction.

1. Feels comfortable
Very
Comfortable |____|____|____|____|____| Uncomfortable

2. Are voices natural?
Very
Natural |____|____|____|____|____| Unnatural

3. Sounds pleasant?
Pleasant |____|____|____|____|____| Unpleasant

4. Does it "make noise" even in quiet?
Too much |____|____|____|____|____| None
5. How many sounds are louder than you can tolerate?
All |____|____|____|____|____| None
6. Is the hearing aid convenient to operate?
Very Convenient |____|____|____|____|____| Very Inconvenient
7. Does the hearing aid help you?
All of the time |____|____|____|____|____| None of the time
8. How would you rate this hearing aid compared to others you have tried?
Best |____|____|____|____|____| Worst

WHAT DID YOU LIKE MOST ABOUT THE HEARING AID? ____________________

WHAT BOTHERS YOU MOST ABOUT THE HEARING AID OR ITS USE? ____________________

WHAT REACTION DID YOU GET FROM OTHERS WHILE WEARING THE HEARING AID ____________________

To be completed by clinician:
Make ____________________
Model ____________________
Ear ____________________
Settings ____________________
Earmold ____________________

APPENDIX B
Reminders for Improving Communication

1. When you communicate, you are trying to determine meaning. It is not necessary to understand every word to get the meaning of a message. Try to relax and let the message wash over you. You'll find that you understand more and better when you are not tense.
2. In communication situations, position yourself so that you can combine hearing with vision. Watch the speaker and listen at the same time; a distance of three to six feet is ideal. Don't watch the lips alone; observe facial expression, gestures, and body movements as well.
3. Try to position yourself so that the speaker's face is well lighted. If the speaker is in

a shadow or if the light source is behind the speaker, the face will not be seen clearly and speech movements will be obscured.

4. Sounds vary in visibility; be able to distinguish them by concentrating on the meaning of the message, rather than each word or sound.
5. People will modify their behavior to help you understand if you give them suggestions or if they know when you are having difficulty. Inform people that you are hearing impaired. Put them at ease by telling them that normal level, natural speech is most helpful. Exaggeration and shouting are difficult to understand. Ask speakers to face you and to get your attention before speaking. Suggest that sources of noise be turned off or removed during communication, if possible. If you need repetition of part of a message, inform the speaker of what you understood and ask what you missed. This will help the speaker determine how to restate the message.

APPENDIX C
Adjusting to Your New World of Sound

We have recommended that you obtain a hearing aid. Our recommendation is based on the knowledge that this hearing aid will provide significant improvement in communication for you. It is important for you to understand, however, that the hearing aid will not restore your hearing to normal, nor will it necessarily allow you to hear in the way you might wish. Those communication situations in which you have had considerable difficulty without a hearing aid will continue to be some problem to you.

Most hearing-impaired people, even though they are unaware of it, have become accustomed to the peace and quiet provided by the hearing loss as a result of not hearing many of the background sounds that are constantly present. At the same time, they would like to be able to hear their friends and relatives when they are speaking. As a result, many find it difficult to adjust to a hearing aid because, in addition to hearing the speech of others, they also hear many background sounds. It is at this point that some people give up the use of a hearing aid, making statements such as "It is too noisy," or "It makes me nervous."

The primary purpose of this brochure is to make you aware of what your first reactions to a hearing aid may be and to provide suggestions to help you become adjusted to your new world of sound.

Become familiar with the care and operation of your hearing aid. The manufacturer will provide a booklet that describes its care and maintenance. Your audiologist should review these matters with you. Make sure you are given instructions in using your hearing aid with the telephone, cleaning the earmold, and setting any external adjustments the aid may have.

The length of time required for you to become adjusted to your hearing aid cannot be predicted, because it varies considerably from person to person. Such factors as age, amount of hearing loss, the length of time the hearing loss has been present, and the way you live will influence your adjustment. Many find that they can satisfactorily adjust to a hearing aid within one month if they follow the procedure outlined.

For the first few days it is suggested that you wear your hearing aid only in quiet familiar situations, preferably in the home. The hearing aid will change the quality of sounds in addition to making them louder. Take as much time as possible to adjust to these amplified sounds. Become familiar with the sounds in your environment that the hearing aid allows you to hear. You have not heard some of these sounds in a long time, and even if you have they will sound a little different. Spend a lot of time listening carefully, trying to identify as many background sounds as possible. For example, listen to water running, footsteps, the vacuum cleaner, kitchen appliances, and the doorbell. Once you become accustomed to hearing these background sounds and can identify them, they will no longer be perceived as noise. To become a satisfied hearing aid user it is *very important* that you become readjusted to hearing background sounds as well as speech.

In the beginning, you may want to wear the hearing aid only for short periods of time because of fatigue or irritation. The aid may be turned off or removed until you are rested. Gradually you will find that each time the hearing aid is turned on you can wear it for a longer period of time. The goal for most hearing aid users is to get to be able to wear the hearing aid all day.

The next step is to wear your hearing aid in simple speech situations, involving conversation with one other person with a minimum of background noise. This can also be accomplished in the home, either by conversing with another member of the family or by listening to the radio or television. During this time you will find yourself experimenting with the volume control of the hearing aid. This is a normal process; eventually you will find a volume setting that is satisfactory for most situations. Once this setting is found, leave it there most of the day. You may also find yourself, during these early stages, wearing your hearing aid at a very low volume setting. This is also very common. You will gradually be able to tolerate higher volume settings as the adjustment process continues.

The next step is to wear your hearing aid in more complicated listening situations, involving interfering background noise. You may also engage in conversations among several people. These situations will probably occur outside of the home, while you are at work, shopping, or dining, for example. At this point you are not fully adjusted to your hearing aid, so you may find yourself using a lower volume setting. Becoming fatigued and irritated is a common occurrence because these complicated listening situations involve many new, and perhaps loud, background noises. There may be a few noisy situations in which the hearing aid is of little benefit. As the adjustment process continues, you should experiment and determine for yourself the amount of help you receive under noisy conditions. Remember, this device is a hearing *aid;* it will make sound louder and improve your hearing, but it will not restore hearing to normal. The important thing to remember is that it can help you significantly in many situations.

If you can derive benefit from your hearing aid in many listening situations, you should try to wear the hearing aid all of the time. If you are going to be a part-time hearing aid user, you might try to become accustomed to leaving the hearing aid in place, even though it may be turned off part of the time. This will allow the most flexible and convenient use of the hearing aid when you need it. Part-time users may never be completely adjusted to hearing aid use because they spend part of their time in the peace and quiet their hearing loss provides and the remainder of the time in a noisy world. As long as you are aware of these facts and your reactions to them, it may be possible for you to satisfactorily adjust to part-time hearing aid use.

If at any time through this adjustment period you have any questions or problems you cannot resolve, do not hesitate to contact this clinic. We encourage you to return to the clinic at the prescribed times, so that we may check your hearing aid and help you with any unresolved problems. There are services available either at this clinic or in other community agencies to help people obtain the maximum use of their hearing, their hearing aid, and the use of visual cues to supplement them.

Glossary

Acoustic reflex (stapedial) Contraction of the stapedius muscle in response to loud acoustic stimulation. The contraction stiffens the mechanical system of the middle ear to protect the ear from damage.

Acoustic trauma Noise-induced permanent threshold shift occurring as a result of a one-time exposure to very high-intensity noise, such as an explosion. Its appearance after one exposure differentiates it from noise-induced hearing loss, which is a more general term for hearing loss developing slowly over time due to daily exposure to rather continuous noise.

Adventitious hearing loss (deafness) Not present at birth; it is a general term concerning time of onset relative to birth that is useful for differentiating those who have never heard normally from those acquiring hearing loss after some normal hearing experience.

ANSI 1969 A standard developed by the American National Standards Institute specifying various parameters of audiometer performance and methods of calibration. ANSI 1969 specified a significant change from the previous American standard (ASA 1951) in the SPL values of O dB HL for the various frequencies.

ASA 1951 A standard developed by the American Standards Association (now known as the American National Standards Institute) specifying various parameters of audiometer performance and methods of calibration. It has been superseded by ANSI 1969. Knowledge of the reference level (ASA 1951 or ANSI 1969) is important because 25 dB thresholds by the two standards are not equally handicapping, but if the reference level differences are utilized data can be transformed to a common reference.

Auditory closure The process by which the meaning of the message as a whole is obtained on the basis of incomplete auditory information. It is usually based on previous experience with the auditory stimulus involved.

Auditory method An educational approach for hearing-impaired children that stresses the use of auditory input alone for the reception of speech.

Bilirubin A pigment found in the blood, an excess of which contributes to jaundice and damage to the central nervous system.

Closed-set response format A test or training situation where the correct response is made available among specified alternatives, as in a multiple-choice task. In hearing evaluation the response alternatives can be in printed or pictorial format.

Conductive loss A condition where hearing thresholds by bone conduction are normal but air conduction thresholds are poorer by 10 dB or more. These losses are caused by some anomaly of the outer or middle ear and are generally amenable to medical/surgical treatment and restoration of hearing at or near bone conduction threshold levels.

Congenital deafness Present at birth; may be due to complications during delivery, in-utero damage, or genetic factors. Congenital sensorineural hearing losses tend to be severe to profound resulting in significant sensory deprivation from the outset.

Cued speech The use of hand signals (cues) as an adjunct to lipreading. The cues have no intrinsic meaning but serve to distinguish between sounds that look alike on the lips.

Dysacusis Faulty hearing caused by a reduction in the clarity of speech beyond that normally associated with a loss of auditory sensitivity. It is caused by cochlear distortion of suprathreshold sound and disturbance of retrocochlear processing. Some authors define the term as presented here, others restrict its use to central problems of an integrative or interpretive nature.

Feedback The squealing sound often heard from any amplification system incorporating a microphone and receiver (loudspeaker). It is a cyclic phenomenon where the amplified input frequencies in the region of the prominent peaks of the response curve on leaving the receiver are reintroduced to the microphone. There are other forms of feedback but the most common is the acoustical feedback described which is associated with a leak in the receiver-ear coupling system.

Frequency resolution Frequency resolution is the ability to resolve, or discriminate among sounds on the basis of their frequencies.

Fundamental frequency In the speech waveform, the fundamental frequency is the frequency at which the vocal folds repeat their vibratory cycle. This frequency ranges from approximately 100 Hz in adult males to approximately 275 Hz in children. Changes in fundamental frequency of the speech waveform usually are perceived as changes in vocal pitch.

Geriatric Relating to the process and problems of aging.

Handicap Is the cumulative interactive effect of severity of impairment, age, time of onset, personality, life-style, and educational or vocational status. Impairment can be audiologically quantified but handicap is rarely describable in objective terms, is highly individual, and the client's assessment is an important valid consideration.

Hearing Level (HL) Since the decibel (dB) is a relative value it is necessary to specify the reference. HL specifies the reference as audiometric zero rather than any of the other common reference levels employed.

High-pass filter A high-pass filter is an electronic device that eliminates energy in the input waveform that is below a certain frequency (the cutoff frequency of the high-pass filter). Thus, the waveform at the output of the filter contains energy only at frequencies *above* the cutoff frequency of the filter.

Homophemes Sounds that look alike on the lips.

Impairment A change for the worse in hearing function. Impairment of hearing is measurable by various tests (i.e., threshold, discrimination, impedance).

ISO 1964 A standard developed by the International Standards Organization specifying various parameters of audiometer performance and methods of calibration. The audiometric zero reference thresholds in SPL specified were utilized in the United States as interim specifications until ANSI 1969 was adopted. The stated SPL values of threshold are very close to those of ANSI 1969.

Lexical Relating to vocabulary and words.

Lipreading (speechreading) The use of visual cues associated with the act of speaking that enables hearing-impaired persons to understand the spoken messages of others. The visual cues include, but are not limited to, lip positions and movements involved in speech production. Depending on the severity and duration of impairment reliance on visual cues may be total or only as a supplement to auditory cues under difficult listening conditions.

Low-pass filter A low-pass filter is an electronic device that eliminates energy in the input waveform that is above a certain frequency (the cutoff frequency of the low-pass filter). Thus, the waveform at the output of the filter contains energy only at frequencies *below* the cutoff frequency of the filter.

Manner of articulation Refers to the general ways in which phonemes are produced by the articulators. Examples are plosives, fricatives, affricates, nasals, and glides.

Manual communication The use of nonoral symbols to represent language; includes fingerspelling, signs, and gestures.

Morpheme Smallest unit of speech that carries meaning. Free morphemes (words) stand alone; bound morphemes (word prefixes, suffixes, and endings) cannot be used alone.

Neooralism An educational approach used in Russia that is similar to the Rochester Method.

Nonlinear distortion The result when changes in frequency or intensity of input signals are not reflected in proportional changes in output. Some specific products of nonlinearity are harmonic and intermodulation distortion.

Nonsegmental Characteristics of speech that spread over several units such as phonemes or words. Intonation and stress are nonsegmental features of speech.

Open-set response format A test or training situation where the correct response to a stimulus is the universe of similar units (monosyllables, spondees, etc.).

Oral method An early educational approach used with hearing-impaired children that stressed the use of lipreading and reading for the reception of language and speech for the expression of language.

Oral-aural method A modification of the oral method to include hearing for the reception of language.

Phonemic regression A term connoting poorer auditory processing performance with speech than would be expected on the basis of severity of the pure-tone loss of sensitivity.

Phonology The study of the sounds of a language.

Place of articulation Refers to the location of the articulators involved in the production of a given phoneme. Examples are bilabial, velar, and linguaalveolar.

Presbycusis Loss of hearing sensitivity and acuity associated with aging.

Prosody The rate, rhythm, and intonation patterns of speech.

Pure-tone average (PTA) The average threshold of hearing usually of 500, 1000, and 2000 Hz for purposes of estimating the threshold of speech.

Recruitment Abnormally rapid growth of loudness as intensity is increased.

Rochester method An educational approach that uses lipreading and fingerspelling for the reception of speech.

Semantics The study of the meaning of words and relations among words.

Sensation level (SL) A dB reference that specifies the level of sound relative to the threshold of the individual involved; 40 dB SL means the signal is presented 40 dB above the pure-tone average or speech reception threshold.

Sensorineural loss Any loss of hearing sensitivity characterized by equal losses of threshold by air and bone conduction testing. Such losses usually involve the peripheral sensory and neural mechanism.

Silica gel An agent used to absorb moisture; placement of a hearing aid in proximity to silica gel in an airtight enclosure will minimize deterioration of components due to moisture.

Simultaneous method An educational approach that uses both speech and manual communication for the reception of language.

Sociocusis Changes for the worse in hearing threshold associated with daily exposure to noise in our social environment including schools, homes, traffic, entertainment, and recreation.

Sound field A sound field is any area in which sound is present. The sound field for the testing of speech perception is usually a sound-treated booth within which a loudspeaker is used for the delivery of the speech stimuli. As an alternative to sound-field testing, speech stimuli may be delivered to the listener via earphones.

Sound-Level meter An instrument for measuring pressure changes in air associated with sound. Modern instruments measure dB level relative to 20 micronewtons per square meter (SPL) or relative to built-in weighting networks (A, B, C). The A scale is the equal-loudness contour developed by comparing the loudness of audible frequencies to a 1000 Hz tone of 40 dB SPL. Measurement of sound pressure employing the A curve provides a good approximation of the perceived loudness of a complex signal and of the level at which noise becomes hazardous to human hearing. The B and C networks correspond to the equal-loudness contours developed in the same way but using 70 and 100 dB SPL references. it is not possible to compare A, B, C, and SPL values without knowledge of the spectral composition of the sound in question.

Sound pressure level (SPL) A dB reference that states that the reference pressure is 20 micronewtons per square meter. There are several other ways of reporting the same reference pressure, such as 0.0002 dynes per square centimeter, or 2×10^{-4} microbars.

Speech reception threshold (SRT) The intensity level at which a person can correctly identify 50 percent of the stimuli presented. Spondees are the speech material most commonly used.

Spondaic words Spondaic words are words consisting of two syllables that are equally stressed. Examples of spondaic words are "baseball," "downtown," and "sidewalk."

Suprasegmental Refers to the prosodic features of rate, rhythm, and intonation.

Syntax The grammatical structure of a language.

Temporal resolution Temporal resolution is the ability to resolve, or discriminate among sounds on the basis of their temporal characteristics. The temporal characteristics of sounds include their durations, as well as more complex aspects such as fluctuation in intensity over time.

Temporary threshold shift (TTS) Temporary change for the worse in threshold due to exposure to loud sound. It is a fatigue of the sensory mechanism of the cochlea and will recover after cessation of the exposure. Continued, prolonged exposure may result in permanent threshold shift (PTS).

Total communication An educational philosophy that encourages the use of all possible input and output modes for the reception and expression of language. Stresses the use of audition, speechreading, fingerspelling, signs, gestures, and so on.

Trochaic words Trochaic words are words of two syllables, the first of which is stressed. Examples of trochaic words are "motion," "factor," and "mother."

Visemes Visually contrastive groups of movements associated with the production of speech sounds. Movements within a viseme category are called homophemes.

Visual closure The process by which the meaning of the message as a whole is obtained on the basis of incomplete visual information.

AUTHOR INDEX

SUBJECT INDEX